Herbs, Spices, and Medicinal Plants

Recent Advances in Botany, Horticulture, and Pharmacology

Volume 2

CONSERVATION AND PRESERVATION NOTES

The paper used in this publication meets the minimum requirements of American National Standard for Information Sciences – Permanence of Paper for Printed Material, ANSI Z39.48-1984.

ABSTRACTING AND INDEXING INFORMATION

The contents of this original book are indexed, abstracted, or summarized in the following indexing, abstracting, or electronic data bases:

- Behavioral Medicine Abstracts
- Bioscience Information Service of Biological Abstracts (BIOSIS)
- CAB Abstracts
- Cambridge Scientific Abstracts
- International Pharmaceutical Abstracts

The above listing was prepared from selection editors of the above reference sources based on pre-publication reviews of the galleys.

Herbs, Spices, and Medicinal Plants

Recent Advances in Botany, Horticulture, and Pharmacology

Volume 2

Lyle E. Craker
James E. Simon
Editors-in-Chief

Food Products Press
An Imprint of The Haworth Press, Inc.
New York • London • Sydney

Originally published by The Oryx Press, © 1987, as part of a series (ISSN 0890-6653).

Food Products Press, 10 Alice Street, Binghamton, NY 13904-1580
EUROSPAN/Food Products Press, 3 Henrietta Street, London WC2E 8LU England
ASTAM/Food Products Press, 162-168 Parramatta Road, Stanmore, Sydney, N.S.W. 2048 Australia

Food Products Press is an imprint of The Haworth Press, Inc., 10 Alice Street, Binghamton, NY 13904-1580

Warning: The medicinal and other uses of herbs described in this volume have been included for informational and study purposes only. The authors and publishers neither advocate nor prescribe the use of any herb for medicinal or other purposes. Please note that some herbs mentioned in this book could be poisonous. The authors and publishers assume no liability for omissions or for use or misuse of information contained herein.

Library of Congress Card Number: 86-646860

Contents

Preface

The support and encouragement we have received from around the world following the publication of Volume 1 has, in a profound way, demonstrated the need for the continuation of this review series. Others, like us, have felt that there is a serious shortage of detailed reviews highlighting current research developments in the field of herbs, spices, and medicinal plants. As our knowledge of the chemistry, biosynthesis, and metabolism of natural plant products expands, and develops new uses for plants and plant compounds, the need to characterize, produce, and extract the basic plant material increases. With many scientific papers being published annually, the demand for up-to-date, accurate reviews of the botany, horticulture, and pharmacology of these plants remains strong.

A major objective of this review series is to forge a link among researchers working in the several disciplines associated with herbs, spices, and medicinal plants. To this end, we have strived to include reviews in a broad range of subject areas to aid in the understanding and appreciation of all the distinct, yet related fields connected with botany, horticulture, and pharmacology. The horticulturalist interested in domestication and commercial cultivation of plants, the ethnobotanist interested in traditional uses of plants within societies, the chemist interested in extraction and purification of natural plant products, the pharmacologist interested in clinical evaluations and efficacy of compounds, the industrial processor interested in provision of plants and plant products to the marketplace, and the many others who have a professional or general interest in these plants and their products will find in these reviews the opportunity to examine the most recent available information.

On behalf of the members of the Editorial Board, we welcome your comments and suggestions of topics for future volumes and on ways that this review series can best meet your scientific and informational needs. If we are successful in meeting our objectives, it is because of the cooperation and assistance of the Board of Editors, contributing scientists, and the many others whose ideas and support have made Volume 2 of *Herbs, Spices, and Medicinal Plants: Recent Advances in Botany, Horticulture, and Pharmacology* possible.

Lyle E. Craker
James E. Simon

Acknowledgments

With Volume 2 of *Herbs, Spices, and Medicinal Plants: Recent Advances in Botany, Horticulture, and Pharmacology*, the editors-in-chief express a special thank you to Jan Krygier, Oryx Press, for her patient and continued encouragement in bringing this volume to fruition. In addition, we give our special thanks to Ms. Lian L. Tan for her typing and organizational skills, to Ms. Alena Chadwick and Mr. John Gancarski for their library support, to Ms. Sarah Craker for her photographic help, and to Dr. Lois Grant and Ms. Karen Craker for proofreading.

Contributors to Volume 2

Fu Shan-Lin — Institute of Medicinal Plant Development, Chinese Academy of Medical Sciences, Beijing, The People's Republic of China

Mohamed Izaddoost — College of Pharmacy, University of Tehran, Tehran, Iran

Richard H.A.M. Janssen — Organic Chemical Laboratory, State University of Utrecht, Utrecht, The Netherlands

Brian M. Lawrence — R.J. Reynolds Tobacco Company, Bowman Gray Technical Center, P.O. Box 2959, Winston-Salem, North Carolina USA

Eli Putievsky — Department of Medicinal, Aromatic and Spice Plants, Agricultural Research Organization, Newe Ya'ar Experiment Station, Haifa, Israel

Michael Raviv — Department of Ornamental Horticulture, Agricultural Research Organization, Newe Ya'ar Experiment Station, Haifa, Israel

Trevor Robinson — Department of Biochemistry, University of Massachusetts, Amherst, Massachusetts USA

Cornelis A. Salemink — Organic Chemical Laboratory, State University of Utrecht, Utrecht, The Netherlands

Hubert G. Theuns — Organic Chemical Laboratory, State University of Utrecht, Utrecht, The Netherlands

Gary A. Thompson — Department of Botany and Plant Pathology, Purdue University, West Lafayette, Indiana USA

Arthur O. Tucker — Department of Agriculture and Natural Resources, Delaware State College, Dover, Delaware USA

Xiao Pei-Gen — Institute of Medicinal Plant Development, Chinese Academy of Medical Sciences, Beijing, The People's Republic of China

Contents of Previous Volumes

Herbs, Spices, and Medicinal Plants:
Recent Advances in Botany, Horticulture, and Pharmacology
Volume 2

Pharmacologically Active Substances of Chinese Traditional and Herbal Medicines

Xiao Pei-Gen and Fu Shan-Lin
Institute of Medicinal Plant Development, Chinese Academy of Medical Sciences, Beijing, The People's Republic of China

CONTENTS

I. INTRODUCTION

In China, traditional and herbal medicines play a role in people's health equal to that of synthetic drugs and antibiotics. The country has an abundance of medicinal plant resources—about 5,500 species—due to the wide variety of geographical and ecological conditions and has accumulated vast experiences with drug plants during a long history in the use of herbal medicines. Recently, an enhanced interdisciplinary and research program with botanical, chemical, pharmacological, and clinical studies has been undertaken by Chinese scientists to explore the potential of Chinese drug plants as a source of new medicines. The contributing institutions include: Institute of Medicinal Plant Development (IMPLAD), Chinese Academy of Medicinal Sciences, Beijing; Institute of Chinese Materia Medica, Chinese Academy of Traditional Chinese Medicine, Beijing; Shanghai Institute of Materia Medica, Academia Sinica, Shanghai; Shanghai Institute of Pharmaceutical Industrial Research, Shanghai; Kunming Institute of Botany, Academia Sinica, Kunming; Guangxi Institute of Chinese Traditional Medical and Pharmaceutical Sciences, Nanning; Institute of Materia Medica, Chinese Academy of Medical Sciences, Beijing; and the several colleges of pharmacy and colleges of traditional Chinese medicine.

Some 250 pharmacologically active compounds have been reported, and approximately 60 new drugs have originated directly or indirectly from these compounds. This report presents details on the pharmacologically active compounds of Chinese traditional and herbal medicine.

II. PHARMACOLOGICALLY ACTIVE COMPOUNDS

A. Alkaloids

1. Ornithine Derived

The most widely used ornithine-derived alkaloids in China are the tropanes anisodamine (Structure 1) and anisodine (Structure 2) that have been isolated from the traditional Tibetan drug plants *Scopolia tangutica* Maxim. (53) and *Przewalskia tangutica* Maxim. (189). Pharmacological studies indicate that both of these alkaloids influence the nervous system. Anisodamine affects the central nervous system similar to, but 6 to 25 times weaker than, that of atropine (53). Anisodine affects the peripheral nervous system but is weaker than both atropine and scopolamine (49). Anisodamine is also known to stimulate microcirculation (48). Clinically, anisodamine is being used for the treatment of septic shock resulting from toxic bacillary dysentery, fulminant epidermic meningitis, and hemorrhagic enteritis (48). Anisodine is also being used for the treatment of migraine headaches and diseases of the fungus occuli caused by vascular spasm. In addition, the compound has been used for treatment of organophosphorus poisoning and acute paralysis caused by accidents to the cerebral vascular system. Interestingly, anisodine is the chief component of traditional Chinese anesthetic preparations (49). Both anisodamine and anisodine are now being commercially produced on a large scale by isolation from natural sources and by synthetic means.

Structure 1. Anisodamine

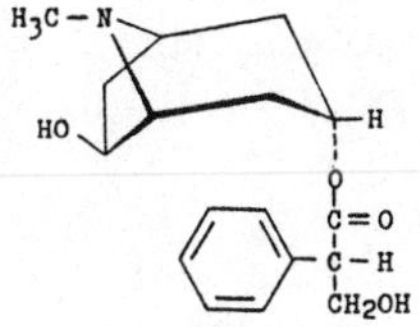

Structure 2. Anisodine

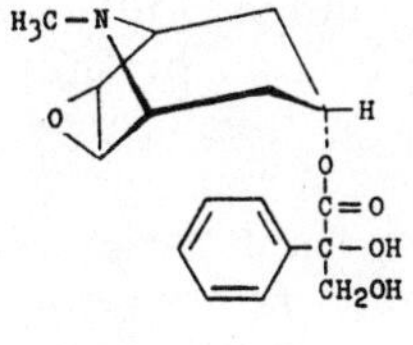

Another ornithine-derived alkaloid is Bao-Gong-Teng A (Structure 3), a myotic agent recently isolated from the stem of *Erycibe obtusifolia* Benth. Clinically, Bao-Gong-Teng A can be used as a substituent for pilocarpine in the treatment of glaucoma (205, 206). The tropane skeleton and activity of this alkaloid may have some significance in the pharmacological studies of receptor theory as other similar compounds are known to have antimydriatic effects.

From a folk remedy using *Crotalaria sessiliflora* L. as an antitumor drug for treatment of skin cancer, 2 ornithine-derived alkaloids have been isolated. The first of these alkaloids is reported to be

Structure 3. Bao-Gong-Teng A

monocrotaline and has demonstrated inhibitory activity against sarcoma 180, leukemia 615, and Walker carcinoma 256. However, hepatic toxicity restricts monocrotaline to external use only. The second alkaloid is identified as a new pyrrolizidine alkaloid from which *trans-trans* platynecic acid and retronecine can be obtained after hydrolysis (77).

2. Lysine Derived

Studies indicate a group of quinolizidine alkaloids isolated from the *Sophora flavescens* Ait., *Sophora tonkinensis* Gagnep. (*Sophora subprostrata* Chun et T. Chen) and *Sophora alopecuroides* L. contain sophocarpine, matrine, and oxymatrine and have marked pharmacological activity. Sophocarpine exhibits *in vitro* activity against ECA cells (111) and *in vivo* activity against transplanted S-180, U-14, W-256, Lio-1, and L-615 in the range of 31 percent to 56 percent based on tumor weights (108). Matrine and oxymatrine are also effective agents against S-180, and oxymatrine will provide protective antihepatotoxic activity in models of mice liver systems damaged by carbon tetrachloride (CCl_4) and D-galacto-samine (15), and against leukopenia induced by ^{60}Co gamma radiation or mitomycin C (218).

Pachycarpine, another quinolizidine alkaloid, has been isolated from *Thermopsis lanceolata* R. Br. This alkaloid markedly strengthened the contraction of the anterior tibialis musculi of anesthetized rabbits and cats and the isolated rat diaphragm (193). The alkaloid piperine (Structure 4) has been discovered to be the active component of an effective, herbal, antiepileptic prescription containing white pepper (*Piper nigrum*) and turnip (*Raphanus sativus*). Piperine has strong anticonvulsive and marked sedative actions (68). Derivatives of piperine have been prepared, and one of them—antiepilepsirine—demonstrates a wide spectrum of anticonvulsive activity with low toxicity. Antiepilepsirine has been approved for commercial production.

Structure 4. Piperine

3. Nicotinic Acid Derived

Ba-Jao-Feng, a folk medicine from the root of *Alangium chinense* (Lour.) Harms, is well known in China as a muscle relaxant. Chemical studies reveal that *dl*-anabasine (Structure 5), a nicotinic acid-derived alkaloid, is the active ingredient. This compound exerts significant neuromuscular blocking effects on isolated rat phrenic nerve-diaphragm preparations and has a depolarizing effect on isolated frog sartorius muscles (203).

Structure 5. *dl*-Anabasine

4. Anthranilic Acid Derived

Several anthranilic acid-derived alkaloids have demonstrated pharmacological activity. Zanthobungeanine (Structure 6), from the root of *Zanthoxylum bungeanum* Maxim, has a broad spectrum of antifungal activity. The traditional Chinese drug Chang-Shan (*Dichroa febrifuga* Lour.) that has long been used as an antimalarial agent contains febrifugine (β-dichroine, Structure 7) as one of the active ingredients. Febrifugine has demonstrated a malariacidal effect on *Plasmodium lophurae* that is 100 times as strong as quinine hydrochloride. This compound also exhibits amebicidal effects stronger than emetine hydrochloride (227). Structural modification of febrifugine has produced changrolin, a quinidine-like antiarrhythmic agent. Clinical trials of changrolin with 489 arrhythmic patients indicate an effectiveness rating of 80.8 percent (35).

Structure 6. Zanthobungeanine

Structure 7. Febrifugine (β-Dichroine)

5. Phenylalanine and Tyrosine Derived

With many varied structure types and large numbers of compounds, the group of alkaloids associated with phenylalanine and tyrosine produce numerous pharmacological responses. Ephedrine, isolated primarily from *Ephedra sinica* Stapf and *Ephedra equisetina* Bge., is an important therapeutic agent used for the treatment of hypotension and bronchial asthma. Securenine, isolated from the leaves of *Securinega suffruticosa* (Pall.) Rehd., is a stimulating agent for the central nervous system. Securenine nitrate is used for the treatment of facial paralysis and sequelae of poliomyelitis (2, 182).

The active cardiac principle of the aconite root, isolated from *Aconitum carmichaeli* Debx. and *Aconitum japonicum* Thunb., has been identified as *dl*-demethylcoclaurine (higenamine, Structure 8). The cardiotonic function of this alkaloid is effected through an isoproterenol-like action (238) and has been demonstrated to be a partial agonist of the β-adrenergic receptor (61). A compound with the same chemical base has been isolated from the stem of *Gnetum parvifolium* (Warb.) C.Y. Cheng, and pharmacological tests of this isolate in guinea pigs reveal an antagonistic activity to bronchial spasms induced by histamine, acetylcholine, and serotonine (52).

Structure 8. *dl*-Demethylcoclaurine (Higenamine)

A number of bisbenzylisoquinolines have neuromuscular blocking activity. Homoaromoline and *l*-curine isolated from *Cyclea barbata* (Wall.) Miers (162), hayatin isolated from *Cissampelos pareira* L. (15), cycleanine isolated from *Stephania Delavayi* Diels (152), dahurisoline isolated from *Menispermum dauricum* DC. (66), and their dimethoiodide, dimethochloride, dimethobromide, and methyl bromide derivatives possess marked muscle relaxant effects.

Dauricine, isolated from the rhizomes of *Menispermum dauricum* DC., exerts an acute hypotensive effect on anesthetized cats and rats when injected intravenously (18). Dauricine also possesses antiarrhythmic activity (103). Tetrandrine and demethyltetrandrine, isolated from the roots of *Stephania tetrandra* S. Moore, exhibit definitive antiphlogistic action on formaldehyde-induced arthritis of rats (129) and analgesic action in mice (226). These 2 alkaloids also produce a profound hypotensive effect in urethan-anesthetized cats, with the activity of demethyltetrandrine being stronger and more sustained than tetrandrine (223). In perfused isolated rabbits' ears, tetrandrine and demethyltetrandrine have direct vasodilating effects (159). Tetrandrine has demonstrated marked anticancer activities (78).

Cepharanthine, reported in *Stephania cepharantha* Hayata and *Stephania epigaea* H.S. Lo (*Stephania Delavayi* auct. non Diels), is claimed to be effective against human tuberculosis (204). This alkaloid is also used for treatment of leukopenia appearing in cancer patients undergoing chemotherapy or radiotherapy (44). Berbamine (Structure 9), an alkaloid obtained from *Berberis poiretii* Schneid. and most other *Berberis* species, has been similarly applied to increase leukocyte content of blood (191, 201).

Structure 9. Berbamine

Thalidasine, an alkaloid in a Chinese meadow rue (*Thalictrum faberi* Ulbr.), has demonstrated antitumor (132) and antibacterial (112) activities. Trilobine, isolated from *Cocculus trilobus* (Thunb.) DC., acts as an analgesic drug. Neither morphine-like tolerance nor physical dependence is evident in treatment with trilobine, and hence, this compound can be considered nonnarcotic (232). A derivative, dimethyltrilobine iodide, can delay the experimental arrhythmias induced by aconitine, ovabain, or chloroform-adrenaline (133). Neferine, an alkaloid obtained from the embryos of *Nelumbo nucifera* Gaertn., has displayed the ability to delay arrhythmia and the effects of calcium (69).

Bicucculine, isolated from *Corydalis repens* Mandl. et Muchld. (*Corydalis humosa* Migo), has strong convulsive action and consequently potential for use in the development of a diagnostic agent for epilepsy (7). Sinomenine, a major alkaloid of the traditional Chinese drug plant *Sinomenium acutum* (Thunb.) Rehd. et Wils., has marked analgesic, anti-inflammatory, hypotensive, and sedative actions (6, 60, 62). This alkaloid and the plant have been used for the treatment of rheumatic and rheumatoid arthritis.

Pharmacological tests with protopine, one of the most widely distributed benzylisoquinoline alkaloids, reveal this compound can increase coronary blood flow and produce antimalarial (230), abortifacient, sedative (235), and bronchodilator effects.

The protoberberine alkaloids berberine and palmatine are being widely used in China today as antimicrobial agents. The relevant derivatives of these alkaloids—tetrahydroberberine (THB, Structure 10) and *dl*-tetrahydropalmatine (THP, Structure 11)—possess sedative, tranquilizing, and analgesic actions. The tetrahydropalmatine is associated with hypnotic and analgesic effects while the *dl*-tetrahydropalmatine is associated with sedative-tranquilizing action (93). Since *dl*-tetrahydropalmatine appears to be nonaddictive, this compound is being commercially manufactured as a sedative and tranquilizer. *l*-Tetrahydropalmatine (rotundine), isolated from *Stephania dielsiana* Y.C. Wu (*Stephania sinica* auct. sin. non Diels), is also being produced as a commercial product and is routinely used for its analgesic and sedative activities (94).

Structure 10. Tetrahydroberberine (R + R$_1$ = -CH$_2$-)
Structure 11. *dl*-tetrahydropalmatine (R = R$_1$ = CH$_3$)

Dehydrocorydaline (DHC, Structure 12) obtained from the traditional Chinese drug Yan-Hu-Suo (*Corydalis yanhusuo* W.T. Wang) improves the tolerance of mice to monobaric and hypobaric hypoxia. Following the administration of DHC, myocardial uptake of ^{86}Rb in mice is increased and protective actions against changes in electrocardiograms induced by pitutrin and experimental myocardial necrosis induced by isoproterenol are observed. These protective actions of DHC undoubtedly account for the use of Yan-Hu-Suo in the treatment of coronary heart disease (84).

Structure 12. Dehydrocorydaline

Although none of them have yet been produced as commercial items, the aporphine alkaloids display a wide range of pharmacological activities. Magnoflorine, isolated from the roots of *Aristolochia debilis* Sieb. et Zucc., displays hypotensive activity. This alkaloid inhibits the N-cholinergic reactive system and has a ganglionic blocking action [probably associated with hypotensive action (5)] of about one-half that of hexamethonium. Stephanine, isolated from *Stephania dielsiana* C.Y. Wu, has demonstrated inhibitory activities against S-180 and Walker 256 cells (143). Identified as the main active principle of *Dicranostigma leptopodum* (Maxim.) Fedde and *Dictylicapnos scandens* (D. Don) Hutch., *d*-isocorydine (Structure 13) possesses marked analgesic and sedative activities and decreases the tonus of the smooth muscle (231). Analgesic and sedative actions are exhibited by *l*-dicentrine (Structure 14), isolated from *Stephania decentrinifera* H.S. Lo et H. Yang (74).

Structure 13. *d*-Isocorydine (R$_1$ = R$_2$ = OCH$_3$, R$_=$ OH, R$_4$ = H)
Structure 14. *l*-Dicentrine (R$_1$ + R$_2$ = O-CH$_2$-O, R$_3$ = H, R$_4$ = OCH$_3$)

Pharmacological and clinical studies of sanguinarine and chelerythrine—compounds isolated from the fruits of *Macleaya cordata* (Willd.) R. Br.—demonstrate antibacterial and antiphlogistical effects, enabling both of them to be used for the treatment of cervicitis (75). Chelerythrine is also reported as the active antibacterial principle of the herb *Eomecon chionantha* Hance (236).

Nitidine chloride and 6-methoxy-5, 6-dihydrochelerythrine—alkaloids isolated from the roots of *Zanthoxylum nitidum* (Roxb.) DC.—increase the life span of mice inoculated with Ehrlich's ascites tumor. Nitidine chloride was effective in the treatment of chronic myelocytic leukemia (79). Corynoline (Structure 15), from the tuber of *Corydalis sheareri* S. Moore, has a marked sedative action on mice treated intraperitoneally at 10 mg/kg of body weight and has an antileptospira effect in a 0.0125 percent solution (235).

Structure 15. Corynoline

Recently, a protective effect of colchicine on chronic liver damage induced in rats by CCl$_4$ has been observed. The results suggest colchicine may inhibit the formation of collagenous fiber in a chronically damaged liver. However, any effect of colchicine on the recovery of liver functions is not conspicuous (23).

The alkaloid lycorine hydrochloride, isolated from *Lycoris radiata* (L'Her.) Herb., has stimulative actions at low concentrations and inhibitory actions at high concentrations on the uteruses of rabbits and guinea pigs (71). Pseudolycorine (an alkaloid isolated from *Narcissus tazetta* var. *chinensis* Roem., *Narcissus papyraceus*, and *Lycoris radiata* Herb.) and the hydrochloride derivative of this alkaloid markedly inhibit, at tolerable doses, the growth of W-256 carcinosarcoma in rats (134).

Anticancer activities displayed by the esters of the cephalotaxine alkaloid isolated from *Cephalotaxus harringtonia* (Forbes) K. Koch have prompted the study of a Chinese species of *Cephalotaxus mannii* Hook. f. (*Cephalotaxus hainanensis* Li). As a result, 11 analogous alkaloids have been isolated. The 4 ester derivatives of cephalotaxine— harringtonine (Structure 16), homoharringtonine (Structure 17), isoharringtonine (Structure 18), and deoxyharringtonine (Structure 19)—demonstrate various degrees of inhibitory activities against transplantable animal tumors. Clinical trials of harringtonine on 165 leukemia patients in 27 separate hospitals indicated a complete remission rate of 20 percent and a total effectiveness rate of 72.7 percent. Among 94 leukemia patients treated with homoharringtonine, a complete remission rate of 22.3 percent and a total effectiveness rate of 63.8 percent was observed (185).

Structure 16. Harringtonine (R_1 = OH, R_2 = H, N = 2)
Structure 17. Homoharringtonine (R_1 = OH, R_2 = H, n = 3)
Structure 18. Isoharringtonine (R_1 = H, R_2 = OH, N = 2)
Structure 19. Deoxyharringtonine (R_1 = H, R_2 = H, n = 2)

$$R = CH_3 - \underset{\underset{CH_3}{|}}{\overset{\overset{R_1}{|}}{C}} - (CH_2)_n - \underset{\underset{C=O}{|}}{\overset{\overset{OH}{|}}{C}} - \underset{}{\overset{\overset{R_2}{|}}{CH}} - \overset{\overset{O}{||}}{C} - OCH_3$$

6. Tryptophan Derived

From the native drug plant *Picrasma quassioides* (D. Don) Bennett, a series of canthin-6-one derivatives have been isolated. Among these derivatives, 4,5-dimethoxycanthin-6-one (Structure 20) and 4-methoxy-5-hydroxycanthin-6-one (Structure 21) have exhibited activity against *Staphylococcus aureus*, including drug-resistant strains. Clinical trials with 4-methoxy-5-hydroxycanthin-6-one confirm the antimicrobial activities (200).

Indirubin (Structure 22) obtained from *Indigofera tinctoria* L. is reported to be an active constituent in the treatment of chronic myelocytic leukemia. Pharmacologically, this tryptophan-derived alkaloid exhibited marked inhibitory activity against Walker carcinosarcoma 256 in rats and against Lewis lung cancer (14, 82). In clinical trials with 314 patients having chronic myelocytic leukemia, 82 patients achieved complete remission, 105 patients had partial remis-

Structure 20. 4,5-Dimethoxycanthin-6-one (R = OCH₃)
Structure 21. 4-Methoxy-5-hydroxycanthin-6-one (R = OH)

sion, and 87 patients displayed beneficial effects following treatment with indirubin for a total effectiveness rating of 87.3 percent. Indirubin now has been officially designated a drug in China and is produced synthetically.

Structure 22. Indirubin

Both the total alkaloid and the rhynchophylline isolated from *Uncaria rhynchophylla* (Maq.) Jackson have demonstrated hypotensive and sedative actions. Preliminary studies on the mechanisms of hypotensive action suggest the central nervous system or vasomotor centers are affected. In addition, the mechanism of rhynchophylline action may involve the function of the sinus nerve and other nerve receptors (166, 219). In clinical trials where the total alkaloids extracted from *Uncaria rhynchophylla* were given orally to 245 hypertensive patients, the overall effectiveness rate for lowering blood pressure was 77.2 percent (167). Hence, the total alkaloids *Uncaria rhynchophylla* have been manufactured commercially.

Rauvolfia verticillata (Lour.) Baill. and *Rauvolfia yunnanensis* Tsiang are the 2 main sources used for extraction of the extensively used hypotensive agent from China, Jiang-Ya-Ling. Along with 10 other alkaloids of known structures, 2 water-soluble alkaloids with strong hypotensive activity have been isolated from *Rauvolfia verticillata*. The first of the active alkaloids is spegatrine (Structure 23), demonstrated to be an α-adrenergic blocking agent. The second active alkaloid (previously unknown) is named verticillatine (Structure 24) and exhibited ganglionic blocking effects (114). Another α-adrenergic blocking alkaloid, sarpagine, has been isolated from the same plant (222). Of the 11 alkaloids isolated from *Rauvolfia yunnanensis*, 2 of these, 19-epiajmaline and the 16, 17-stereoisomer of pseudoreserpine, were new ones. The 16, 17-stereoisomer of pseudoreserpine has demonstrated hypotensive activity similar to that of reserpine.

Camptothecine isolated from *Campotheca acuminata* Decsne exhibits very high antitumor activity in the L-1210 system, and 2 other

Structure 23. Spegatrine

Structure 24. Verticillatine

alkaloids isolated from the same plant—10-hydroxycamptothecine and 10-methoxy-camptothecine—demonstrate even higher antitumor activities (150, 153). Both camptothecine and 10-hydroxycamptothecine are being used in China as antitumor agents.

7. Isoprenoid Derived

Gentianine, obtained from *Gentiana macrophylla* Pall., exerts hypotensive, anti-inflammatory, and weak analgesic actions (21, 160). Lappaconitine (Structure 25), isolated from the roots of *Aconitum sinomontanum* Nakai, demonstrates analgesic effects during the hot plate test in mice and the tail-flick test in rats. Anesthesia tests on rabbit corneas reveal the surface anesthetic potency of lappaconitine to be 8 times stronger than that of cocaine. The local anesthetic activities of lappaconitine in sciatic nerve block tests in mice and intracutaneous wheal tests in guinea pigs were about 5 times as great and about the same, respectively, in activity as cocaine (164). Lappaconitine is currently being used as a nonaddictive analgesic agent (13).

Structure 25. Lappaconitine

An isoprenoid pathway-derived alkaloid isolated from the roots of *Aconitum flavum* Hand.-Mazz. and *Aconitum pendulum* Busch, 3-acetylaconitine has stronger analgesic action than that of aconitine. Local anesthetic activity of 3-acetylaconitine on the sciatic nerve block test in mice and the intracutaneous wheal test in guinea pigs were 92 and 53 times, respectively, as active as cocaine (161). Increased vascular permeability induced by acetic acid or histamine is considerably inhibited by 3-acetylaconitine. Edema produced by carrageenin or fresh egg white is also markedly inhibited by 3-acetylaconitine (163).

Delsoline has proved to be an active principle in *Aconitum finetianum* Hand.-Mazz. This alkaloid displays a relaxant action on intestinal smooth muscles (8). From the same plant, N-deacetylfinaconitine, N-deacetylranaconitine, and N-deacetylappaconitine have also been isolated, and all 3 of these alkaloids have been proven to have analgesic activities (83). Dedudatine, a known base originally obtained from *Delphinium denudatum* and now known to occur in *Aconitum jinyangense* W.T. Wang and *Aconitum pseudohuiliense* Chang et W.T. Wang, exhibits curing and prophylactic effects against the arrhythmia elicited by aconitine in rats (89).

Cycloviribuxine D, isolated from *Buxus sinica* (Rend. et Wils.) Cheng, increases coronary blood flow, decreases oxygen consumption, and demonstrates antiarrhythmic and cardiotonic action. Clinically, this alkaloid is being used for the treatment of rheumatic cardiopathia and coronary heart diseases (59). Pingpeimine A (Structure 26), isolated from *Fritillaria ussuriensis* Maxim., exhibits expectorant and hypotensive effects (195).

Structure 26. Pingpeimine A

8. Miscellaneous Alkaloids

Leonurine, isolated from the traditional Chinese drug plant *Leonurus artemisia* (Lour.) S.Y. Hu (Structure Leonurus heterophyllus Sweet), stimulates contraction of the uterine smooth muscle (210). Tetramethylpyrazine (TMPZ) is the active ingredient of the traditional Chinese drug Chuan-Xiong (Structure Ligusticam chuanxiong Hort.).

Pharmacological and clinical studies reveal that TMPZ hydrochloride can improve microcirculation in the mesenteroids of rabbits and, *in vitro*, dilate capillary vessels. TMPZ not only will inhibit platelet aggregation caused by ADP but will also separate aggregated platelets. Clinically, this alkaloid has been satisfactorily used for the treatment of occlusive cerebral blood vessel diseases, such as cerebral embolism (3).

A water-soluble preparation from *Ganoderma capense* (Lloyd) Teng has been clinically demonstrated to produce satisfactory effects on progressive muscular dystrophy and atrophic myotonia. Since hyperaldolasemia is one of the biochemical indicators of muscular dystrophy, the effect of *Ganoderma* on experimental aldolasemia caused by the administration of 2,4-dichlorophenoxy acetic acid in mice has been studied. Results of these studies indicate uracil and uridine, among other alkaloids occurring in the water-soluble preparation, are responsible for the specified actions (124, 214).

B. Terpenes

1. Monoterpenes and Sesquiterpenes

Linalool, isolated from *Thymus quinquecostatus* Celak. and *Lonicera japonica* Thunb., exhibits anti-inflammatory action. Ankle joint swelling of the rat hind leg, caused by injection of egg white, can be significantly reduced by treatment with linalool (107). Linalool has also proved to be an antimicrobial agent.

The essential oil from the fruits of *Phellodendron amurense* Rupr. and the main components of oil, α- and β-myrcene, have marked expectorant effect and some antitussive activity (105). From the leaves of the traditional Chinese drug plant *Artemisia argyi Level*. et Vant., several antiasthmatic ingredients have been isolated. These include the terpenes trans-carveol, αterpineol (33), terpinen-4-ol, and β -caryophyllene (34). Preparations of the essential oil from *Artemisia argyi* have been recommended for clinical trials.

Juniper camphor, isolated from the essential oil of *Rhododendron anthopogonides* Maxim., is reported to possess expectorant activity, while limonene and neofuranodiene (Structure 27) isolated from the same source exhibit antitussive effects (126). Germacrone, isolated from the leaves of *Rhododendron dauricum* L., has also exhibited antitussive effects (220). In the essential oil of *Rhododendron tsinghaiense* Ching, d-γ-cadinene, α-cadinol, and bulnesol possess expectorant activity and guaiol and bulnesol possess antitussive activity (125). In addition, β-pinene isolated from *Rhododendron capitatum* Maxim. displays expectorant activity (127).

Piperitone, the major constituent of the essential oil from *Cymbopogon distanus* (Nees) A. Camus, has pharmacological

Structure 27. Neofuranodiene

antiasthmatic, antitussive, and antimicrobial activities. Clinically, this terpine has been used for the treatment of chronic bronchitis with a total effectiveness rating of about 80 percent (139). Carvone, isolated from the fruits of *Carum carvi* L., displays antiasthmatic, antitussive, and antispasmolytic effects (220).

The juice squeezed from fresh *Apium graveolens* L. has long been used in southeastern China for the treatment of epilepsy. The anticonvulsant components 3-*n*-butylphthalide (Ag-1, Structure 28) and 3-*n*-butyl-4,5-dihydrophthalide (Ag-2, Structure 29) have been isolated from the juice and clinically evaluated. Both of these compounds produced protective action against the maximal electroshock seizure test, the minimal electroshock threshold test, the metrazol seizure threshold test, and the maximal audiogenic seizure response in mice and rats with doses lower than the dose for minimal toxic signs in 50 percent of the animals (TD_{50}) (215, 216).

Structure 28. 3-*n*-Butylphthalide

Structure 29. 3-*n*-Butyl-4,5-dihydrophthalide

The essential oil of the traditional Chinese drug plant *Angelica sinensis* (Oliv.) Diels contains 2 major components—ligustilide and butylidene phthalide. Ligustilide has been demonstrated to have a remarkable antiasthmatic effect on guinea pigs that have been injected with acetylcholine or histamine. Ligustilide also has an antispasmodic effect on isolated guinea pig trachea strips that were contracted by acetylcholine, histamine, and barium chloride, and a relaxation effect on trachea strips under normal tension (165). Similarly, butylidene phthalide has provided considerable antiasthmatic relief in experimental asthmatic guinea pigs and a relaxation effect on trachea strips (39).

Isolated from *Mentha haplocalyx* Briq., *d*-8-acetoxycarvotanacetone acts as a good repellent to the mosquito, biting midge, buffalo gnat, and horsefly (221). Curcumol (Structure 30) and curdione (Structure 31), isolated from the essential oil of *Curcuma aromatica* Salisb., have demonstrated inhibitory effects on S-37, U-14, and ECA tumor development in mice. Clinically, the essential oil as well as curcumol and curdione are being used for the treatment of the early stages of cervical cancer (142, 149).

Structure 30. Curcumol

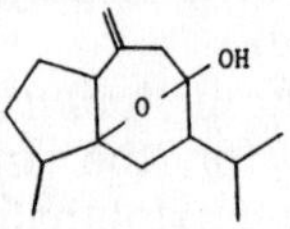

Structure 31. Curdione

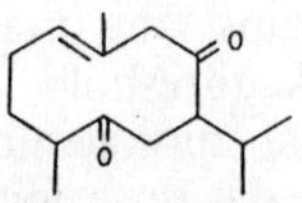

After a systematic investigation of the traditional Chinese antimalarial drug plant *Artemisia annua* L., the active component was identified as qinghaosu (Structure 32). Essentially, patients were all cured in clinical trials on 2,099 cases of *Plasmodium vivax* and *Plasmodium falciparum* malaria treated with qinghaosu preparations (38). An acid isolated from the same plant, designated as qinghaoic acid, demonstrated antibacterial activities on *Staphylococcus aureus*, *Escherichia coli*, *Solmonella typhosa*, and other microrganisms (240).

Structure 32. Qinghaosu

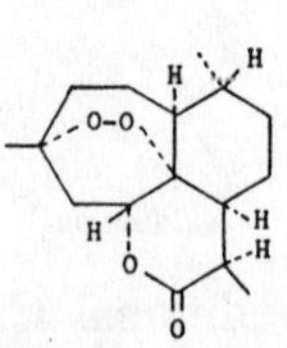

The root of *Artabotrys hexapetallus* (L. f.) Bhandari is a folk remedy for malaria. Yingzhaosu A (Structure 33) has been extracted from the roots and demonstrated to be the active ingredient of this herb (110). Paeoniflorin, isolated from the traditional Chinese drug plant *Paeonia lactiflora* Pall., has a marked effect against acute myocardial ischemia caused by pituitrin and inhibits platelet aggregation caused by adenosine diphosphate (ADP). In addition, paeoniflorin possesses sedative, hypotensive, and anti-inflammatory activities; has protective effects on stress ulcers; and initiates the dilation of coronary vessels.

Structure 33. Yingzhaosu A

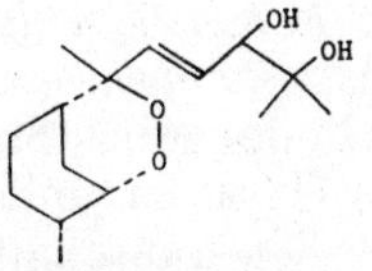

Swertiamarin, isolated from *Swertia patens* Burk., has displayed inhibition of the central nervous system, and anodyne has sedative and spasmolytic effects (99, 100). Of the 6 compounds isolated from the leaves of *Syringa oblata* Lindl., tyrosol, E-*p*-hydrocinnamic acid, 3,4-dihydroxyphenethyl alcohol, 3,4-dihydroxybenzoic acid, and aglucone of syringopicroside have bacteriostatic activity. The strongest of these compounds in action appears to be 3,4-dihydroxyphenethyl alcohol with the minimum bacteriostatic concentration against *Shigella flexneri* being 6.25 μg/ml. In addition, the aglucone of syringopicroside has a prominent cholecystagogic effect (172). Tutin (Structure 34), isolated from *Loranthus parasiticus* (L.) Merr., a parasite on *Coriaria sinica* Maxim., has been demonstrated to be effective in the treatment of schizophrenia (217). Pogostone (Structure 35) isolated from *Pogostemon cablin* (Blanco) Benth. has antifungal activities (96).

Structure 34. Tutin

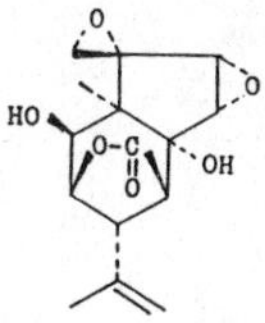

Structure 35. Pogostone

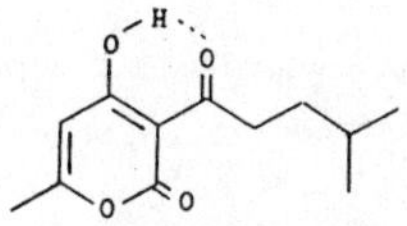

2. Diterpenes

Several diterpene bitter principles that occur in one genus *Rabdosia* (Fam. Labiatae) have displayed antitumor or antimicrobial activities. Rabdosin A (Structure 36) and B (Structure 37) isolated from *Rabdosia japonica* (Burm. f.) Hara are significantly cytotoxic on ECA tumor cells and L-1210 (104). Rabdophyllin G (rabdosin C, Structure 38), isolated from *Rabdosia macrophylla* (Migo) C.Y. Wu et H. W. Li and *Rabdosia japonica* (Burm. f.) Hara, lengthens the survival time of mice with Ehrlich ascites tumor and is cytotoxic to liver cancer cells *in vitro* (31, 118). The new diterpenes sculponeata A (Structure 39) and B (Structure 40), isolated from *Rabdosia sculponeata* (Vaniot) Hara, have antibacterial activities against *Staphylococcus aureus, Shigella flexneri*, and *Bacillus grass* (178). Ludongnin (Structure 41), isolated from *Rabdosia rubescens* (Hemsl.) Hara, has inhibitory activities against the growth of ECA, S-180, and P-388 transplantable animal tumors (233).

Structure 36. Rabdosin A (R$_1$ = H, R$_2$ = OCH$_3$, R$_3$ = ---OH)
Structure 42. Macrocalin A (R$_1$ = AcO, R$_2$ = OH, R$_3$ = ---OAc)

Structure 37. Rabdosin B (R = Ac)
Structure 38. Rabdophyllin G (Rabdosin C) (R = H)

Structure 39. Sculponeata A

Structure 40. Sculponeata B

Macrocalin A (Structure 42) and B (Structure 43), 2 new diterpenoids isolated from *Rabdosia macrocalyx* (Dunn) Hara, exert

Structure 41. Ludongnin

cytotoxic effects *in vitro* against cultures of Hela cells (27). Amethystoidin A (Structure 44), isolated from *Rabdosia amethystoides* (Benth.) Hara, has inhibitory action *in vivo* on experimental tumors and *in vitro* on hepatoma cells and *Staphylococcus aureus* (30). Lasiodonin (Structure 45) and lasiokaurin (Structure 46), isolated from the leaves of *Rabdosia macrophylla* (Migo) C.Y. Wu et H.W. Li, have demonstrated, respectively, cytotoxicity against *in vitro* cultures of hepatoma cells (28) and the ability to prolong the survival time of mice inoculated with Ehrlich ascites carcinoma (10 mg/kg/d for 7d, ip) or hepatoma ascites carcinoma (10 mg/kg/d for 7d, ip) (118). The increase in the survival rate of mice with Ehrlich and hepatoma ascites carcinoma and treated with lasiokaurin was 70.6 percent and 109.6 percent, respectively, longer than controls (118).

Structure 42. Appears with Structure 36.

Structure 43. Macrocalin B (R_1 = OH, R_2 = H)
Structure 48. Ponicidine (Rubescensine B) (R_1 = H, R_2 = OH)

Structure 44. Amethystoidin A

Oridonin (rubescensine A, Structure 47), isolated from *Rabdosia rubescens* (Hemsl.) C.Y. Wu et Hsuen and *Rabdosia macrophylla* (Migo) C.Y. Wu et H. W. Li, exhibits significant cytotoxicity on hepatoma cells, inhibitory tumor activity against Ehrlich ascites carcinoma in mice, and bactericidal effect against *Staphyloccoccus aurea* (29). Oridonin also displays various degrees of inhibitory activity against transplantable animal tumors. This compound has been used

Structure 45. Lasiodonin (R$_1$ = R$_2$ = OH, R$_3$ = H)
Structure 46. Lasiokaurin (R$_1$ = AcO, R$_2$ = H, R$_3$ = OH)
Structure 47. Oridonin (Rubescensine A) (R$_1$ = R$_3$ = OH, R$_2$ = H)

for the treatment of esophageal cancer (51). Ponicidine (rubescensine B, Structure 48), isolated from *Rabdosia rubescens* (Hemsl.) C. Y. Wu et Hsuen, has exhibited significant inhibitory activities against Ehrlich ascites carcinoma, S-180 cells, hepatoma ascites carcinoma, and L-1 ascites carcinoma in mice (Table 1) (224) with an increase in the survival rate.

Structure 48. Appears with Structure 43.

TABLE 1. Carcinoma Inhibitory Activity of Ponicidine in Mice

Tumor Type	Ponicidine Treatment	Increase in Survival Longevity
Ehrlich ascites	10 mg/kg/d for 7d,ip	+ 101.7
S-180 cells	20 mg/kg/d for 7d,ip	+ 232.7
Hepatoma ascites	20 mg/kg/d for 7d,ip	+ 64.5
L-1 ascites	20 mg/kg/d for 7d,ip	+ 136.1

Data taken from Zhang et al. (224).

Roots of *Daphne Genkwa* Sieb. et Zucc. are used as an abortifacient in folklore medicine. Yuanhuacine (Structure 49) and yuanhuadine (Structure 50), 2 new diterpenes isolated from the root, elicit abortion in monkeys. Clinically, these compounds have been used in the abortifacients at a dose of 70 to 80 μg yuanhuacine or 60 μg yuanhuadine through intraamniotic injection (171, 212).

Triptolide (Structure 51) and tripdiolide (Structure 52), isolated from *Triptergium wilfordii* Hook or *Triptergium hypoglaucum* (Levl.) Hutch., demonstrated significant tumor inhibitory activity against leukemias in mice and KB cells (97). Triptolide markedly prolonged the survival time of L-615-bearing mice with some living for more than one month. When the long-term survivors were rechallanged with leukemic cells, no further disease was induced. Triptolide acted as a depressant on humoral-mediated immunity (225).

Structure 49. Yuanhuacine (R = ⬡) 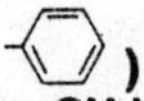
Structure 50. Yuanhuadine (R = —CH₃)

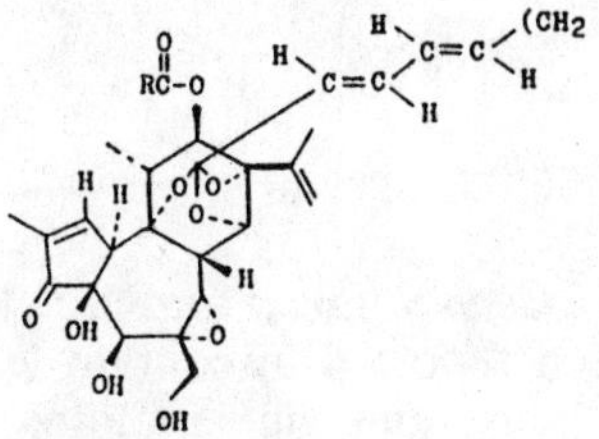

Structure 51. Triptolide (R = H)
Structure 52. Tripdiolide (R = OH)

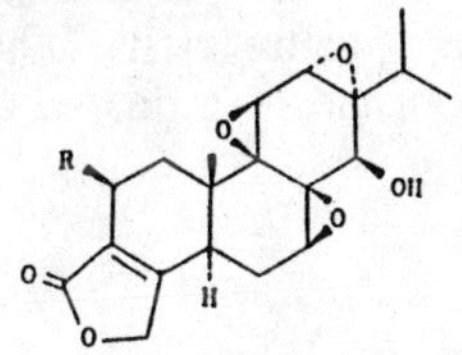

The fruit of *Brucea javanica* (L.) Merr. is a traditional Chinese drug with noted toxicity to humans. However, among the series of quassinoides that have been isolated from this plant, brusatal (Structure 53) is active against sarcoma 180. In addition, bruceine D (Structure 54) and bruceine E (Structure 55) are active against malaria (113).

Structure 53. Brusatal

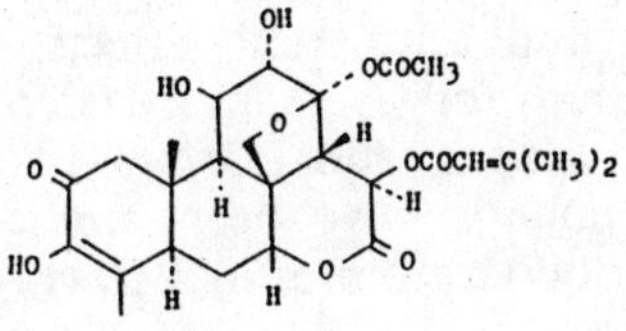

Structure 54. Bruceine D

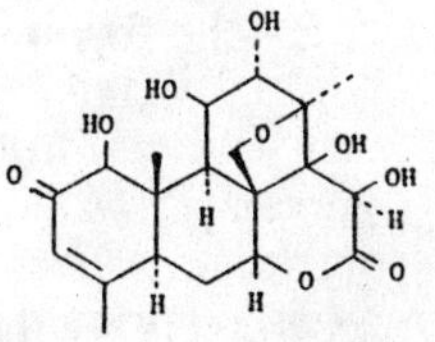

Structure 55. Bruceine E

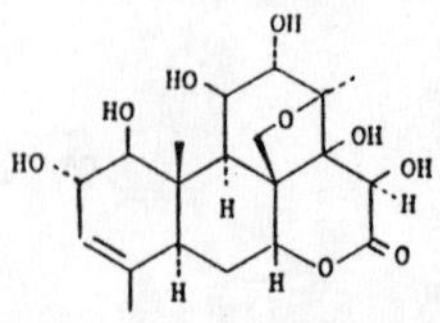

The alkaloid-rich *Cephalotaxus mannii* Hook. f. (*Cephalotaxus hainanensis* Li) has been reported to contain 2 new diterpene lactones: hainanolide (Structure 56) and hainanolidol. Hainanolide is active against sarcoma 180, Walker carcinosarcoma 256, Lewis lung carcinoma, L-615 leukemia, P-388 leukemia, and L-1210 leukemia (159). Hainanolide is active in tissue culture against plaque formation by influenza virus type A (WS), Newcastle disease virus, Japanese B encephalitis virus (AZ), and vaccina virus. The zone of inhibition for hainanolide activity against viruses extends to about 15 to 50 mm wide (91).

Structure 56. Hainanolide

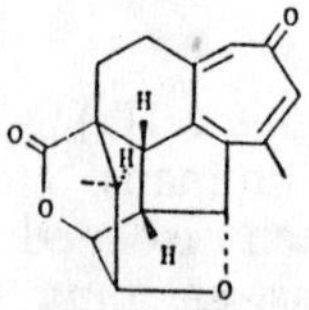

Isolated from the herbal drug plant *Andrographis paniculata* (Burm. f.) Nees, the lactones deoxyandrographolide (Structure 57), andrographolide (Structure 58), neoandrographolide (Structure 59), and deoxydidehydroandrographolide (Structure 60) possess various degrees of anti-inflammatory and antipyretic effects. Deoxydidehydroandrographolide displays the strongest activity, deoxyandrographolide and neoandrographolide the next, and andrographolide the least activity. Clinically, these compounds have been applied in the treatment of infectious diseases of the gastrointestinal tract, respiratory organs, and urinary system (42).

The bark of *Pseudolarix kaempferi* Gord. is known as an antifungal agent. Of the new diterpenes characterized in the bark—pseudolarix A and pseudolarix B—the former has antifungal activity.

3. Triterpenes

Curcurbitacin B and curcurbitacin E (elaterin), isolated from the fruit stalk of *Cucumis melo* L., possess activity against hepatitis (70, 144). A mixture of curcurbitacin IIa (Structure 61) and curcurbitacin

Structure 57. Deoxyandrographolide

Structure 58. Andrographolide

Structure 59. Neoandrographolide

Structure 60. Deoxydidehydroandrographolide

IIb (Structure 62), 2 new tetracyclic triterpenes isolated from the tuber
of *Hemsleya amabilis* Diels have a marked and broad antibacterial

spectrum. Clinically, the mixture of these 2 triterpenes is being used for the treatment of bacterial dysentery, bronchitis, tonsillitis, and tuberculosis (19). Ursolic acid and oleanolic acid, 2 widely distributed triterpenes isolated from *Incarvillea arguta* Royle, *Amphicome arguta* *Swertia mussotii* Franch., and *Swertia chinensis* Franch, have proved effective in the prevention of experimental liver injury induced by CCl_4 and in lowering the SGPT level of rats (131, 202).

Structure 61. Cucurbitacin IIa (R = COCH₃)
Structure 62. Cucurbitacin IIb (R = H)

Astramembrannin I (astragalus saponin I, Structure 63), isolated from Huang-Qi (the traditional Chinese drug plant *Astragalus membranaceus* Bge.) (4) has anti-inflammatory action and lowers blood pressure. When given intravenously (5 mg/kg) or orally (50 mg/kg), astramembrannin inhibits any increase in vascular permeability caused by 5-hydroxy-tryptamine and histamine. A lowering of blood pressure by astramembrannin was demonstrated in anesthetized rats or cats by intravenous treatments of 10 and 15 mg/kg (229). Astramembrannin also induces accumulation of cAMP in rabbit plasma following intraperitoneal injection (10 mg/kg) and is known to enhance the incorporation of [³H] TdR into the regenerating liver of mice (228).

Structure 63. Astramembrannin I (Astragalus Saponin I)

The esculentosides A, B, C, D, E, and F have been isolated from *Phytolacca esculenta* Van Houtte. The total saponins as well as the esculentoside A exert considerable enhancement of phygocytic function of leucocytes and promote DNA synthesis in mice. The aglycone jaligonic acid of esculentoside E has been considered to have good anti-inflammatory action (180). A great number of papers on triterpenoid glucosides isolated from *Panax ginseng* C.A. Mey. have been published, and thus, information on that area will not be presented here.

4. Cardiac Glucosides

The inotropic and toxic effects of peruvoside and neriifolin, isolated from the kernels of *Thevetia peruvians* (Pers.) K. Schum., have been studied in anesthetized cats and guinea pigs. The maximum effect of these 2 compounds is similar to that of ouabain and strophanthin K, but the safety margin of pervoside treatment is about twice the other 3 glucosides (92). A mixture (known as neriperside) of peruvoside, neriifolin, and cerberin has been clinically used for the treatment of heart failure (186). Diacetylneriifolin, a derivative of neriifolin, displays a sedative effect in small doses and induces hypnosis or anesthesia in large doses (209).

C. Phenolic Compounds

1. Quinones

Irisquinone (Structure 64) is an antitumor principle isolated from the seeds of *Iris pallasii* Fisch. var. *chinensis* Fisch. Injected intraperitoneally, irisquinone has proven to be effective against U-14 and lymphosarcoma and significantly inhibitory to hepatic and Ehrlich ascite cancer. The LD_{50} of irisquinone in mice was 25.4 $\pm$ 1.9 mg/kg (ip) and 2.8 $\pm$ 0.3 g/kg (po). The subacute toxicities in both rats and dogs are low, and no signs of inhibition of bone marrow development have been observed (102).

Structure 64. Irisquinone

$$H_3CO \quad (CH_2)_9CH=CH(CH_2)_5CH_3$$

The naphthoquinone derivatives acetylshikonin and β,β-dimethylacrylshikonin are active ingredients in the traditional Chinese drug Zi-Cao [*Arnebia euchroma* (Royle) Johnst.]. Both of these compounds inhibit the usual increase of capillary permeability induced in rats by histamine and have significant anti-inflammatory effects in rats on edema of the paws induced by acute exposure to formalin (115, 116).

Plumbagin, reported in *Drosera peltata* Smith var. *lunata* Clark and *Ceratostigma plumbaginoides* Bge., has demonstrated anti-inflammatory, antitussive, and antibacterial effects (148). This compound also significantly inhibits growth of *Mycobacterium tuberculosis* (187).

Eleutherol (Structure 65), elutherin (Structure 66), and isoeleutherin (Structure 67) isolated from *Eleutherine americana* Merr. er Heyne markedly increase the bloodflow of atreriae coronaria (26).

Structure 65. Eleutherol

Structure 66. Elutherin (R = ---H)
Structure 67. Isoeleutherin (R =◄H)

A series of anthraquinone derivatives isolated from Chinese rhubarb, *Rheum palmatum* L., and other *Rheum* species demonstrate various pharmacological activities. Rhein, emodin, and aloeemodin were proven active against *Bacillus anthracis*, *Bacillus substilis*, *Corynebacterium diptheriae*, *Salmonella paratyphi*, *Shigella dysenteriae*, *Staphylococci*, and *Streptococci* (11). *Salmonella typhi* was sensitive to rhein only (11), and *Leptospiri* (*in vitro*) was sensitive to emodin only (196). Emodin and rhein markedly inhibit the growth of melanoma (76% and 73% respectively). In addition, emodin inhibits growth of mammary carcinoma, and rhein inhibits growth of Ehrlich ascites carcinoma (10). Emodin and rhein are also reported to exhibit strong inhibitory effects on the respiration and glycolysis, respectively, of Ehrlich ascites carcinoma cells (12). Sennosides exhibit purgative activity regarded as the main active ingredients in Chinese rhubarb (190).

Chrysophanol isolated from *Rumex crispus* L. shortens the time of blood coagulation (88). Physcion, an antibacterial ingredient isolated from the herbal drug *Polygonum multiflorum* Thunb. var. *cilinerve* Steward, exhibits strong activity against the growth of *Staphylococcus aureus*, *Escherichia coli*, and *Pseudomonas aeruginosa* (47).

A series of phenanthrenequinone derivatives has been discovered in the traditional Chinese drug Dan-Shen (*Salvia miltiorrhiza* Bge.). This herbal drug is described as being able to mobilize the blood circulation, removing stasis. The medicinal mixture known as tanshinone, as well as ingredients of the mixture such as cryptotanshinone (Structure 68), dihydrotanshinone I (Structure 69), hydroxytanshinone II-A (Structure 70), methyl tanshinate, and tanshinone II-B, display bacteriostatic action, particularly on regular and drug-resistant strains of *Staphylococcus aureus*. Tanshinone has also demonstrated inhibitory activity against *Mycobacterium tuberculosis* H 37 Rv and 2 related dermatophytes. Tablets and ointment of tanshinone provided satisfactory clinical results in 455 cases of infection with mainly *Staphylococcus aureus* (63). Sodium tanshinone II-A sulfonate is a water-soluble derivative and exhibits marked cardiovascular activity. This derivative has been used for the treatment of cardiovascular diseases, cerebral thromoboembolism, and thromoboangitis obliterans where anginal pain and the feeling of chest tightness were ameliorated and ischemic alterations in the electrocardiogram were improved (20).

Structure 68. Cryptotanshinone

Structure 69. Dihydrotanshinone I

Structure 70. Hydroxytanshinone II-A ($_1$ = OH, R_2 = CH_3)
Structure 71. Przewaquinone A (R_1 = H, R_2 = CH_2OH)

Przewaquinone A (Structure 71), a strong bacteriostatic component isolated from *Salvia przewalskii* Maxim. var. *mandarinorum* Stib., has demonstrated the ability to inhibit Lewis lung carcinoma and melonoma B-16. The survival time of P-388-infected mice treated with przewaquinone can be lengthened by more than 100 percent (199).

2. Flavonoids

One of the most widely distributed flavonols is quercetin, isolated from plants like *Euphorbia lunulata* Bge. (67) and *Hypericum ascyron* L., which exhibits pharmacologically antitussive, antiasthmatic, and antiallergic effects (181). Another commonly occurring flavonol is kaempferol obtained from plants like *Euphorbia lunulata* Bge. and *Thesium chinense* Turcz. This flavonol has displayed antitussive and antibacterial activities (67, 145). Even rutin, a common flavonoid, has been demonstrated to be one of the active ingredients of *Berchemia polyphylla* Wall. and has exhibited antitussive, antiasthmatic, and expectorant activities (37).

Luteolin, isolated from *Ajuga decumbens* Thunb., has demonstrated antitussive, expectorant, and antibacterial activities (135). Unexpectedly, luteolin also affected acute hypotension in animals and increased their coronary blood flow (183). Hyperin has been demonstrated to be an active principle in many herbal antibronchitis remedies, like the use of *Rhododendron dauricaum* L. (128), *Euphorbia helioscopia* L. (22), and *Hypericumascycon* L. (163). Clinically, hyperin has been used as an antitussive agent.

Heliosin (quercetin-3-digalactoside) isolated from *Euphorbia helioscopia* L. has been clinically tested on 286 bronchitis patients with the results indicating this compound is a satisfactory drug for antitussive treatment (22). Farrerol isolated from the leaves of *Rhododendron dauricum* L. has displayed good expectorant activity (146).

A flavone, nevadensin (lysionotin, Structure 72), active against tuberculosis, has been identified in the herb *Lysionotus pauciflora* Maxim. At concentrations of 200 µg/ml, nevadensin displayed inhibitory activity against the growth of *Mycobacterium tuberculosis in vitro* (197). From a traditionally used Chinese drug plant, *Scutellaria baicalensis* Georgi, baicalein and baicalin have been isolated. Baicalein exhibits a marked antibacteriological effect and baicalin exhibits sedative, antipyretic, hypotensive, and diuretic effects (50). Baicalin has been used in clinics for the treatment of infectious hepatitis (136).

Structure 72. Nevadensin (Lysionotin)

Scutellarin, isolated from *Erigeron breviscapus* (Vant.) Hand.-Mazz., increases cerebral blood flow, decreases the resistance of cerebral vessels, and inhibits platelet aggregation caused by ADP (65). Clinically this compound has been used for the treatment of occlusive cerebral blood vessel diseases, such as paralysis caused by a cerebral embolism (176).

The flavonol glucoside crytophyllin, an ingredient of *Clerodendron cyrtophyllum* Turcz., manifested marked diuretic and anti-inflammatory effects in rats (130). Swertiajaponin, obtained from *Swertia mileensis* T.N. He et W.L. Shi, lowers the elevated serum glutamic pyruvic transaminase (SGPT) level caused by CCl_4 (109). An ingredient with antitussive and expectorant properties, hydroxygenkwanin has been extracted from the flower bud of *Daphne Gènkwa* Sieb. et Zucc. (36).

A new chalcone, corylifolinin (Structure 73), was isolated from *Psoralea corylifolia* L. and has been reported to inhibit growth of Hela cells and increase coronary blood flow in isolated guinea pig hearts (239). Icariin, the major flavonoid glucoside found in *Epimedium sagittatum* (Sieb. et Zucc.) Maxim., *Epimedium brevicornum* Maxim., and *Epimedium koreanum* Nakai, is reported to inhibit inotropism of heart ventricles (119).

Structure 73. Corylifolinin

Several isoflavones—daidzein (Structure 74), daidzin (Structure 75), puerarin (Structure 76), and daidzein-4',7-diglucoside (Structure 77)—have been isolated from the traditional Chinese drug plant *Pueraria lobata* (Willd.) Ohwi. Pharmacological studies indicate that a mixture of all of the isolated isoflavones or daidzein or puerarin individually, was capable of increasing cerebral and coronary blood flow, decreasing oxygen consumption of the myocardium, increasing the blood oxygen supply, and depressing the production of lactic acid by an oxygen-deficient heart muscle. Clinically, these isoflavones have been used for the relief of hypertensive disease, angina pectoris, migraine headaches, and sudden deafness (57, 168).

Structure 74. Daidzein ($R_1 = R_2 = R_3 = H$)
Structure 75. Daidzin ($R_1 = R_3 = H$, $R_2 =$ Glucopyranose)
Structure 76. Peurarin ($R_2 = R_3 = H$, $R_1 =$ Glucopyranose)
Structure 77. Daidzein-4', 7-diglucoside ($R_1 = H$, $R_2 = R_3 =$ Glucose)

Hemerocallone isolated from *Hemerocallis minor* Mill. exhibits a diuretic effect in rats (194).

3. Xanthones

An extract of the total xanthones and the single xanthone mangiferin from *Swertia mussotii* Franch. have demonstrated protective effects against acute liver injury caused by hypoxia (55). Isomangiferin, isolated from *Pyrrosia sheareri* (Bak.) Ching, displays antitussive and expectorant properties (151).

4. Phenyl Propanoids

Elemicin and *trans*-isomethyleugenol, obtained from *Asarum forbesii* Maxim., provide analgesic effects on mice, rabbits, cats, and dogs when injected intravenously (117). Another active principle, methyl-eugenol, from the same plant potentiates the hypnotic action of pentobarbital and thiopental; the central depressant effect of chlorpromazine; and a narcotic effect in rabbits, cats, dogs, and monkeys (85).

From the volatile oil of a traditional Chinese drug plant, *Acorus gramineus* Soland, several active principles have been isolated. Spasmolytic action was discovered to be initiated by α-asarone, β-asarone, and 1-allyl-2,4,5-trimethoxybenzene on isolated guinea pigs' tracheas and ileums (123). The phenylpropanoid 4-allyl-veratrole acts as a depressant on the central nervous system and, *in vitro*, as a bacteriocide against *Staphylococcus aureus* and *Diplococcus pneumoniae* (140).

Dang-Gui, [*Angelica sinensis* (Oliv.) Diels.] a commonly used traditional Chinese drug, has been used with favorable results for the treatment of thromboangitis obliterans and acute cerebral thrombolic diseases. Of the active ingredients, ferulic acid and sodium salt of ferulic acid inhibit rat platelet aggregation induced by ADP or collagen. The sodium salt of ferulic acid also has been observed to promote the release of ^{3}H-5HT-labelled platelets and inhibit platelet aggregation induced by thrombin in rats (211).

Chlorogenic acid isolated from *Cirsium segetum* Bge. and *Artemisiascoparia* Waldst et Kit. and the hydrolyzed chlorogenic acid product caffeic acid exhibit hemostatic and choleretic effects (72, 106). One of the bacteriostatic ingredients from the leaves of *Syringa oblata* Lindl. is *p*-coumaric acid. This compound inhibits, in various degrees, activity against *Staphylococcus aureus*, *Shigella flexneri*, *Escherichia coli*, and *Pseudomonas aeruginosa* (172). Syringin, isolated from *Daphne Giraldii* Nitshe and *Ilex rotunda* Thunb., has been proved pharmacologically and clinically hemostatic (175, 237).

From the water-soluble fraction of *Salvia miltiorrhiza* Bge., an active principle, danshensuan B (Structure 78), was isolated. This compound promotes fibrinolysis and increases coronary blood flow (24).

Structure 78. Danshensuan B

5. Coumarins

The coumarins esculetin, esculin, fraxetin, and fraxin have been reported in *Fraxinus rhynchophylla* Hance. Esculetin exhibits a fair antiasthmatic effect, esculin demonstrates antitussive activity, and both have expectorant and antibacterial effects (64). In addition, esculetin and esculin inhibit the increase in permeability of capillary vessels induced by histamine (16). These compounds are also reported to prolong the duration of sleep when administered with pentobarbital (73).

Daphnetin, isolated from herbal drug plants *Daphne Giraldii* Nitsche, *Daphne tangutica* Maxim., and *Daphne koreana* Nakai, has displayed analgesic and sedative effects in a series of animal tests (86). Daphnetin also exhibits significant anti-inflammatory effects on acute albumin or dextrose-induced edema of hind paws in rats (122). This coumarin has considerable cardiovascular activities, increasing the tolerance to monobaric and hypobaric hypoxia in mice and enhancing the coronary venous flow in anesthetized open-chest cats (138). Clinically, daphnetin has been used in the treatment of thromboangitis obliterans, angina pectoris, and rhematism (86).

An active principle isolated from *Wikstroemia indica* C. A. Mey., daphnoretin, has been observed to significantly increase the myocardial uptake of ^{86}Rb into the blood of mice, following the administration of 2.6 mg/0.25 ml/10 g (45). Scopoletin and scoplin, obtained from *Erycibe obtusifolia* Benth., demonstrated anti-inflammatory activity against acute albumin- or histamine-induced edema of hind paws and acute subacute joint swelling caused by formaldehyde. Both compounds also exhibit analgesic effects (207, 241). Isofraxidine, obtained from *Sarcandra glabra* (Thunb.) Nakai, inhibits tranplanted S-180 cells in mice (170).

Scoparone (6,7-dimethoxycoumarin), one of the active ingredients isolated from the traditional Chinese drug plant *Artemisia capillaris* Thunb., has several pharmacological actions, including choleretic (1), hypotensive, and antiasthmatic effects (184). Scoparone also increases coronary blood flow. Armillarisin A (Structure 79), a new coumarin derivative, was isolated from the ethanol extracts of the culture medium of the fungus *Armillariella tabescens* (Scop. ex Fr.) Sing. This compound markedly increases the bile secretion in experimental rats and dogs (158).

Structure 79. Armillarisin A

Several new coumarins isolated from the traditional Chinese drug plant *Peucedanum praeruptorum* Dunn have been demonstrated to have pharmacological effects. (+)-Praeruptorin A (Structure 80) increases coronary blood flow in isolated guinea pig hearts (25), and (+)-praeruptorin E (Structure 81) increases the tolerance of mice to anoxia (208).

Structure 80. (+)-Praeruptorin A (R = -C-CH$_3$)
Structure 81. (+)-Praeruptorin E (R = -C-CH$_2$-CH-CH$_3$-(CH$_3$)

Psoralen, a rather common coumarin isolated from *Psoralea corylifolia* L., has a photosensitizing effect and hence has been used for the treatment of leukoderma. This compound also has a hemostatic effect and is used for the treatment of several hemorrhagic diseases in obstetrics and gynecology (141). Another rather common coumarin, bergapten, obtained from the herbal drug plant *Pseudostreblus indica* Bur., promotes blood coagulation in rabbits (95). An isocoumarin derivative, bergenin, isolated from *Ardisia japonica* (Thunb.) Bl., has antitussive effects (147).

6. Lignans

A number of lignan compounds (Structures 82 and 83) (Table 2) isolated from the kernels of genus *Schisandra* lower elevated SGPT

TABLE 2. Actions of Lignans from the Kernals of *Schisandra*

Structure	Compounds	Plants	Actions
82-1	Deoxyschizandrin (wuweizisu A) $R_1=R_2=R_3=R_4=R_6=O-CH_3$ $R_5=H$	S. chinensis S. sphenanthera S. rubriflora	lower SGPT level analgesic
82-2	γ-Schizandrin (wuweizisu B) $R_1=R_2=R_6=O-CH_3$ $R_3=R_4=O-CH_2-O$, $R_5=H$	S. chinensis S. rubriflora	lower SGPT level
82-3	Wuweizisu C $R_1-R_2=R_3-R_4=O-CH_2-O$ $R_5=H$, $R_6=O-CH_3$	S. chinensis	lower SGPT level depress CNS
82-4	Schizandrin (wuweizichun A) $R_1=R_2=R_3=R_4=R_6=O-CH_3$ $R_5=OH$	S. chinensis	lower SGPT level analgesic action depress CNS decrease heart rate
82-5	Gomisin (wuweizichun B) $R_1=R_2=O-CH_2-O$ $R_3=R_4=R_6=O-CH_3$, $R_5=OH$	S. chinensis	lower SGPT level depress CNS antitussive action
82-6	Gomisin C (schizantherin A) $R_1=R_2=R_6=O-CH_3$ $R_3=R_4=O-CH_2-O$ $R_5=O-CO-\bigcirc$	S. chinensis S. sphenanthera	lower SGPT level
82-7	Gomisin B (schizantherin B) $R_1=R_2=R_6O-CH_3$ $R_3=R_4O-CH_2O$ $R_5=O-OC$	S. chinensis S. sphenanthera S. rubriflora	lower SGPT level
82-8	Shizantherin C $R_1=R_2=R_6=O-CH_3$ $R_3=R_4=O-CH_2O$ $R_5=O-OC$	S. sphenanthera	lower SGPT level
82-9	Schizantherin D $R_1=R_2=R_3=R_4=O-CH_2O$ $R_5=O-OC-\bigcirc$, $R_6=O-CH_3$	S. sphenanthera	lower SGPT level
82-10	Schizandronol (wuweizifen) $R_1=R_2=R_3=R_4=O-CH_3$ $R_5=H$, $R_6=OH$	S. henryi S. rubriflora	lower SGPT level
83-1	Schisanhenrin $R_1=OH$, $R_3=O-CH_3$ $R_2=O-OC$	S. henryi	lower SGPT level
83-2	(−)-Rubschisandrin $R_1=R_2=H$, $R_3=O-CH_3$	S. rubriflora	lower SGPT level
83-3	Schisanhenol B $R_1=R_2=R_3=H$	S. rubriflora	lower SGPT level

levels and help CNS depression (157, 173). In this connection, various herbal medicine Wu-Wei-Zi [*Schisandra chinensis* (Turcz.) Baill.] preparations have been tested on over 5,000 cases of hepatitis patients with total effectiveness rating for lowering SGPT levels of 84 to 97.9 percent (198).

Structure 82. Deoxyschizendrin and Related Compounds (Table 2)

Structure 83. Schisanhenrin and Related Compounds (Table 2)

7. Other Phenolic Types

Pinitol, obtained from *Lespedeza cuneata* G. Don or *L. sericea* Miq., displayed antitussive activity in clinical trials (80).

Acer ginnala Maxim., used as a bacteriostatic and anti-inflammatory herbal remedy, has 3 strongly bacteriostatic constitutents—chaotiaoqisu A (Structure 84), B (Structure 85), and C (Structure 86)—that have been isolated (156). Gastrodin (Structure 87) is a phenol-glucoside obtained from *Gastrodia elata* Blume (Fam. Orchidaceae) for which pharmacological tests indicate active sedative and anticonvulsive properties. Clinically, gastrodin has been used for the treatment of neurasthenia, insomnia, and headache (40).

Structure 84. Chaotiaoqisu A

Structure 85. Chaotiaoqisu B

Structure 86. Chaotiaoqisu C

Hemerocallin (Structure 88), a very toxic compound isolated from *Hemerocallis minor* Mill., has demonstrated remarkable inhibitory ac-

Structure 87. Gastrodin

tivity against *Schistosoma japonica* in mice. Gossypol (Structure 89) obtained from the seed oil cotton *Gossypium hirsutum* L. or *Gossypium herbaceum* L. is used as an antifertility agent for males and has been clinically demonstrated as an effective antifertility drug in a 6-month trial with over 8,000 healthy men (188).

Structure 88. Hemerocallin

Structure 89. Gossypol

Agrimorphol (Structure 90), isolated from the winter bud of *Agrimonia pilosa* Ledeb. (Gemma Agrimoniae), has a confirmed *in vitro* taeniacidal effect on *Taenia solium*. When submitted to clinical trials, the efficacy of agrimorphol was fully substantiated. This drug enjoys the advantages of only mild side effects with high anthelmintic action and thus is widely used (188). Agrimorphol also displays strong, direct action *in vitro* against *Schistosoma japonica* (213).

Structure 90. Agrimorphol

Robustanol A (Structure 91) obtained from *Eucalyptus rubusta* Smith has been reported to have inhibitory activity against malaria in mice (137). *Syringa oblata* Lindl., used as a bacteriostatic herbal drug, has a highly effective bacteriostatic ingredient (3,4-dihydroxyphenethyl alcohol) that is active against *Shigella flexner* at a minimum concentration of 6.25 µg/ml. (172). Obtained from *Artemisia scoparia* Waldst et Kit., *p*-hydroxyacetophenone displayed cholecystagogic activity in rats (81). Isolated from the leaves of *Ilex pubescens* Hook. et Arn. var. *glaber* Chang, 3,4-dihydroxyacetophenone can significantly increase coronary blood flow in dogs (179).

Structure 91. Robustanol A

Both a crude extract of *Gastrodia elata* Bl. and the ingredients vanillin and vanillyl alcohol demonstrate antiepileptic effects and elevate the electric shock threshold for producing convulsive seizures in rabbits (87). Vanillin and vanillyn alcohol also display anticonvulsive activity in mice treated with pentylenetetrazol (121). *Ardisia japonica* (Hornsted) Blume, used as a herbal drug for tuberculosis, has 2 phenols—ardisinol I (Structure 92) and II (Structure 93)—that are responsible for the specific activity. The minimum bacteriostatic concentrations of ardisinol I and II against *Mycobacterium tuberculosis* were 12.5 µg/ml and 25 to 50 µg/ml, respectively (76).

Structure 92. Ardisinol I (R = CH₃)
Structure 93. Ardisinol II (R = H)

When rhapontin, a stilbene glycoside obtained from *Rheum hotaoense* C.Y. Cheng et Kao, is given orally to normal and hyperlipidemic rabbits, decreases in the levels of lipid, total cholesterol, triglyceride, β-lippoprotein, and pre-β-lippoprotein in serum are measured (101). Another stilbene glycoside, polydatin, isolated from *Polygonum cuspidatum* Sieb. et Zucc., is also reported to lower serum lipid level (120).

The active constituents of *Citrus aurantium* L., N-methyltyramine (Structure 94) and synephrine (Structure 95) have been demonstrated to increase blood pressure (46). Paeonol, obtained from the traditional Chinese drug Mu-Dan-Pi (the root bark of *Paeonia suffruticosa* Andr.), has bacteriostatic, anti-inflammatory, and CNS depressive effects.

Clinically, an injection of 5 percent paeonol sulfonate displayed analgesic action (234).

Structure 94. N-Methyltyramine (R = H)
Structure 95. Synephrine (R = OH)

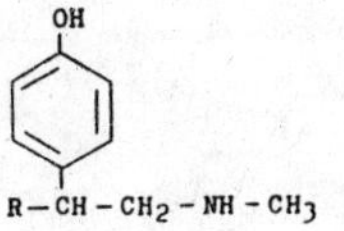

$$R-CH-CH_2-NH-CH_3$$

with OH group on benzene ring

D. Acids

An anthelmintic, quisqualic acid (Structure 96) has been isolated from the traditional Chinese drug Shi-Jun-Zi (fruits of *Quisquilis indica* L.). In clinic trials, potassium quisqualate at doses of 0.125 g were anthelmintic without any laxative side effects. The percentage of patients who excreted ascarids approached that of those who received santonin (56).

Structure 96. Quisqualic Acid

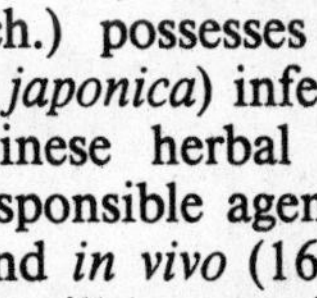

$$CH_2-\overset{H}{\underset{NH_2}{C}}-COOH$$

Cucurbitine (Structure 97) obtained from the pumpkin seeds (*Cucurbite moschata* Duch.) possesses a protective activity against schistosomal (*Schistosoma japonica*) infections (155). Fumaric acid and succinic acid in the Chinese herbal drug plant *Sarcandra glabra* (Thunb.) Nakai are the responsible agents for the bacteriostatic activities of the drug *in vitro* and *in vivo* (169). In addition, intraperitoneal injection of succinic acid will cause significant decreases in spontaneous activity, decreases in hypothermia, and significant increases in sleeping time induced in mice by pentobarbital treatment (90).

Structure 97. Cucurbitine

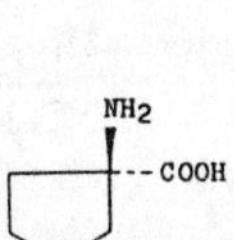

$$NH_2 \quad --COOH$$

Danshensu, β(3,4-dihydroxyphenyl)-lactic acid (Structure 98), obtained from the water-soluble fraction of *Salvia miltiorrhiza* Bge., is reported to dilate the coronary artery and significantly antagonize the constricting responses elicited by morphine and propranolol (54).

Plumbagic acid (Structure 99) isolated from *Plambago zeylanica* L. displays expectorant and bacteriostatic activities. Both *p*-hydroxybenzoic acid (Structure 100) obtained from *Lobelia chinensis* Lour. and protocatechuic acid (Structure 101) obtained from *Cryptolepsis sinensis* (Lour.) Merr. provide protective activities against cobra venom administered to mice (43). *Conyza canadensis* (L.) Cronq. is an antidysenteric herbal remedy from which vanillic acid (Structure 102) and syringic acid (Structure 103) are the major bacteriostatic constituents (174). Rubia naphaic acid (Structure 104) and the glycoside of this acid (Structure 105) isolated from *Rubia cordifolia* L. increase leucocyte numbers (192). Aristolochic acid (Structure 106) obtained from *Aristolochia debilis* Sieb. et Zucc. and *Aristolochia mollissima* Hance possess phagocyte stimulating action (32). Given orally (3.7 mg/kg) or intra-amniotically (30 mg/kg) to mice, this aristolochic acid displayed significant anti-implantation and abortifacient effects (177).

Structure 98. Danshensu [β(3,4-dihydroxyphenyl)-lactic acid]

Structure 99. Plumbagic Acid

Structure 100. *p*-Hydroxybenzoic Acid (R_1 = R_2 = H)
Structure 101. Protocatechuic Acid (R_1 = H, R_2 = OH)
Structure 102. Vanillic Acid (R_1 = OCH$_3$, R_2 = H)
Structure 103. Syringic Acid (R_1 = R_2 = OCH$_3$)

Structure 104. Rubia Naphaic Acid (R = H)
Structure 105. Rubia Naphaic Acid Glycoside (R = Glucose + xylose + rhamnose)

Structure 106. Aristolochic Acid

E. Miscellaneous Compounds

Rorifone (Structure 107) isolated from the herbal plant *Roripa montana* (Wall) Small has demonstrated expectorant and antitussive activities (188). Sarmentosin (Structure 108), demonstrated as an active principle of *Sedum sarmentosum* Bge., is able to lower the SGPT level in humans and is used for treatment of hepatitis (58). The volatile oil of *Houttynia cordata* Thunb. contains an antimicrobial principle decanoylacetaldehyde (Structure 109) that also possesses immuno-stimulating action. Hence, decanoylacetaldehyde has been synthetically produced for commercial use (41). The bacteriostatic ingredient diallyl thiosulfonate (Structure 110), first isolated from *Allium sativum* L. and then synthesized as a commercial product, has been clinically tested for use in treatment of infections of respiratory and digestive systems (98, 154).

Structure 107. Rorifone

$$CH_3 - SO_2 - CH_2 - (CH_2)_7 - CH_2CN$$

Structure 108. Sarmentosin

Structure 109. Decanoylacetaldehyde

$$CH_3 - (CH_2)_8 - \overset{O}{\overset{\|}{C}} - CH_2 - \overset{H}{\overset{|}{C}} = O$$

Structure 110. Diallyl Thiosulfonate

$$CH_2 = CH - CH_2 - \overset{O}{\underset{O}{\overset{\uparrow}{\underset{\downarrow}{S}}}} - S - CH_2 - CH = CH_2$$

III. DISCUSSION

Almost all pharmacologically active compounds belong to the secondary metabolites of plants. Selection and use of these metabolites can be regarded as an evolutionary process for humankind combating the harmful side of nature. Even though humans have reached the "atomic age," the precious ethnopharmacologic information gathered throughout history can still be used in eliminating human suffering. Isolation and elucidation of the chemical structure of the active principles in medicinal herbs, followed by synthesis and chemical modification through modern drug design, provides impetus in the development of therapeutic agents.

Of the pharmacologically active substances described in this review, alkaloids are of major importance with the benzylisoquinoline type potentially serving as the basis of new drugs for analgesic, sedative, antimicrobial, and cardiovascular ailments. The tropane-type alkaloid such as anisodamine and anisodine isolated from *Scopolia* is attractive for its effect on microcirculatory systems. The diterpene-type alkaloid isolated from *Aconitum* and *Delphinium* provides a starting point in the quest for more effective anodyne, arrhythmia, and cardionic drugs. The alkaloids related to harringtonine provide for antileukemic action.

In the phenolic compounds, several flavonoids (such as scutellarin, icariin, isorhamnetin, and puerarin) and the coumarins (such as daphnetin and daphnoretin) need to be considered for their cardiovascular activity. Within the terpenoids, many monoterpenes display efficacy against respiratory problems and can perhaps be used in the development of more favorable remedial medicines. Several peroxide substances, such as quinghuosu and yingzhaosu A, hold promise as antimalarial agents.

A recent survey has indicated that approximately 60 new drugs in China originated directly or indirectly from Chinese traditional and herbal medicines, providing evidence of the important role the medicinal plant plays in the exhaustive search for formulation of active compounds for use in new drugs.

Acknowledgements

Our grateful thanks are due to Professor Sung Wei-Liang of our institute for his valuable suggestions and help in preparing this manuscript.

IV. REFERENCES

1. Anonymous. 1973. The active constituents of Ying-Chen, *Artemisia capillaris* Thunb. or *A. scoparia* Waldst. et Kit. Chinese Medical Journal 53(8):471.

2. Anonymous. 1978. Securenine nitrate. National Medical Journal of China 58(6):379.

3. Cai, X.L. and Y.P. Li. 1979. Determination of the influence of tetramethylpyrazine on nourishing myocardial blood flow in mice by ^{86}Rb. Zhongcaoyao Tongxun (1):33-34.

4. Cao, Z.Z., J.H. Yu, L.X. Gan, and Y.Q. Chen. 1985. The structure of astramembrannins. Acta Chim. Sinica 43(6):581-585.

5. Chang, J.Q., J.G. Wang, C.C. Li, Y.D. Shao, Y.Q. Pei, M.Y. Jiang, T. Li, and D.Z. Xu. 1964. Pharmacological studies on magnoflorine, a hypotensive principle from Tu-Qing-Mu-Xiang. Acta Pharm. Sinica 11(1):42-49.

6. Chang, S.S., S.X. Fu, Y.S. Li, and N.C. Wang. 1960. The pharmacology of sabianine A. I. The analgesic and antiphlogistic actions and acute toxicity. Acta Pharm. Sinica 8(4):177-180.

7. Chao, S.H., J.S. Hsu, and J.H. Chu. 1966. The alkaloids of the Chinese drug Yen-Hu-So, the tubers of *Corydalis humosa* Migo. Acta Pharm. Sinica 13(1):6-13.

8. Chen, B.R., Y.F. Yang, R.M. Tian, C.P. Zhang, Y.Z. Xiao, and M.X. Liu. 1981. Alkaloids of *Aconitum finetianum* Hand.-Mazz. I. Isolation and identification of alkaloids from *Aconitum finetianum* Hand.-Mazz. Acta Pharm. Sinica 16(1):70-72.

9. Chen, C., X.Y. Zhang, Y.F. Quian, S.H. Xiao, B.R. Shao, and L.S. Huang. 1962. Studies on *Hemerocallis thunbeprgii* Baker. III. Isolation and characterization of active principle against *Schistosomiasis japonica*. Acta Pharm. Sinica 9(10):579-586.

10. Chen, C.H., Y.C. Chao, and D.D. Li. 1966. Studies of Chinese rhubarb. IX. The effect of rhein and emodin on transplantable tumors in animals. Acta Pharm. Sinica 13(5):363-366.

11. Chen, C.H., W.F. Cheng, H.L. Su, and W.S. Lai. 1962. Studies on Chineserhubarb. I. Preliminary study on the antibacterial activity of anthraquinone derivatives of Chinese rhubarb (*Rhuem palmatum* L.). Acta Pharm. Sinica 9(12):757-762.

12. Chen, C.H., C.Y. Liu, and C.H. Qiu. 1980. Studies of Chinese rhubarb. XII. Effect of anthraquinone derivatives on the respiration and glycolysis of Ehrlich ascites carcinoma cell. Acta Pharm. Sinica 15(2):65-70.

13. Chen, D.H., 1984. Biological activities and medicinal potentialities of diterpene alkaloids. Chinese Traditional and Herbal Drugs 15(4):180-184.

14. Chen, D.H., R.F. Li, and H.P. Yi. 1979. The synthesis of indirubin. Zhongcaoyao Tongxun (3):103-105.

15. Chen, J.H., H.P. Yu, C.Q. Luo, F.J. Xie, M.L. Ding, and Z.Y. Lu. 1980. Thirty years of studies on the pharmacologically active constituents in Chinese traditional and herbal medicines. Chinese Traditional and Herbal Drugs 11(1):3 p.

16. Chen, J.Y. 1983. The bark of *Fraxinus*. *In* Wang Yu-Sheng, ed. *The Pharmacology and Usage of Traditional Chinese Drugs*. People's Medical Publishing House, Beijing. 858 p.

17. Chen, J.Y., W.Y. Xiang, G.L. Zhou, G. Yu, and Z.L. Wang. 1983. Studies on the protective action of oxymatine in experimental liver damage. Chin. Pharm. Bull. 18(7):407-409.

18. Chen, S.H. and C.J. Hu. 1982. The hypotensive effect of dauricine and preliminary analysis of its mechanism. Acta Academiae Medicinae Wuhan 11(3):75-79.

19. Chen, W.S., S.L. Nieh, Y.C. Chen, and K.M. Hsia. 1975. The structure of cucurbitacin IIa and IIb from *Hemsleya amabilis*. Acta Chim. Sinica 33(1):49-56.

20. Chen, W.Z., Y.L. Dong, C.G. Wang, and G.S. Ting. 1979. Pharmacological studies of sodium tanshinon II-A sulfonate. Acta Pharm. Sinica 14(5):277-283.

21. Chen, X.Y. 1959. The pharmacology of gentianine. IV. Action on central nervous system. Acta Pharm. Sinica 23(4):311-317.

22. Chen, Y., Z.J. Tang, F.X. Jiang, X.X. Zhang, and A.N. Lao. 1979. Studies on the active principles of Ze-Qi, *Euphorbia heliopscopia* L., a drug used for chronic bronchitis (I). Acta Pharm. Sinica 14(2):91-95.

23. Chen, Y.X., Y. Zhang, Q.Y. Cai, J.P. Zhou, Pen Han-Lin, X.K. Xiong, S.B. Li, W.X. Tang, and J.Y. Guo. 1984. The effect of treatment of colchicine on chronic liver damage induced by CCl$_4$ in rats: an observation of morphology. Acta Academiae Medicinae Wuhan 13(5):316-320.

24. Chen, Z.X., W.H. Gu, H.Z. Huang, X.M. Yang, C.J. Sun, W.Z. Chen, Y.L. Dong, and H.L. Ma. 1981. Studies on the water soluble phenolic acid of *Salvia miltiorrhiza*. Chin. Pharm. Bull. 16(9):536-537.

25. Chen, Z.X., B.S. Huang, Q.L. She, and G.F. Zeng. 1979. The chemical constituents of Bai-Hua-Qian-Hu, the root of *Peucedanum praeruptorum* Dunn. - four new coumarins. Acta Pharm. Sinica 14(8):486-496.

26. Chen, Z.X., H.Z. Huang, C.R. Wang, Y.H. Li, and J.M. Ding. 1981. Studies on the active constituents of Hong-Cong (rhizome of *Eleutherine americana*). Chinese Traditional and Herbal Drugs 12(11):484.

27. Cheng, P.Y., Y.L. Lin, and G.Y. Xu. 1984. New diterpenoids of *Rabdosia macrocalyx*: the structure of macrocalin A and macrocalin B. Acta Pharm. Sinica 19(8):593-598.

28. Cheng, P.Y., M.J. Xu, and Y.L. Lin. 1984. Studies on the antitumor principles of large leaf rabdosia (*Rabdosia macrophylla*) (III). Chinese Traditional and Herbal Drugs 15(2):53-54.

29. Cheng, P.Y., M.J. Xu, Y.L. Lin, and J.C. Shi. 1981. The antitumor constituents of *Rabdosia macrophylla*. Acta Pharm. Sinica 16(10):796-797.

30. Cheng, P.Y., M.J. Xu, Y.L. Lin, and J.C. Shi. 1982. The antitumor constituents of *Rabdosia amethystiods*. Acta Pharm. Sinica 17(1):33-37.

31. Cheng, P.Y., M.J. Xu, Y.L. Lin, and J.C. Shi. 1982. The structure of rabdophyllin G, an antitumor constituent of *Rabdosia macrophylla* (II). Acta Pharm. Sinica 17(12):917-921.

32. Cheng, Z.L., B.S. Huang, D.Y. Zhu, and M.L. Yin. 1981. Studies on the active principles of *aristolochia debilis*. II. 7-Hydroxy aristolochic acid-A and 7-methoxy aristolochic acid-A. Acta Chim. Sinica 39(3):237-242.

33. Coordinating Research Group of Antiasthmatica in Zhejang. 1982. New antiasthmatic principles in the essential oil from leaves of *Artemisia argyi*. Chinese Traditional and Herbal Drugs 13(6):241-245.

34. Coordinating Research Group on Artemisia Oil for Chronic Bronchitis. 1977. Studies on the antiasthmatic constituents of *Artemisia* oil. Yi Yoa Gong Ye (10):8-23.

35. Coordinating Research Group on Changrolin. 1978. Clinical observations on changrolin, an antiarrhythmic drug. National Medical Journal of China 58(2):84-86.

36. Coordinating Research Group on Chronic Tracheitis, Nanjing P.L.A. Units. 1973. The preliminary pharmaceutical studies and therapeutic effect of the flower bud of *Daphne Gènkwa* on chronic tracheitis. Zhongcaoyao Tongxun (5):263-279.

37. Coordinating Research Group on Chronic Tracheitis in Shaoyang Region, Huan. 1974. The effect of *Berchemia polyphlla* on chronic tracheitis in 231 cases. Zhongcaoyao Tongxun (1):39-42.

38. Coordinating Research Group on Qinghaosu. 1979. Antimalaria studies on qingaosu. Chinese Medical Journal 92(12):811-816.

39. Cui, Z.G., Y.T. Song, W.L. Wang, W.Q. Cheng, and X.Y. Wang. 1982. Antiasthmatic action of *n*-butenyl phthalide from Dang-Gui and some other synthetic derivatives of phthalide. Chinese Traditional and Herbal Drugs 13(2):65-69.

40. Deng, S.X. and Y.J. Mo. 1979. Pharmacological studies on *Gastrodia elata* Blume. I. The sedative and anticonvulsant effect of synthetic gastrodin and its genin. Acta Botanica Yunnanica 1(2):66-73.

41. Deng, W.L. 1983. *Houttuynia cordata* Thunb. In Wang Yu-Sheng, ed. *The Pharmacology and Usage of Traditional Chinese Drugs*. People's Medical Publishing House, Beijing. pp. 709-718.

42. Deng, W.L., R.J. Nie, and J.Y. Liu. 1982. Pharmacological comparison of four kinds of andrographolides. Chin. Pharm. Bull. 17(14):195-198.

43. Department No 4, Hunan Institute of Medicinal Industry and Research Group of Anti-snake-venom, Guangzhou P.L.A. Units. 1978. Studies on the anti-cobra venom active constituents. Zhongcaoyao Tongxun (9):385-390.

44. Department No 5, Shanghai Institute of Materia Medica, Academia Sinica. 1978. Chemical studies on *Stephania delavayi* (II). The pharmacology and clinic trial of cepharanthine. Zhongcaoyao Tongxun (9):410-414.

45. Department of Chinese Traditional and Herbal Drugs, Guangzhou Institute of Drug Control. 1978. The isolation and identification of daphnoretin from *Wikstroemia indica*. Zhongcaoyao Tongxun (3):97-101.

46. Department of Internal Medicine, Second Affiliated Hospital of Hunan Medical College, Institute of Medical Industry, Department of Pharmacology, and Department of Pharmacy. 1978. Pharmacological investigation of the pressor action of *Citrus aurantium* L. Kexue Tongbao 23(1):58-62, 37.

47. Department of Materia Medica, Shaanxi Institute of Traditional Chinese Medicine. 1972. The isolation and identification of the antibacterial principles of *Polygonum multiflorum* Thunb. var. *cilinerve* Steward. Shanxi Xinyiyao (5):36-39.

48. Department of Pediatrics, Beijing Friendship Hospital, Department of Pharmacology, Institute Materia Medica, Chinese Academy of Medical Sciences and Laboratory No. 1. 1973. Studies on the treatment of

anisodamine on acute microcircular blocking diseases. National Medical Journal of China 53(5): 259-263.

49. Department of Pharmacology, Institute of Materia Medica, Chinese Academy of Medical Sciences. 1975. Comparison of the pharmacological actions of anisodine and scopolamine. National Medical Journal of China 55(11):795-798.

50. Department of Pharmacology, Xi'an Medical College. 1958. The pharmacology of baicalinum. Acta Instituti Medicinalis Sinici (5):30-34.

51. Department of Pharmacology and Pharmaceutico-Chemistry, Institute of Medical Science, Honan, Department of Chemistry, Honan Medical College, Laboratory of Phytochemistry, Institute of Botany, Yunnan and Chengchow Chemicopharmaceutical Plant. 1978. A new antitumor substance - rubescensin. Kexue Tongbao 23(1):53-56.

52. Department of Pharmacy II, Fujian Institute of Medica and Medicina, Fuzhou, Department of Pharmacy, Military Medical Research Institute of P.L.A. Units, Fuzhou and Department of Phytochemistry, Shanghai Institute of Materia Medica, Academia Sinica. 1980. Studies on antiasthmatic principles of *Gnetum parvifolium* (Warb.) C.Y. Cheng. Acta Pharm. Sinica 15(7):434-436.

53. Department of Phytochemistry, Institute of Materia Medica, Chinese Academy of Medical Sciences and Institute of Medical Science, Chinghai. 1976. Chemical studies on anisodamine. Acta Chim. Sinica 34(1):39-44.

54. Dong, Z.T. and W.D. Jiang. 1982. Effect of danshensu on isolated swine coronary artery perfusion preparation. Acta Pharm. Sininca 17(3):226-228.

55. Du, J.Z., Q.F. Li, and X.G. Chen. 1983. Protective effects of *Swertia mussotii* on liver damage induced by hypoxia. Acta Pharm. Sinica 18(3):174-178.

56. Duan, Y.C., C.H. Li, and S.Y. Chen. 1957. A preliminary study of anthelmintic action of potassium quisqualate. Acta Pharm. Sinica 5(2):87-91.

57. Fan, L.L., G.Y. Zen, Y.P. Zhou, L.Y. Zhang, and Y.S. Cheng. 1975. Pharmacological effects of isoflavones of *Pueraria lobata* on coronary circulation, myocardial hemodynamics and myocardial metabolism in dogs. National Medical Journal of China 5:724-727.

58. Fang, S.D., X.Q. Yan, C.F. Li, Z.Y. Fan, X.Y. Xu, and J.S. Xu. 1979. The isolation and structure of the active principles of sarmentosin. Kexue Tongbao 24(9):431-432.

59. Fang, T.H., J.S. Wu, and S.W. Zhang. 1981. Experimental antiarrhythmic study of cyclovirobuxine D. Chin. Pharm. Bull. 16(4):246.

60. Feng, C.I. and S.S. Chang. 1965. The pharmacological action of sinomenine on the central nervous system. Acta Pharm. Sinica 12(2):81-85.

61. Feng, Y.P., H.J. Jia, L.Y. Zhang, and G.Y. Zeng. 1982. Effects of *dl*-demethylcoclaurine on β-adrenergic receptors and adenylate cyclase in turkey erythrocyte membrane. Acta Pharm. Sinica 17(9):642-646.

62. Fu, S.X., S.S. Chang, Y.S. Li, and N.C. Wang. 1963. The toxicity and general pharmacological actions of sinomenine. Acta Pharm. Sinica 10(11): 673-676.

63. Gao, Y.G., Y.M. Song, Y.Y. Yang, W.F. Liu, and J.X. Tang. 1979. Pharmacology of tanshinone. Acta Pharm. Sinica 14(2):75-82.

64. General Hospital, Shenyang P.L.A. Units. 1973. Studies on chemistry, toxicology and toxicity of Chinese drug Qin-Pi, the bark of *Fraxinus rhynchophylla*. Zhongcaoyao Tongxun (6):349-357.

65. Gong, B.Q. 1980. A news report of scutellarin for paralysis. Chinese Traditional and Herbal Drugs 11(10):480.

66. Gong, T. and Z.Y. Wu. 1979. Some pharmacologic actions of the dahurisoline methyl bromide, a preliminary report. Acta Pharm. Sinica 14(7): 439-442.

67. Group of Investigation, The Public Health Faculty and Coordinating Research Group on *Euphorbia lunulata* in Baoding Region, Hobei. 1974. Studies on the active constituents of *E. lunulata*. Zhongcaoyao Tongxun (3):142-149.

68. Group of Pharmacology, Beijing Medical College. 1974. Anticonvulsive and sedative actions of piperine. Journal of Beijing Medical College (4): 217-220.

69. Guo, M.D. and L.G. Chen. 1984. Studies on the alkaloids of embryo nelumbins (*Nelumbo nucifera*) in the Chinese mainland. Chinese Traditional and Herbal Drugs 15(7):291-293.

70. Han, D.W., X.H. Ma, Y.C. Zhao, and L.M. Zhou. 1979. Effects of cucurbitacin B on experimental hepatitis and cirrhosis. National Medical Journal of China 59(4):206-209.

71. He, G.B., S.H. Deng, M.T. Wang, T.C. Wang, and Y.C. Mao. 1964. The action of lycorine hydrochloride on the uterus. Acta Pharm. Sinica 11(8): 562-564.

72. Hu, R.S., B.Z. Li, and M. Chen. 1965. Choleretic principles of *Artemisia scoparia*. I. Water soluble fraction of its extract. Acta pharm. Sinica 12(5):289-294.

73. Hu, Y.H. and M.Y. Wang. 1975. The main pharmacological actions of esculetin and esculin. Xingyiyao Zazhi (8):377-378.

74. Hu, Z.B., R.S. Xu, G.J. Chen, and S.X. Wu. 1979. The structure identification and pharmacological actions of *l*-dicentrine. Chin. Pharm. Bull. 14(3):110-111.

75. Hu, Z.B., Y. Xu, S.C. Feng, and G.J. Fan. 1979. Studies on the active principles of the fruits of *Macleaya cordata* (Willd.) R. Br. Acta Pharm. Sinica 14(9):535-540.

76. Huang, B.H., W.S. Chen, Y. Hu, C.B. Qiu, W.J. Zhang, and B.L. Liang. 1981. A study on the chemical constituents of *Ardisia japonica* (Hornsted) Blume. Acta Pharm. Sinica 16(1):27-30.

77. Huang, L., K.M. Wu, Z. Xue, J.C. Cheng, L.Z. Xu, S.P. Xu, and Y.G. Xi. 1980. The isolation of an antitumor active principle of *Crotalaria sessiliflora* and synthesis of its derivatives. Acta Pharm. Sinica 15(5): 278-283.

78. Huang, X.Y. 1979. Pharmacological and clinical studies on the anticancer actions of tetrandrine in foreign countries. Shanghai Journal of Traditional Chinese Medicine (4):44-45.

79. Huang, Z.X. and Z.H. Li. 1980. Studies on the antitumor constitutes of *Zanthoxylum nitidum* (Roxb.) DC. Acta Chim. Sinica 38(6):535-542.

80. Hunan Institute of Medicinal Industry. 1972. Studies on the active constituents of *Lespedeza cuneata* G. (or *L. sericea*) for chronic tracheitis. Zhongcaoyao Tongxun (1):16-18.

81. Hunan Institute of Medicinal Industry. 1974. The pharmacology of
p-hydroxyacetophenone, an active principle of *Artemisia scoparia* Waldst et
Kit Chinese Medical Journal 54(2):101-103.

82. Ji, X.J., F.R. Zhang, J.L. Lei, and Y.T. Xu. 1981. Studies on the
antineoplastic action and toxicity of synthetic indirubin. Acta Pharm. Sinica
16(2):146-148.

83. Jiang, S.H., Y.L. Zhu, Z.Y. Zhao, and R.H. Zhu. 1982. Studies on
Aconitum finetianum Hand.-Mazz.(II). Chinese Traditional and Herbal Drugs
13(2):53.

84. Jiang, X.R., Q.X. Wu, H.L. Shi, W.P. Chen, S.Q. Chang, S.Y. Zhao,
X.Y. Tian, L.F. Zhou, S.M. Guo, and Y.J. Li. 1982. Pharmacological actions
of dehydrocorydaline on the cardiovascular system. Acta Pharm. Sinica
17(1):61-65.

85. Jiang, Y., G.Q. Liu, J.R. Ma, L. Xie, and H.Q. Wu. 1982. The
pharmacological studies on methyl-eugenol. Acta Pharm. Sinica 17(2):87-92.

86. Jiang, Y., Z.C. Zhao, and F. Li. 1984. The relationship between
daphnetin analgesia and central neurotransmitters of the monoamincs. Acta
Pharm. Sinica 19(9):647-650.

87. Jiang, Z.Y. and T.H. Chang. 1961. Antiepileptic effects of *Gastrodia
elata* and vanillin. Acta Physiol. Sinica 24(3-4):187-195.

88. Jiangsu New Medical College. 1977. *Dictionary of Traditional Chinese Drugs*. People's Publishing House, Shanghai. 105 p.

89. Jin, L.S., Y.P. Zhou, and G.Y. Zeng. 1982. Effects of denudatine on
experimental arrhythmia and heart functions. Acta Pharm. Sinica
3(2):104-108.

90. Jin, Y. and S.S. Zhang. 1980. The inhibitory effect of succinic acid
on the central nervous system. Acta Pharm. Sinica 15(12):761-763.

91. Kang, S.Q., S.Y. Cai, and L. Teng. 1981. The antiviral effect of
hainanolide, a compound isolated from *Cephalotaxus hainanensis*. Acta
Pharm. Sinica 16(11):867-868.

92. Kao, S.J. and G.Y. Zeng. 1983. Cardiotonic and toxic effects of
peruvoside and neriifolin. Acta Pharm. Sinica 18(8):572-578.

93. Kin, K.C., S.Y. Tsoch, X.C. Tang, and B. Hsu. 1962. Pharmacological actions of tetrahydroberberine on the central nervous system. Acta
Physiol. Sinica 25(3):182-190.

94. Kin, K.C., Y.E. Wang, and B. Hsu. 1964. Some neuropharmacological actions of rotundine. Acta Pharm. Sinica 11(11): 754-761.

95. Kuenming Pharmaceutical Factory. 1975. Chemical and pharmacological studies on *Pseudostreblus indica*. Zhongcaoyao Tongxun (1):18-24.

96. Laboratory No 1, Kwangtung Institute of Analysis and Section of
Chinese Medical Herbs, Canton Institute of Drug Control. 1977. Isolation and
structure of pogostone - an antifungal component from the Chinese drug
Kwang-Ho-Hsiang, *Pogostemon cablin* (Blanco) Benth. Kexue Tongbao
22(7):318-320.

97. Laboratory of Phytochemistry, Yunnan Institute of Botany and
Pharmacologic Laboratory, Honan Institute of Medical Science. 1977.
Diterpenoid triepoxides, antitumor principles from *Tripterygium hypoglaucum*
and *T. wilfordii*. Kexue Tongbao 22(10):436, 458-460.

98. Lang, Y.J. and X.D. Zhang. 1981. Studies on the active principles
of garlic. Chinese Traditional and Herbal Drugs 12(1):4-6.

99. Lei, W.Y., S.T. Shi, and C.C. Yu. 1982. Effects of swertiamarin on the central nervous system. Chin. Pharm. Bull. 17(5):305.

100. Lei, W.Y., S.T. Shi, and C.C. Yu. 1982. Antispastic effects of swertiamarin. Chinese Traditional and Herbal Drugs 13(10):464-466.

101. Li, C.L. and Y.W. Ye. 1981. Effects of rhapontin of *Rheum hotaoense* on lipid and lippoprotein level serum. Acta Pharm. Sinica 16(9):699-702.

102. Li, D.H., X.G. Hao, S.K. Zhang, S.X. Wang, R.Y. Liu, K.S. Ma, S.P. Yu, H. Jiang, and J.F. Guan. 1981. Antitumor action and toxicity of irisquinone. Acta Pharmacol. Sinica 2(2):131-134.

103. Li, G.R., D.C. Fang, C.J. Hu, and F.H. Lu. 1984. Effects of dauricine on physiologic properties of myocardium. Acta Pharmacol. Sinica 5(1):20-22.

104. Li, J.C., C.J. Liu, X.Z. An, M.T. Wang, T.Z. Zhao, S.Z. Yu, G.S. Zhao, and K.F. Chen. 1982. Studies on the antitumor constituent of *Rabdosia japonica* (Burm. f.) Hara. I. The structures of rabdosin A and B. Acta Pharm. Sinica 17(9):682-687.

105. Li, L.Y. and J.M. Ye. 1982. Expectorant activity of volatile oil and myrcene in the fruit of *Phellodendron amurense*. Chin. Pharm. Bull. 17(5):304.

106. Li, Q.H. 1982. Studies on the hemostatic principles of Xiao-Ji (*Cirsium segetum*). Chinese Traditional and Herbal Drugs 13(9):393-396.

107. Li, S.R., D.M. Luan, and X.Z. Xue. 1982. Antioncotic effect on joints by the volatile oil of *Thymus quinquicostatus*. Chin. Pharm. Bull. 17(5):305.

108. Li, X.M., L.Z. Li, S.L. Chen, X.H. Qiu, Y.H. Yu, D.X. Pan, L.L. Zou, and Z.L. Yang. 1984. Inhibitory effects of sophocarpine on animal tumors. Acta Pharmacol. Sinica 5(2):125-130.

109. Liang, Q.X. and X.Y. Gao. 1979. Studies on the antihepatitis flavonoids of *Swertia mileensis*. Zhongcaoyao Tongxun (9):385-388.

110. Liang, X.T., D.Q. Yu, W.L. Wu, and H.C. Deng. 1979. The structure of yingzhaosu A. Acta Chim. Sinica 37(3):231-240.

111. Liao, C.S. 1980. A news report of sophocarpine for malignant Hydalidoform Mole. Chin. Pharm. Bull. 15(2):58.

112. Lin, L.Z., C.Q. Song, Z.Y. Fan, C.F. Du, M.L. Zhou, Z.Q. Ma, and R.S. Xu. 1980. Studies on the chemical constituents of *Thalictrum faberi*. Chin. Pharm. Bull. 15(7):334.

113. Lin, L.Z., J.S. Zhang, Z.L. Chen, and R.S. Xu. 1982. Studies on chemical constituents of *Brucea javanica* (l.) Merr. I. Isolation and identification of bruceaketolic acid and four other quassinoids. Acta Chim. Sinica 40(1):73-78.

114. Lin, M., D.Q. Yu, X. Lin, F.Y. Fu, Q.T. Zheng, C.H. He, G.H. Bao, and C.F. Xu. 1985. Chemical studies on the quaternary alkaloids of *Rauvolfia verticillata* (Lour.) Baill. f. *ruberocarpa* H. T. Chang, Mss. Acta Pharm. Sinica 20(3):198-202.

115. Lin, Z.B., B.L. Chai, P. Wang, Q.X. Guo, F.S. Lu, and G.Q. Xiang. 1980. Studies on the anti-inflammatory effect of chemical principle of Zi-Cao, *Arnebia euchroma* (Royle) Johnst. Journal of Beijing Medical College 12(2):101-110.

116. Lin, Z.B., P. Wang, Y. Ruan, and Q.X. Guo. 1980. Anti-inflammatory effect of β,β-dimethylacrylshikonin. Acta Pharmacol. Sinica 1(1):60-63.

117. Lin, Z.D., C.J. Liu, X.Z. Zhu, P. Zhao, and F.Y. Shi. 1978. Studies on the anesthetic constituents of *Asarum forbesii*. Zhongcaoyao Tongxun (9):391-395.

118. Liu, C.J., J.C. Li, X.Z. An, R.M. Cheng, F.Z. Shen, Y.L. Xu, and D.Z. Wang. 1982. Studies on the antitumor diterpenoid constituents of *Rabdosia japonica* (Burm. f.) Hara. II. The structure of rabdosin C. Acta Pharm. Sinica 17(10):750-754.

119. Liu, C.M., Q.H. Yu, and L.M. Zhang. 1982. Effects of icarin on heart. Chinese Traditional and Herbal Drugs 13(9):414, 416.

120. Liu, C.W. 1983. *Polygonum cuspidatum* Sieb. et Zucc. *in* Wang Yu-Sheng, ed. *The Pharmacology and Usage of Traditional Chinese Drugs*. People's Medical Publishing House, Beijing. 654 p.

121. Liu, G.Q., D.Z. Dai, J.L. Rao, H.S. Cai, and F.B. Xu. 1974. Neuro-pharmacological studies on vanillyl alcohol, a constituent of *Gastrodia elata*. Zhongcaoyao Tongxun (5):305-308.

122. Liu, G.Q., Y. Jiang, Q.J. Wang, and E.X. Yang. 1977. Pharmacological studies on daphnetin. Zhongcaoyao Tongxun (3):117-120.

123. Liu, G.Q., J.N. Sun, Z.Z. He, and Y. Jiang. 1983. Spasmolytic actions of active principles of volatile oil of *Acorus gramineus*. Acta Pharm. Sinica 4(2):95-97.

124. Liu, G.T., H.L. Wei, T.T. Bao, and Z.Y. Song. 1980. The effect of *Ganodermas* on elevated serum aldolase levels induced by 2,4-dichlorophenoxyacetic acid (2,4-D) in mice. Acta Pharm. Sinica 15(3):142-146.

125. Liu, Y.L., F.Y. Fu, T.H. Hsie, and S.L. Chang. 1976. Studies on the constituents of Man-Shan-Hong (*Rhododendron dauricum* L.) part I. Acta Chim. Sinica 34(3):211-221.

126. Lu, Y.C. 1980. Studies on the constituents of the essential oil of *Rhododendron tsinghaiense* Ching. Acta Chim. Sinica 38(3):241-249.

127. Lu, Y.C., Y.L. Wang, and Y.F. Bai. 1980. A study on the chemical composition of essential oil *Rhododendron anthopogonoides* Maxim. Acta Chim. Sinica 38(2):140-148.

128. Lu, Y.C., J.P. Xing, and R.L. Wei. 1981. Studies on the constituents of *Rhododendron capitatum* (I). Chin. Pharm. Bull. 16(1):54.

129. Lue, F.H., T.M. Chang, and T.C. Fong. 1957. The antiphlogistic and antianaphylactic shock actions of tetrandrine and demethyltetrandrine. Acta Pharm. Sinica 5(2):113-122.

130. Ma, J.Z., L.D. Ma, X.Y. Sun, and L.R. Pan. 1980. Pharmacological study on cyrtophyllin. Chinese Traditional and Herbal Drugs 11(6):268.

131. Ma, X.H., Y.C. Zhao, L. Yin, D.W. Han, and C.X. Ji. 1982. Studies on the effect of oleanolic acid on experimental liver injury. Acta Pharm. Sinica 17(2):93-97.

132. Ma, Z.Q. 1980. The antitumor effect and preclinical pharmacological studies of thalidasine. Chin. Pharm. Bull. 15(7):334.

133. Ming, Z. and G.S. Zhao. 1984. The effect of dimethyltrilobine iodide on experimental arrhythmia and its electrophysiological action on myocardium. Acta Pharm. Sinica 19(1):12-15.

134. Pan, Q.C., X.J. Chen, Z.C. Liu, Z.M. Meng, and Q.L. She. 1979. The antitumoral and pharmacological studies of pseudolycorine. Acta Pharm. Sinica 14(12):705-709.

135. Peng, H.M., S.Y. Xiang, and Z.Q. Bi. 1981. Pharmacological studies on the antitussive, expectorant and antiasthmatic effects of luteolin, an active principle of *Ajuga decumbens*. Chin. Pharm. Bull. 16(2):75-77.

136. Qi, T.P., B.S. Li, and Y.C. Yu. 1973. Effect of baicalin on infectious hepatitis. Xinyiyaoxue Zazhi (8):304-306.

137. Qin, G.W., Z.X. Chen, H.C. Wang, and M.K. Qian. 1981. The structure and synthesis of robustaol A. Acta Chim. Sinica 39(1):83-89.

138. Qu, S.Y. 1980. The effects of daphnetin on experimental acute myocardial ischemia and cardiovascular system in rabbit. Journal of Traditional Chinese Medicine 21(6):43.

139. Quan, Y.Z. 1983. *Cymbopogon distans* (Nees) A. Camus. *In* Wang Yu-Sheng, ed. *The Pharmacology and Usage of Traditional Chinese Drugs.* People's Medical Publishing House, Beijing. 499 p.

140. Research Group of Chinese Traditional Herbal Anesthesia, Nanjing College of Pharmacy. 1978. The preliminary studies on the volatile oil of *Acorus gramineus*. (I). Zhongcaoyao Tongxun (6):241-245.

141. Research Group on Contraceptive Drugs, Department of Obstetrics and Gynecology, The Affiliated Hospital of Tianjing Medical College. 1978. The hemostatic effect of psoralen. Zhongcaoyao Tongxun (5):217-218.

142. Research Group on *Curcuma aromatica*, Luda Hospital for Obstetrics and Gynecology. 1977. The clinical observation of *Curcuma aromatica* on cervical carcinoma. Xinyiyaoxue Zazhi(3):109-111.

143. Research Group on Drugs, Guangzhou Institute of Medicine and Health. 1978. The preliminary studies on the antitumor actions of stephanine. Zhongcaoyao Tongxun (9):409.

144. Research Group on Hepatitis, Department of Pharmacology, Hunan Institute of Medical Industry. 1979. The pharmacology of the active constituents of the fruit stalk of *Cucumis melo*. Zhongcaoyao Tongxun (9):414-416.

145. Research Group on *Thesium chinense*, Department of Phytochemistry, Anhui Institute of Medical Sciences. 1976. Chemical studies on active constituents of *Thesium chinense* (I). Zhongcaoyao Tongxun (8):342-348.

146. Research Group on Tracheitis, Department of Pharmacology, Institute of Materia Medica, Chinese Academy of Medical Sciences. 1975. Studies on the expectorant action of farrerol. National Medical Journal of China 55(12):856-859.

147. Research Group on Tracheitis, First Affiliated Hospital of Hunan Medical College. 1973. The clinical observation of bergenin for chronic tracheitis. Chinese Medical Journal 53(12):710.

148. Research Group on Tracheitis, Sichuan Institute of Traditional Chinese Drugs. 1973. The isolation and pharmacology of plumbagin from *Ceratostigma plumbaginoider* Bge. Zhongcaoyao Tongxun (5):208-283.

149. Research Group on Tumors, Department of Traditional Chinese Medicine, Liaonin College of Traditional Chinese Medicine, Department of Chinese Traditional and Herbal Drugs, Shengyang College of Pharmacy and Department of Electronmicroscope, Shenyany Medical College. 1976. Studies on the antitumor action of the active constituents of *Curcuma aromatica*. Xinyiyaoxue Zazhi (12):556-560.

150. Shanghai Fifth Pharmaceutical Plant, Shanghai Twelfth Pharmaceutical Plant, Institute of Pharmaceutical Industrial Research and Shanghai Institute of Materia Medica. 1977. Total synthesis of *dl*-10-hydroxy-camptothecin and *dl*-10-methoxy-camptothecin. Kexue Tongbao 22(6):269-270.

151. Shanghai First Medical College and Its Affiliated Zhongshan Hospital, Shanghai Institute of Medicinal Industry, Shanghai Second Plant for Chinese Medicine and Institute of Drug Control, Shanghai Health Bureau. 1973. Studies of the active constituents of *Pyrrosia sheareri* on chronic tracheitis. Yi Yao Gong Ye (6):1-13.

152. Shanghai Institute of Materia Medica, Academia Sinica. 1975. Chemical studies on *Stephania delayayi* (I). Zhongcaoyao Tongxun (5):266-270.

153. Shanghai Institute of Materia Medica, Academia Sinica. 1978. Studies on the anticancerous action of 10-hydroxycamptothecin. National Medical Journal of China 58(10):598-602.

154. Shen, L.C., Y.Y. Wang, and L.H. Feng. 1983. Preparation of allicin microcapsule. Chinese Traditional and Herbal Drugs 14(4):161-164.

155. Shia, S.H., B.R. Shao, Y.S. Ho, and Y.C. Yang. 1962. Prophylatico-therapeutic studies of curcurbitine in *Schistosomiasis japonica* in mice. Acta Pharm. Sinica. 9(6):327-332.

156. Song, C.Q., R.S. Xu, G.Q. Song, S.H. Hong, N. Zhang, F.J. Zhang, and Y. Shen. 1981. Effective constituents of *Acer ginnala*. Chin. Pharm. Bull. 16(12):756.

157. Song, W.Z. and P.G. Xiao. 1982. Medicinal plants of Chinese Schisandraceae and their lignan components. Chinese Traditional and Herbal Drugs 13(1):40-48.

158. Sun, F.Z., J.D. Su, and H. Zhen. 1981. Studies on pharmacological activities and toxicities of armillarisin A, a new choleretic drug. Acta Pharm. Sinica 16(6):401-406.

159. Sun, N.J., Z. Xue, X.T. Liang, and L. Huang. 1979. Studies on the structure of a new antitumor agent-hainanolide. Acta Pharm. Sinica 14(1):39-44.

160. Sung, C.Y., H.C. Chi, and K.T. Liu. 1958. The pharmacology of gentianine. I. Antiphlogistic effect and action on pituitary-adrenal function of the rat. Acta Physiol. Sinica 22(3):201-205.

161. Tang, X.C. and J. Feng. 1981. Analgesic actions and local anesthetic activity of 3-acetyl-aconitine hydrobromide. Acta Pharmacol. Sinica 2(2):82-84.

162. Tang, X.C., G.Z. Jin, J. Feng, Z.D. Zhang, and Y.F. Han. 1980. Studies on the neuromuscular blocking activity of alkaloids of *Cyclea barbata* (Wall.) Miers. Acta Pharm. Sinica. 15(9):513-519.

163. Tang, X.C., Z.G. Lin, W. Cai, N. Chen, and L. Shen. 1984. Antiinflammatory effect of 3-acetylaconitine. Acta Pharmacol. Sinica 5(2):85-89.

164. Tang, X.C., M.Y. Zhu, J. Feng, and Y.E. Wang. 1983. Studies on pharmacologic actions of lappaconitine hydrobromide. Acta Pharm. Sinica 18(8):579-584.

165. Tao, J.Y., Y.P. Ruan, Q.B. Mei, A. Liu, Q.L. Tian, Y.Z. Chen, H.D. Zhang, and Z.X. Duan. 1984. Studies on the antiasthmatic action of

ligustilide of Dang-Gui, *Angelica sinensis* (Oliv.) Diels. Acta Pharm. 19(8)Sinica 19(8):561-565.

166. Tientsin Institute of Materia Medica. 1974. Extraction of hypotensive constituents and pharmacological research of *Uncaria rhynchophylla*. Zhongcaoyao Tongxun (4):216-227.

167. Tientsin Institute of Materia Medica. 1976. A news report of total alkaloids of *Uncaria*. Zhongcaoyao Tongxun (7):333-334.

168. Tseng, K.Y., Y.P. Chou, L.Y. Chang, and L.L. Fan. 1974. Pharmacologic studies on *Radix puerariae*. I. Its effects on dog arterial pressure, vascular reactivity, cerebral and peripheral circulation. Chinese Medical Journal 54:265-270.

169. Wang, A.Q. and X.R. Ma. 1979. A preliminary study on active constituents of *Sarcandra glabra*. Zhongcaoyao Tongxun (4):152-153.

170. Wang, A.Q., P. Xie, and Y.H. Yi. 1983. Studies on the coumarin components in Zhong-Jie-Feng (*Sarcandra glabra*). Chinese Traditional and Herbal Drugs 14(6):277.

171. Wang, C.R., Z.X. Chen, B.P. Ying, B.N. Zhou, J.S. Liu, and B.C. Pan. 1981. Studies on the active principles of the root of Yuan-Hua (*Daphne genkwa*). II. Isolation and structure of an new antifertile diterpene yuanhuadine. Acta Chim. Sinica 39(5):421-426.

172. Wang, D.D., S.Q. Liu, Y.J. Chen, L.J. Wu, J.Y. Sun, and T.R. Zhu. 1982. Studies on the active constituents of *Syringa oblata* Lindl. Acta Pharm. Sinica 17(12):951-954.

173. Wang, H.J. and Y.Y. Chen. 1985. Studies of lignans from *Schiasandra rubriflora* Rhed. et Wils. Acta Pharm. Sinica 20(11):837-841.

174. Wang, J.X., R.S. Gong, and T.G. Huang. 1983. Antibacterial constituents of *Conyza canadensis*. Chin. Pharm. Bull. 18(2):91-92.

175. Wang, M.S. 1980. Studies on the chemical constituents of Zu-Shi-Ma (*Daphne giraldii*) (III). Chinese Traditional and Herbal Drugs 11(9):389-390.

176. Wang, S., S.Y. Yang, and Y. Li. 1983. Treatment of postapoplectic paralysis with breviscapin injection (a report of 469 cases). Chinese Traditional and Herbal Drugs 14(1):33-34.

177. Wang, W.H. and J.H. Zheng. 1984. The pregnancy terminating effect and toxicity of an active constituent of *Aristolochia mollissima* Hance, aristolochic acid A. Acta Pharm. Sinica 19(6):405-409.

178. Wang, X.R., Z.Q. Wang, and J.G. Dong. 1982. A new diterpene from Huang-Hua-Xiang-Cha-Cai (*Robodosia sculponeata*). Chinese Traditional and Herbal Drugs 13(11):491-492.

179. Wang, Y.X., X. Yan, H. Li, and Y.Z. Tan. 1981. Effect of 3,4-dihydroxyacetophenone on coronary collateral blood flow of regional myocardial isochemia in anesthetized dogs. Chin. Pharm. Bull. 16(8):501.

180. Wang, Z.L. and Y.H. Yi. 1984. Studies on the active principles of the Chinese drug Shang-Lu (*Phytolacca esculenta* van Houtte). Acta Pharm. Sinica 19(11):825-829.

181. Wang, Z.Q. and X.R. Wang. 1980. Studies on the constituents of Hong-Han-Lian *Hypericum ascyron* L. Acta Pharm. Sinica 15(6):365-367.

182. Wang, Z.Y., B.Z. Zhu, and H.Y. Zhang. 1974. The clinical observation of point-injection of securentine nitrate. Xinyiyaoxue Zazhi (4):162-165.

183. Wei, J.X., S.Q. Yu, Z.T. Kou, X.X. He, and J.F. Mo. 1980. Studies on the active principles of the shells of *Arachis hypogaea*. Chin. Pharm. Bull. 15(8):380.

184. Wu, C.R. 1983. *Artemisia capillaris* Thunb. *In* Wang Yu-Sheng, ed. The pharmacology and usage of traditional Chinese drugs. People's Medical Publishing House, Beijing. pp. 757-766.

185. Wu, T.K. 1983. *Cephalotaxus fortunei* Hook. f. *In* Wang Yu-Sheng, ed. *The Pharmacology and Usage of Traditional Chinese Drugs*. People's Medical Publishing House, Beijing. 54 p.

186. Xia, D.Y. 1976. The clinical observation of neriperside on treatment of congestive heart failure in 32 Keshan disease patients. National Medical Journal of China 56(4):233-234.

187. Xiangtan Institute of Drug Control, Hunan. 1978. The isolation of plumbagin from *Drosera peltata* Smith. var. *lunata* Clarke and its action against *Mycobacterium tuberculosis*. Zhongcaoyao Tongxun (1):16-17.

188. Xiao, P.G. 1981. Traditional experience of Chinese herb medicine. Its application in drug research and new drug searching. *In* J. Beal and E. Reinhard, eds. Natural products as medicinal agents. Hippokrates Verlag, Stuttgart, pp. 351-394.

189. Xiao, P.G. and L.Y. He. 1982. *Przewalskia tangutica*—A tropane alkaloid-containing plant. Planta Med. 45(2):112-115.

190. Xiao, P.G., L.Y. He, and L.W. Wang. 1984. Ethnopharmacologic study of Chinese Rhubarb. J. Ethnopharm. 10(3):275-293.

191. Xiao, P.G., G.S. Liu, B.Z. Chen, and W.Z. Song. 1979. Utilization of *Berberis* sources in China. Chin. Pharm. Bull. 14(8):381-382.

192. Xiao, P.G., Y.Y. Tong, S.R. Luo, B.Z. Chen, L.W. Wang, and J.H. Shang.1982. Qian-Cao (*Rubia cordifolia* L.). In *Chinese Materia Medica* (New edit.) II. People's Medical Publishing House, Beijing. pp. 149-159.

193. Xie, R.M., A.R. Miao, Z.P. Zhu, P.F. Zhou, Y.Q. Shen, G.J. Chen, Q.Y. Xu, and S.D. Ma. 1982. The excitation effect of pachycarpine on skeletal muscles. Acta Pharm. Sinica 17(6):462-465.

194. Xiu, S.B., H.L. Ma, X.S. Wan, J.S. Shi, and Y. Zhuang. 1982. Active constituents of Xiao-Xuan-Cao (*Hemerocallis minor*). Chinese Traditional and Herbal Drugs 13(2):49-52.

195. Xu, D.M., B. Zhang, H.R. Li, and M.L. Xu. 1982. Isolation and identification of alkaloids from *Fritillaria ussuruensis* Maxim. Acta Pharm. Sinica 17(5):355-359.

196. Xu, Q.F. 1981. Preliminary study on active constituents of *Polygonum aubertii*. Chin. Pharm. Bull. 16(9):567.

197. Xu, Y., Z.B. Hu, S.C. Feng, and G.J. Fan. 1979. Studies on the antituberculosis principles from *Lysionotus pauciflora* Maxim. I. Isolation and identification of nevadensin. Acta Pharm. Sinica 14(7):447-448.

198. Xue, C.S. 1983. *Schizandra chinensis* (Turcz.) Baill. *In* Wang Yu-Sheng, ed. *The Pharmacology and Usage of Traditional Chinese Drugs*. People's Medical Publishing House, Beijing. 183 p.

199. Yang, B.J., M.K. Qian, G.W. Qin, and Z.X. Chen. 1981. Studies on the active principle of Dan-Shen. V. Isolation and structures of przewaquinone A and B. Acta Pharm. Sinica 16(11):837-841.

200. Yang, J.S., S.R. Luo, X.L. Shen, and Y.X. Li. 1979. Chemical investigation of the alkaloids of Ku-Mu [*Picrasma quassioides* (D. Don) Benn.]. Acta Pharm. Sinica 14(3):167-177.

201. Yang, K., X.L. Zhao, P.G. Xiao, and G.S. Liu. 1982. Clinical trial of berbamine in 405 leucopenia patients. Chin. Pharm. Bull. 17(4):213-214.

202. Yang, M.K., Y.S. Tang, R.H. Liao, Z.M. Huang, C.X. Ran, Q.L. Yang, and L.M. Cai. 1981. Chemical constituents of Ma-Tong-Hua (*Incavillea arguta*). Chinese Traditional and Herbal Drugs 12(11):489-490.

203. Yang, Q.Z., H.D. Shu, and L.R. Lin. 1981. The blocking action of anabasin of the neuromuscular junction. Acta Pharm. Sinica 2(2):84-88.

204. Yang, T.C. and C.S. Chang. 1949. The antituberculous effect and pharmacology of stepharanthine (cepharanthine). National Medical Journal of China 35(6):239-250.

205. Yao, T.R. and Z.N. Chen. 1979. Chemical investigation of Chinese medicinal herb, Bao-Gong-Teng. I. The isolation and preliminary study of a new myotic constituent, Bao-Gong-Teng A. Acta Pharm. Sinica 14(12):731-735.

206. Yao, T.R., Z.N. Chen, D.N. Yi, and G.Y. Xu. 1981. Chemical investigation of Bao-Gong-Teng (*Erycibe obtusifolia* Benth.). II. The structure of Bao-Gong-Teng A, a new myotic agent. Acta Pharm. Sinica 16(8):582-588.

207. Ye, H.Z., Y.X. Fan, Z.W. Liu, and Y.S. Jing. 1981. Studies on the antirheumatic constituents of Ding-Gong-Teng (*Erycibe obtusifolia*). Chinese Traditional and Herbal Drugs 12(5):197-199.

208. Ye, J.S., H.Q. Zhang, and C.Q. Yuan. 1982. Isolation and identification of coumarin praeruption E from the root of Chinese drug *Peucedanum praeruptorum* Dunn. Acta Pharm. Sinica 17(6):431-434.

209. Yeau, K.L., C.K. Wong, D.S. Young, and H. Whong. 1964. The cardiac and sedative effects of diacetylneriifolin. Acta Pharm. Sinica 11(10):673-679.

210. Yeung, H.W., Y.C. Kong, W.P. Lay, and K.F. Cheng. 1977. The structure and biological effect of leonurine, a uterotonic principle from Chinese drug I-Mu-Ts'ao. Planta Med. 31(1):51-56.

211. Yin, Z.Z., L.Y. Zhang, and L.N. Xu. 1980. The effect of Dang-Gui (*Angelica sinensis*) and its ingredient ferulic acid on rat platelet aggregation and release of 5-HT. Acta Pharm. Sinica 15(6):321-326.

212. Ying, B.P., C.R. Wang, P.N. Chou, P.C. Pan, and J.S. Liu. 1977. Studies on the active principles of the root of Yuan-Hua (*Daphne genkwa*). I. Isolation and structure of yuanhuacine. Acta Chim. Sinica 35(1,2):103-108.

213. You, J.Q., W.J. Le, and J.Y. Mei. 1982. The *in vitro* effect of agrimophol on *Schistosoma japonicum*. Acta Pharm. Sinica 17(9):663-666.

214. Yu, J.G. and Y.F. Zhai. 1979. Studies on the constituents of *Ganoderma capens* (part I). Acta Pharm. Sinica 14(6):374-378.

215. Yu, S.R. and S.Q. You. 1984. The anticonvulsant action of 3-*n*-butylphalide (Ag-1) and 3-*n*-butyl-4,5-dihydrophthalide (Ag-2). Acta Pharm. Sinica 19(8):566-570.

216. Yu, S.R., S.Q. You, and H.Y. Chen. 1984. The pharmacological action of 3-*n*-butylphthalide (Ag-1). Acta Pharm. Sinica 19(7):486-490.

217. Yuan, D.J. 1979. Clinical observations on the effects of lactoni *Coriariae* and tutin in the treatment of schizophrenia (report of 140 cases). Chinese Journal of Neurology and Psychiatry 12(4):196-200.

218. Yuan, W. 1983. *Sophora flavescens* Ait. *In* Wang Yu-Sheng, ed. *The Pharmacology and Usage of Traditional Chinese Drugs.* People's Medical Publishing House, Beijing. pp. 637-644.

219. Yuan, W.X. and I. Chang. 1962. The sedative and hypotensive action of *Uncaria rhynchophylla.* Acta Physiol. Sinica 25(6):161-170.

220. Yunnan Institute of Botany, Kuenming Pharmaceutical Factory and Kuenming Medical College. 1973. The chemical and pharmacological studies on germacrone and its derivatives. Zhongcaoyao Tongxun (1):23-28.

221. Yunnan Institute of Botany, Military Medical Research Institute of Kuenming P.L.A. Units, Yunnan Institute of Tropical Plant, Shanghai Institute of Daily Chemical Industry and Anti-Labour Hygiene Occupational Disease Institute, Shanghai. 1975. Studies on *d*-8-acetoxycarvotanacetone, a new repellent. Acta Botanica Yunnanica (1):1-14.

222. Zen, G.Y., Y.P. Zhou, L.Y. Zhang, and L.L. Fan. 1977. Pharmacological studies of *Rauvolfia verticillata* in China. VIII. The hypotensive and hemodynamic effects of sarpagine in anesthetic dogs. National Medical Journal of China 57(1):56-58.

223. Zhang, T.M., K.C. Chao, and F.H. Lue. 1958. The cardiovascular effects of tetrandine and demethyletetrandine. Acta Pharm. Sinica 6(3):147-154.

224. Zhang, T.M., Z.Y. Chen, J.H. Chao, Q.Z. Zhao, H.D. Sun, and Z.W. Lin. 1980. Rubescensine B, another antitumor constituent of *Rubdosia rubescens.* Kexue Tongbao 25 (22):1051-1054.

225. Zhang, T.M., Z.Y. Chen, and C. Lin. 1981. Antineoplastic action of triptolide and its effect on the immunologic functions in mice. Acta Pharm. Sinica 2(2):128-131.

226. Zhang, T.M., T.C. Fong, and F.H. Lue. 1957. The potentiating effect of diphenhydramine upon the analgesic action of Han-Fang-Chi and some other analgesics. Acta Physiol. Sinica 21(2):133-141.

227. Zhang, T.M., F.H. Lue, and Department of Pharmacology, Wuhan Medical College, Hankow. 1958. Studies of β-dichroine, chloroguanide, cyclochloroquininide and baicalin on amebicides. Acta Academiae Medicinae Wuhan (1):11-16.

228. Zhang, Y.D., J.P. Shen, J. Song, Y.L. Wang, Y.N. Shao, C.F. Li, S.H. Zhou, Y.F. Li, and D.X. Li. 1984. Effects of astragalus saponin I on cAMP and cGMP level in plasma and DNA synthesis in regenerating liver. Acta Pharm. Sinica 19(8):619-621.

229. Zhang, Y.D., Y.L. Wang, J.P. Shen, and D.X. Li. 1984. Effects on blood pressure and inflammation of astragalus saponin I, a principle isolated from *astragalus membranaceus* Bge. Acta Pharm. Sinica 19(5):333-337.

230. Zhao, Y., J.J. Zheng, S.Y. Huang, X.J. Li, Q.Y. Lin, and J.X. Zhang. 1981. Studies on the antimalarial activity of protopine derivatives. Chin. Pharm. Bull. 16(6):327-330.

231. Zhao, Z.H., L.H. Chen, Y.J. Wang, and D.Y. Liang. 1981. Inhibitory actions of *d*-isocorydine from Tu-Chuang-Hua (*Dicranostigma leptopodum*) on the central nervous system and smooth muscles. Chinese Traditional and Herbal Drugs 12(9):402-405.

232. Zheng, L.Z., J.Q. Tan, and X.C. Tang. 1984. Analgesic and antipyretic effects and no physical dependence of trilobine hydrochloride. Acta Pharm. Sinica 5(1):11-14.

233. Zheng, X.R., Z.Y. Gao, H.D. Sun, and Z.W. Lin. 1984. The structure of ludongnin. Acta Botanica Yunnanica 6(3):316-320.

234. Zheng, Y.X. 1984. Clinical observations of the analgesic action of paeonol sulfanate injection. Chinese Traditional and Herbal Drugs 15(10):460.

235. Zhou, J.M., Z.Q. Yu, Y. Cao, B.Z. Zhou, and C.Y. Liu. 1981. Active principles in She-Han-Qi (*Corydalis sheareri*). Chinese Traditional and Herbal Drugs 12(3):99-100, 107.

236. Zhou, T.D. and X.X. Zhou. 1981. Studies on the structure of an antibacterial constituent from Xie-Shui-Cao (*Eomecon chionantha*). Chinese Traditional and Herbal Drugs 12(1):1-3.

237. Zhou, Y.N. 1980. The hemostatic effects of syringin injection. Xinyiyao Tongxun (3):24-25.

238. Zhou, Y.P., L.L. Fan, L.Y. Zhang, and G.Y. Zeng. 1978. The effect of higenamine on the cardiovascular system. National Medical Journal of China 58(11):664-669.

239. Zhu, D.Y., Z.X. Chen, B.N. Zhou, J.S. Liu, B.S. Huang, Y.Y. Xie, and G.F. Zeng. 1979. Studies on chemical constituents of Bu-Gu-Zhi, the seeds of *Psoralea corylifolia* L. Acta Pharm. Sinica 14(10):605-611.

240. Zhu, D.Y., S.G. Zhang, B.N. Liu, G.J. Fan, J. Liu, and R.S. Xu. 1982. Studies on the antibacterial constituents of *Artemisia annua*. Chinese Traditional and Herbal Drugs 13(2):6.

241. Zhu, H.L. and J.C. Huang. 1984. Anti-inflammatory action of scopoletin. Chinese Traditional and Herbal Drugs 15(10):462-465.

The Alkaloids of the *Papaver* section *Oxytona* Bernh.

Hubert G. Theuns, Richard H.A.M. Janssen, and Cornelis A. Salemink
Organic Chemical Laboratory, State University of
Utrecht, Utrecht, The Netherlands

CONTENTS

I. INTRODUCTION

During the years 1971 to 1974, the cultivation of the opium poppy *Papaver somniferum* L. was temporarily suppressed in Turkey in order to cut down on the illegal availability of heroin, the diacetyl-derivative of natural (–)-morphine. At that time, fear of a possible shortage of medically useful opiates, especially codeine, arose (37, 38), and attention was focused on new natural sources of the morphinan alkaloids as substitutes for the opium poppy.

Among the potential substitutes were plants of the *Papaver* species sect. *Oxytona* Bernh. (*Macrantha* Elk.). In particular, the species *Papaver bracteatum* Lindl. proved most promising. The species *Papaver bracteatum* contains, almost exclusively, the alkaloid thebaine, which can serve as an excellent substitute for morphine as a starting material for chemical conversion into codeine (145) (Figure 1). Yet, chemical conversion of thebaine into drugs that can be abused is considered unlikely by United Nations experts (149). Thebaine abuse has never been reported and would probably not be expected even if heroin should cease to be available (153). In addition, the abuse potential of minor alkaloids from *Papaver bracteatum* is considered negligible (61, 62). Therefore, substitution of *Papaver bracteatum* for *Papaver somniferum* as a source of opiates may contribute to a curtailment of the heroin market.

Figure 1. Structures of Important Alkaloids in the Introduction of a New Natural Source of Morphinans

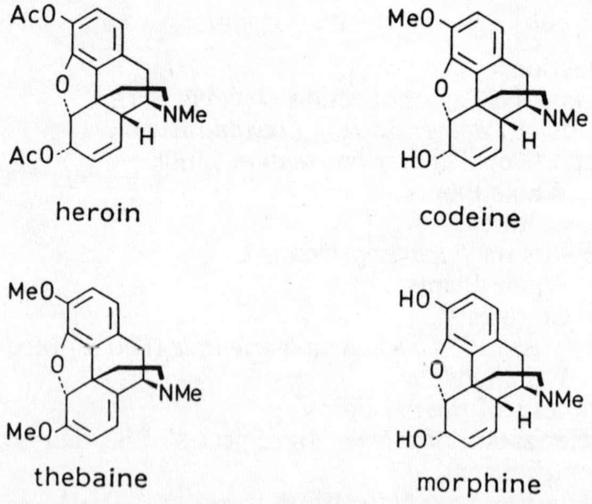

heroin

codeine

thebaine

morphine

Partly due to the restoration of opium poppy cultivation in Turkey and partly due to the fear of negative economic consequences for countries traditionally growing *Papaver somniferum*, large-scale cultivation of *Papaver bracteatum* has not been introduced into the industrial countries of the Western Hemisphere, and promotion of commercial cultivation of *Papaver bracteatum* has been stopped in most countries. Research on this species, however, is continuing in several countries (118, 150). Since permanent suppression of safer opiate-yielding species is unlikely (2), the socioeconomical implications associated with the introduction of new species need to be considered.

Some of the problems connected with introducing new natural sources of opiates were recently discussed (146).

This review deals with the alkaloids of the *Papaver* species sect. *Oxytona* Bernh. Due to insufficient characterization of these species in botanical and chemical literature, there has been considerable confusion over the alkaloid compositions of these plants. Several divergent alkaloid compositions have been reported, and the presence of certain alkaloids in certain plant species has often been reported but not confirmed. Indeed, the reports of some investigators have been questioned even by other investigators. Generally, the confusion on data has arisen from several causes, including:

1. The research was not performed on identical plant material [due to incorrect identification of species, chemical varieties, or chemical races within a species; due to sampling of different parts (morphogenetic variability) or different stages of development (ontogenetic variability); due to variability in source of germplasm].
2. Some alkaloids can decompose during isolation.
3. Different extraction methods and procedures can give contradictory results.
4. Differences in origin of the plant material (habitat, soil condition, nutrition, climatic environment) alter the contents.

II. SPECIES OF THE *PAPAVER* SECTION *OXYTONA* BERNH.

The genus *Papaver* L., belonging to the tribe *Papavereae*, the subfamily *Papaveroideae*, the family *Papaveraceae*, and the order *Papaverales*, is comprised of about 100 species. Native plants of this genus are usually found in the temperate regions of the Northern Hemisphere. The genus *Papaver* has been divided into 10 sections, based on taxonomic botanical properties (31, 99). Recently, the section *Mecones* Bernh. was further divided by Preininger *et al.* (99) into the sections *Glauca* J. Novák and *Mecones* Bernh. to account for differences in chemical, cytological, and morphological characteristics. The plants in each of these sections contain large numbers of alkaloids that have a wide variety of structures. Most of the compounds, however, are biogenetically derived from the amino acids phenylalanine, tyrosine, and 3,4-dihydroxyphenylalanine (Scheme 1). Enzymes present in different *Papaver* plants have the potential to construct many different alkaloid skeletons.

Due to confusion on the botanical identification of the *Papaver* species sect. *Oxytona*, Goldblatt (36) reinvestigated the biosystematics of this section and treated the section as comprised of 3 species

SCHEME 1. Early Alkaloid Precursors and Major Types of *Papaver* section *Oxytona* Alkaloids

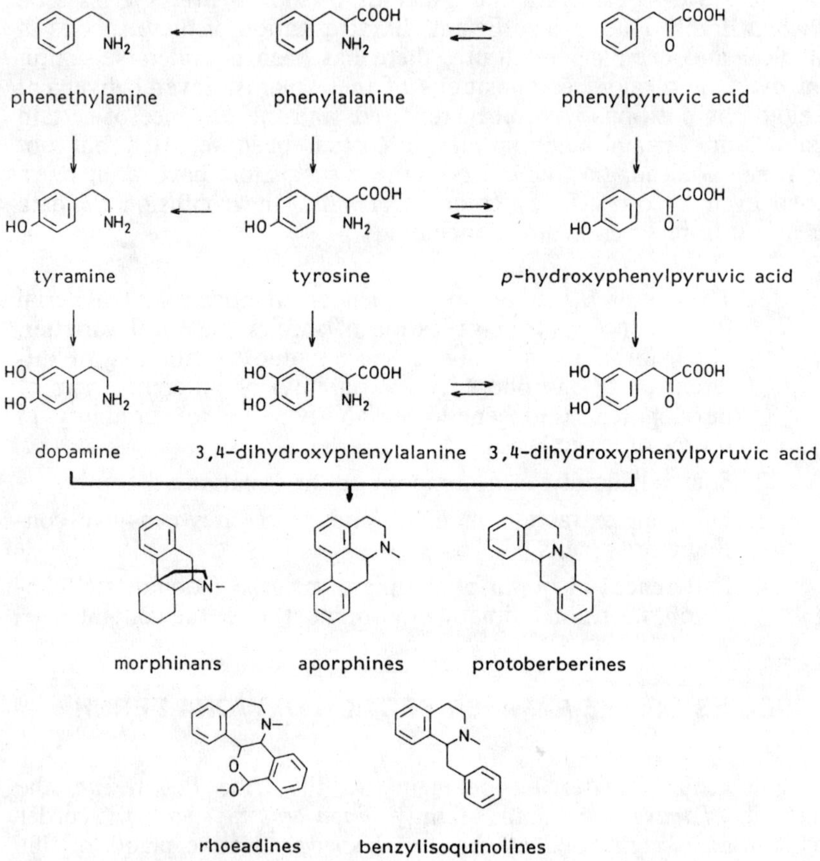

phenethylamine   phenylalanine   phenylpyruvic acid

tyramine   tyrosine   p-hydroxyphenylpyruvic acid

dopamine   3,4-dihydroxyphenylalanine   3,4-dihydroxyphenylpyruvic acid

morphinans   aporphines   protoberberines

rhoeadines   benzylisoquinolines

differing in ecological, botanical, and chemical characteristics (Table 1). The ploidy level is highly indicative for identification of the species and is preferred over other botanical or chemical characteristics. Identification by botanical characteristics is very difficult even for a botanist who is specialized in this particular field. Among other reasons, chemical profiles vary within species and with age of plant. Surprisingly, chromosome counting is not included among the methods recommended in the literature for plant identification.

Unfortunately, the wild plants of the *Papaver* species sect. *Oxytona* growing in the U.S.S.R. were not included in Goldblatt's (36) systematics study. Several reports indicate the occurrence of unusual alkaloid profiles in specimens of those plants. However, correct species identification of plants is usually quite obscure.

TABLE 1. The Biosystematics of the *Papaver* Species Sect. *Oxytona**

Papaver bracteatum Lindl. -- a robust plant; dark-red marked
       petals; numerous large floral bracts.
  Ecology: The species is found in three separate areas:
    the Alborz Mountains north of Tehran (Iran),
    Iranian Kurdistan, and in widely separated areas
    on the north slope of the Caucasus in the
    U.S.S.R.; shows a preference for comparatively dry
    situations.
  Cytology: Diploid (2n = 14).
  Chemistry: Dominant alkaloid thebaine, sometimes
    accompanied by alpinigenine.
  Synonym: Papaver lasiothrix Fedde.

Papaver orientale L. -- a slender plant; pale orange flowers
    with light to no petal markings; no floral
    bracts.
  Ecology: The species is found in northwestern Iran,
    northeastern Turkey, and transcaucasian U.S.S.R.;
    shows a preference for alpine conditions and
    likes more moist situations than Papaver bracteatum.
  Cytology: Tetraploid (2n = 28).
  Chemistry: Dominant alkaloid oripavine, sometimes
    accompanied by traces of thebaine and/or
    isothebaine, and several unidentified alkaloids.
  Synonyms: Papaver paucifoliatum (Trautv.) Fedde;
    Papaver orientale var. paucifoliatum Trautv.;
    Papaver orientale var. parviflora Busch.

Papaver pseudo-orientale (Fedde) Medw. -- a medium to
    large plant; deep orange flowers that often have
    heavy black markings; frequently has bracteate
    flowers.
  Ecology: The species is widespread in northwestern
    Iran, central and eastern Turkey, and southern
    Transcaucasus; usually associated with moist
    conditions.
  Cytology: Hexaploid (2n = 42).
  Chemistry: Dominant alkaloid isothebaine, sometimes
    accompanied by oripavine, thebaine, or
    alpinigenine, and other trace alkaloids.
  Synonyms: Papaver intermedium DC.; Papaver bracteatum
    var. pseudo-orientale Fedde.

* As described by Goldblatt (36)

    The alkaloid concentrations mentioned in this survey were taken from literature or calculated from extracted quantities. In view of the many different analytical methods used, the different extraction procedures employed, the different parts of the plants analyzed, the differing stages of plant development, the inevitable losses in purifications, and other associated technical problems, only the order of magnitude and, to a lesser degree, the relative proportions of the alkaloids should be considered to have meaning.

Literature reports on alkaloids of plants of the *Papaver* species sect. *Oxytona* are rather extensive and variable due to previously described problems concerning identification. Böhm (16) should be credited with the first attempt to select reliable literature references concerning the constituents of *Papaver bracteatum*. However, his work needs to be extended, as more recent information on these plants is now available. In contrast to Böhm's view (16), chemical races do exist within the species *Papaver bracteatum*. Furthermore, due to confusing reports on their alkaloidal constituents, the data on both of the other species of the *Papaver* sect. *Oxytona* need to be reevaluated. Such an evaluation of the other species will affect the data of *Papaver bracteatum* as reclassification of some plants reported in literature as *Papaver orientale* or *Papaver pseudo-orientale* is necessary. Tragically, confusion caused by faulty plant identification and thus incorrect interpretation of results still persists. An attempt is made in the last part of this review to arrange the data according to corrected plant identifications (Table 2).

TABLE 2. Alkaloids and Synonymic Names

Alkaloid	Synonym
alborine	alkaloid PO-5 = alkaloid R-K
alpinigenine	alkaloid E
arypavine	11-demethylmecambridine
bracteine	? (+)-bracteoline = ? glaucidine
glaucidine	? (+)-bracteoline = ? bracteine
(±)-laudanidine	laudanine
mecambridine	oreophiline
orientalidine	bractavine
(-)-stylopine	(-)-tetrahydrocoptisine
thebaine N̲-oxide major isomer*	α-thebaine-N-oxide*
thebaine N̲-oxide minor isomer*	β-thebaine-N̲-oxide*

*The structures of the thebaine N̲-oxides were revised by Theuns e̲t̲ a̲l̲. (137). In view of the confusion that may be caused by synonymic names, the use of α- and β- indications is not recommended.

III. ALKALOIDS OF *PAPAVER* SECTION *OXYTONA* BERNH.

A. Reports on *Papaver bracteatum* Lindl.

1. Whole Plants

In 1948, Kiselev and Konovalova (64) described the isolation of 4 alkaloids from Transcaucasian *Papaver bracteatum*. The total alkaloid content was 0.15 to 0.18 percent with isothebaine (Figure 2) the major alkaloid (0.04% to 0.07%). The minor alkaloids isolated were oripavine (0% to 0.003%), bracteine (0.001% to 0.003%), and bractamine (0% to

Figure 2. Structures of Some Important Alkaloids of *Papaver* Species Section *Oxytona* Bernh.

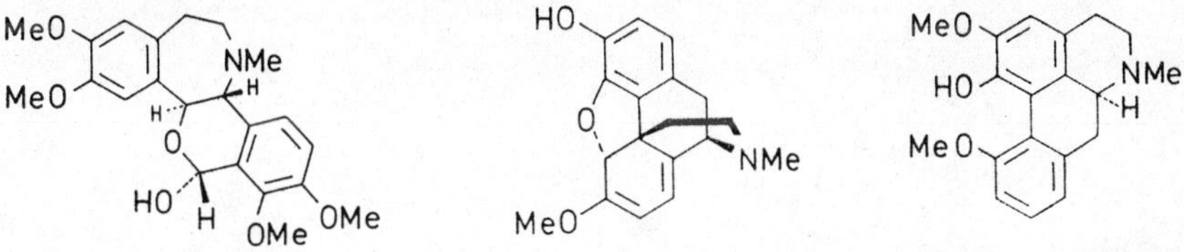

alpinigenine   oripavine   isothebaine

0.001%). Kiselev and Konovalova (64) assumed in their report that bractamine was an isomer of corypalline [demonstrated unlikely by Theuns *et al.* (145)] and that bracteine could be isomeric to corytuberine. In later reports, Heydenreich and Pfeifer (47) proposed that bracteine was identical to (+)-orientalinone, and Kühn *et al.* (69) considered bracteine as probably identical to bracteoline (Figure 3).

Neubauer and Mothes (87) were the first to report on a chemical race of *Papaver bracteatum* var. *Halle III* that contained almost exclusively (98%) thebaine. The thebaine content in the roots was 0.7 to 1.3 percent. This alkaloid profile was confirmed by Sharghi and Lalezari (127) from a collection of wild plants growing in the Alborz mountains in northern Iran. The latex of the Iranian plants contained 26 percent thebaine. No morphine was found.

In 1965, Böhm (11) reported a trace of protopine along with the major alkaloid thebaine in *Papaver bracteatum* var. *Halle III* plants. In some of the plants analyzed, the presence of another alkaloid, named alkaloid E [later proved to be identical to alpinigenine (17, 79)], was also readily recognizable. The constitution and absolute configuration of alpinigenine have been thoroughly studied (41, 106).

The alkaloid profile of *Papaver bracteatum* var. *Halle III* plants containing only thebaine (thebaine-type) or containing thebaine as well

Figure 3. Proposed Structures of Some *Papaver bracteatum* Alkaloids

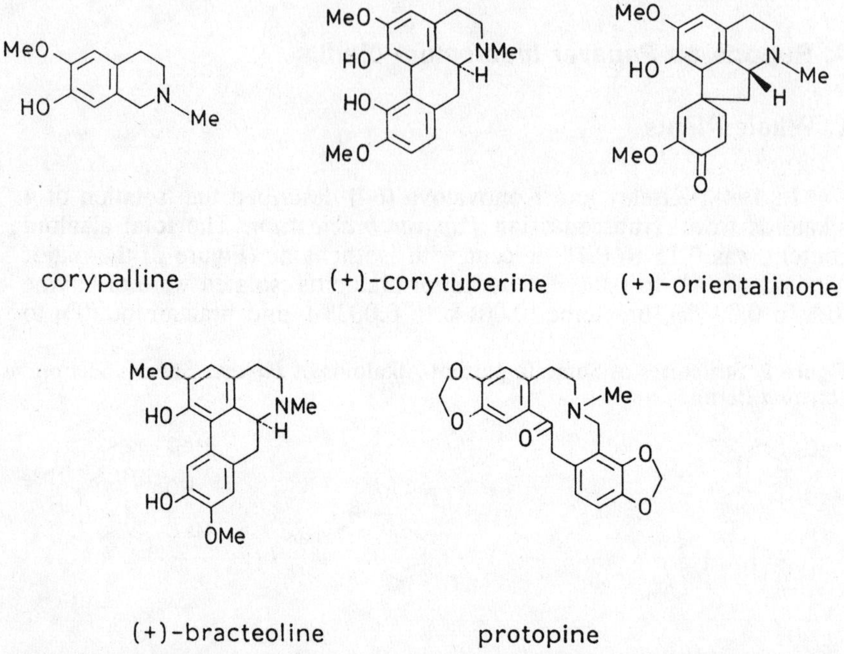

corypalline   (+)-corytuberine   (+)-orientalinone

(+)-bracteoline   protopine

as alpinigenine (E-type) was studied during plant development by Böhm (12) in 1967. Not surprisingly, seedlings proved to have a much wider alkaloid spectrum than mature plants. Thebaine-type seedlings contained 6 to 8 alkaloids at the age of 2 weeks. Usually, thebaine was not dominant, isothebaine was only present in traces, and alpinigenine was distinctly detectable. An additional 2 weeks' growth by the plants led to increased concentrations of all 3 of the above alkaloids. Following another month's growth, one of the unknown alkaloids disappeared, and the alpinigenine concentration decreased. No alpinigenine was detectable in plants of this type at the age of 3 months. Isothebaine disappeared suddenly, within 3 days, just before the plant reached the age of 4 months. Throughout the further life of the plant, 2 of the other 3 minor alkaloids remained, and the thebaine concentration continued to increase. Mature plants yielded mainly thebaine.

E-type seedlings basically resemble thebaine-type seedlings in their alkaloid profile. Alpinigenine remains present during the development of the plant, and isothebaine is generally absent in mature plants and disappears very slowly (sometimes not until the second year). Traces of isothebaine occasionally are found in older E-type plants. Böhm (15) and Gröger (39) have also reported on a selection of a type of *Papaver bracteatum* never containing alpinigenine.

Thus for the occurrence of alpinigenine, 3 types of plants can be distinguished:

1. e$^+$ thebaine always accompanied by alpinigenine
2. e^{h-} thebaine accompanied by alpinigenine only in young stages of plant growth
3. e$^-$ thebaine never accompanied by alpinigenine

The presence of alpinigenine in *Papaver bracteatum* was confirmed by Lalezari *et al.* (71), who isolated this alkaloid (2.3%) and thebaine (28%) from the latex. Fairbairn and Hakim (27) reported alpinigenine as the major alkaloid (18% to 19% of the total alkaloids in latex) along with thebaine (12.4% of the fresh latex). Minor alkaloids similar to those reported by Böhm (15) were observed at young stages in plant development (Figure 4).

Figure 4. *Papaver bracteatum* Alkaloids (46, 47, 48)

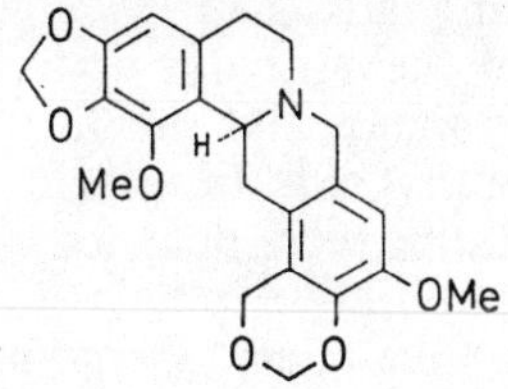

orientalidine

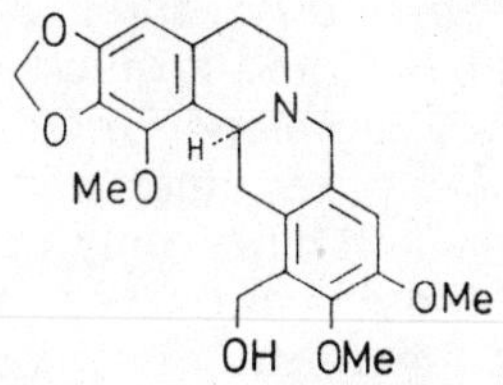

mecambridine

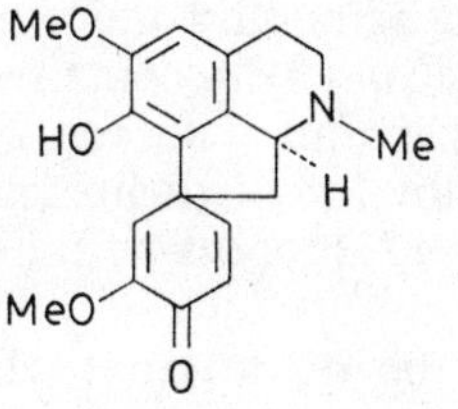

(-)-orientalinone

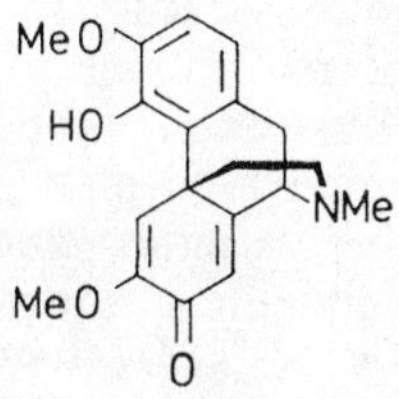

salutaridine

The presence of trace amounts of isothebaine in mature plants of the E-type was reported by Rönsch *et al.* (106). The total alkaloid content was 1.1 percent and the thebaine and alpinigenine concentrations were 0.55 and 0.28 percent, respectively.

Plants studied by Heydenreich and Pfeifer (46) contained isothebaine as the major alkaloid. Only traces of thebaine and protopine were detected, and bractavine (orientalidine) was isolated as the minor alkaloid present in the highest concentration (0.02% to 0.03%). The isolation of (–)-orientalinone, salutaridine, and oreophiline (mecambridine) was reported in 1966 (47), and the isolation of small amounts of bracteoline was reported in 1967 (48).

Preininger and Šantavý (101) isolated isothebaine (as the major alkaloid at 0.061%), orientalidine (0.01%), nuciferine (0.0006%), mecambridine (0.003%), protopine (0.00006%), and oxysanguinarine from plants. The presence of salutaridine; coptisine; the papaverrubines B, D, and E; and an unknown alkaloid was demonstrated by thin-layer chromatography (TLC) (Figure 5). The papaverrubines had been detected earlier by Pfeifer (94) and Pfeifer and Banerjee (95), who indicated that papaverrubine D was the major papaverrubine present. The other 2 papaverrubines, B and E, were present only in trace amounts, and the presence of papaverrubine F could not be ensured. Kühn *et al.* (69) also mentioned the presence of papaverrubine C in the plant.

Cheng (21) obtained a 66 percent yield of thebaine from the latex of *Papaver bracteatum*. Roots of Iranian plants had orientalidine, no isothebaine, and an increasing content of thebaine during the development of the plant. Orientalidine was the major alkaloid (about 2%) in 2-week-old seedlings and plants 3 months old. In plants at age 4 months and older, only traces of orientalidine were detected.

In an investigation on roots of 7-month-old plants grown from seeds obtained from various sources, the East German *Papaver bracteatum* var. *Halle III* was superior in thebaine content (1.3%) to all other varieties tested, including those from Iran. The East German *Papaver bracteatum* var. *Halle III* was the only one having neither orientalidine nor isothebaine. With 2 exceptions, other 7-month-old types of plants contained orientalidine, thebaine, and isothebaine as major alkaloids. A Russian type had orientalidine and thebaine in the roots, but no isothebaine in the leaves. A second type contained traces of orientalidine and isothebaine, but no thebaine. The var. *Halle III* and the Iranian type plants were clearly superior in thebaine content. None of the varieties studied by Cheng (21) contained detectable amounts of codeine or morphine.

Smith *et al.* (131) have reported on the quantitative chromatographic determination of thebaine in poppy plants and revealed the presence of isothebaine as a major alkaloid along with thebaine. The studied plant material was of Iranian origin and tentatively identified as *Papaver bracteatum*. The thebaine content of mature capsules from the plants was determined at 1.4 percent to 1.6 percent.

Fairbairn and Helliwell (28) have suggested the presence of "bound thebaine" as an explanation for differences observed between alkaline and acidic extraction methods. Analyses indicated latex was free from the "bound" forms, but the bled capsule had significant amounts of this form. The "bound" form represents 18 percent to 36 percent of the total thebaine in unripe capsules but is lacking in ripe capsules (29).

Figure 5. Papaverrubines and Other Alkaloids Reported for *Papaver bracteatum*

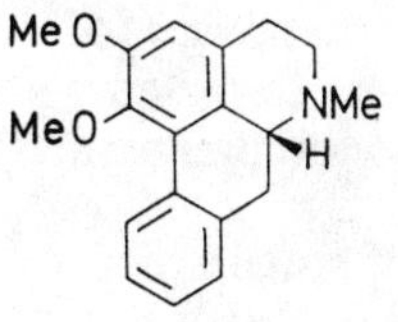

(-)-nuciferine

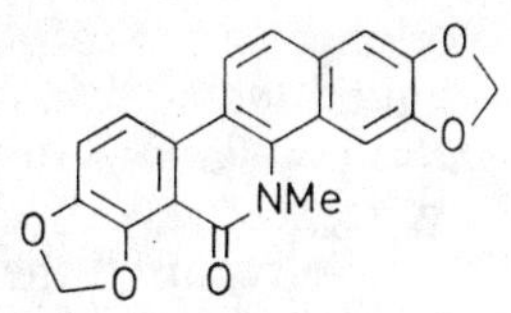

oxysanguinarine

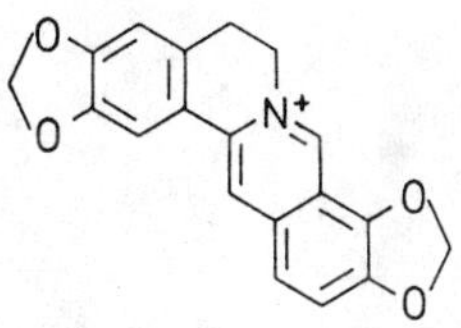

coptisine

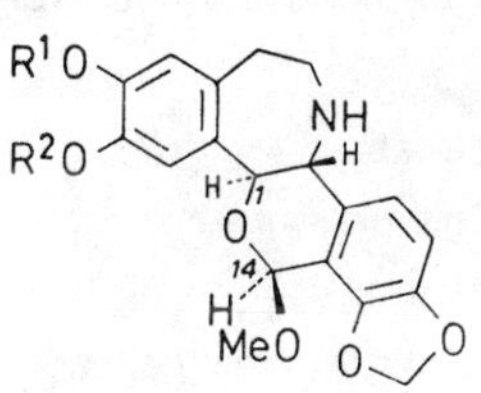

papaverrubines

B	$R^1 = R^2 = Me$	
D	$R^1 = Me;$	$R^2 = H$
C	$R^1 = Me;$	$R^2 = H;$ 14-epi
F	$R^1 = R^2 = Me;$ 1-epi	
E	$R^1, R^2 = -CH_2-;$ 1-epi	

Bled latex, representing only 46 percent of the total thebaine of the capsule, contained 28 percent to 53 percent thebaine. The capsules had 0.5 percent to 3.0 percent thebaine. A study on variations in thebaine content of bled latex indicated that a maximum thebaine content of 1.5 times the minimum was reached at about 3 p.m. local time. Minima content of thebaine were observed at about 1 a.m., 9 a.m., and 7 p.m. local time.

Phillipson *et al.* (97) first reported the isolation of thebaine *N*-oxides from *Papaver bracteatum*. The major isomer gave a yield of 0.015 percent, and the minor isomer gave a yield of 0.002 percent of fresh capsule. The total alkaloid content was 0.33 percent with thebaine being the major alkaloid. The correct structures for these *N*-oxides were reported by Theuns *et al.* (137) in 1984.

In 1974, a high thebaine-yielding (3.6%) variety, *Papaver bracteatum* var. *Arya II,* was discovered in Mahabad (western Iran) by Lalezari *et al* (71). No other alkaloids were detected in these plants. In 1973, the Second Working Group of the United Nations (148) on *Papaver bracteatum* adopted the additional indications *Arya I* and *Arya II* for *Papaver bracteatum* populations in the Alborz Mountains and the Mahabad region of Iran, respectively.

Küppers *et al.* (70) have reported the presence of small amounts of codeine (0.004%), neopine (0.003%), and alpinine (0.022%), along with thebaine (1.72%) in *Papaver bracteatum,* var. *Arya I* (Figure 6). The correct structure of this "alpinine" was presented by Theuns *et al.* (140).

Figure 6. Structures of Alpinine and Some Morphinans from *Papaver bracteatum*

thebaine *N*-oxides
major isomer $R^1 = O^-$; $R^2 = Me$
minor isomer $R^1 = Me$; $R^2 = O^-$
(structures corrected by Theuns et al., 1984e)

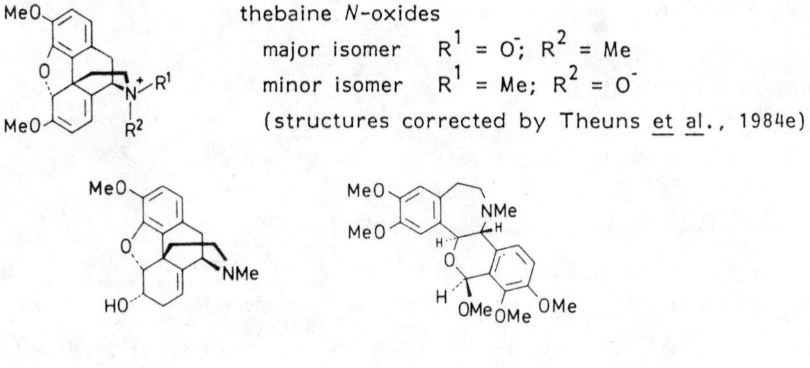

neopine   alpinine

In 1977, Denisenko *et al.* (25) isolated 12 alkaloids from *Papaver bracteatum* plants collected in the area of Besjtaw Mountains in the North Caucasus (Pjatigorsk). The total alkaloid content of the tissue was 0.6 percent, and the major alkaloids were thebaine (0.24%), oripavine (0.17%), mecambridine (0.087%), and isothebaine (0.061%). Minor alkaloids identified in the plants were alpinigenine (0.017%), orientalidine (0.011%), alpinine (0.0042%), floripavidine (0.0013%), bracteoline (0.0013%), salutaridine (0.0008%), and 2 unknown alkaloids (0.00017% and 0.00013%). The correct structure of this alpinine was presented by Theuns *et al.* (146). Floripavidine isolated from *Papaver bracteatum* collected in the environs of Mineral'nye Vody (Caucasus) was reported by Israilov *et al.* (55) to be a glycosidic alkaloid of the aporphine series.

In a study on the biosynthesis of alpigenine in *Papaver bracteatum,* Rönsch demonstrated the presence of tetrahydropalmatine, tetrahydropalmatinemetho salt, and muramine by use of tracer dilution techniques (104) (Figure 7).

Figure 7. Some Minor Alkaloids Reported for *Papaver bracteatum*

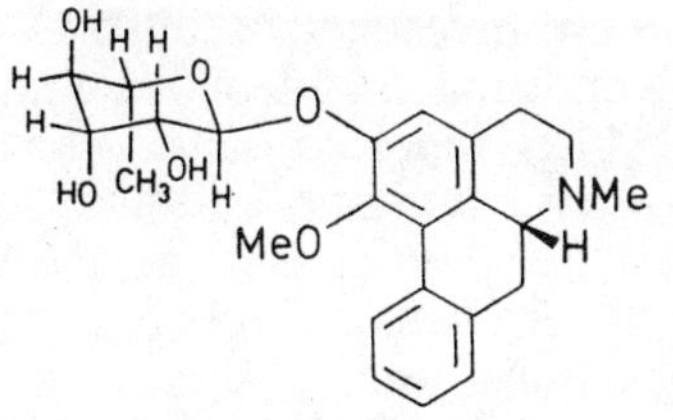

floripavidine

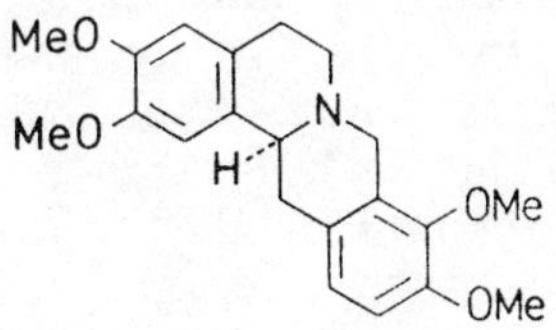

tetrahydropalmatine

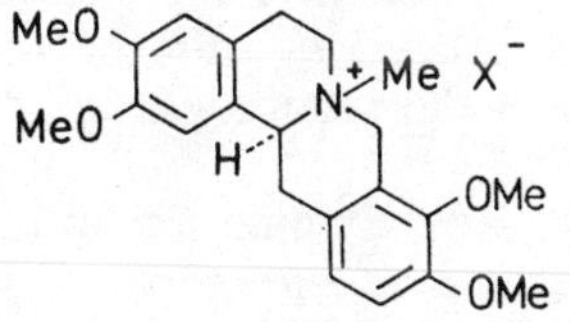

tetrahydropalmatine metho salt

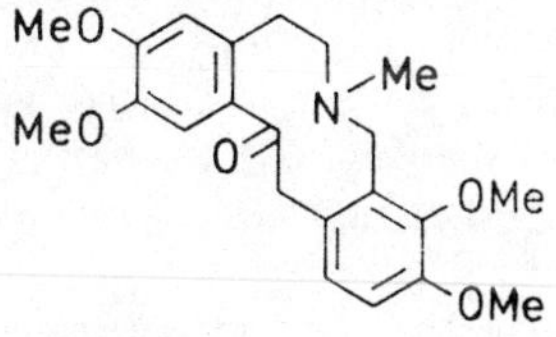

muramine

Sárkány *et al.* (116), in studies on *Papaver bracteatum* plants of Iranian and other origins, indicated that the latter varieties consistently contained isothebaine (1.0% to 6.0%) besides thebaine (0.6% to 1.0%). Isothebaine was absent in plants of Iranian origin; however, these plants did contain 7 percent to 12 percent thebaine. Morphine was not found in any of these plants. A nomenclature for these plants based on botanical and phytochemical characteristics was proposed as *Papaver eu-orientale, Papaver pseudo-orientale,* and *Papaver pseudo-bracteatum.*

Rönsch and Schade (107) reported in 1979 on the isolation of thebaine methochloride (0.14%) from *Papaver bracteatum.* The crude alkaloid content was 0.48 percent, and the tertiary alkaloid content was 0.26 percent in the material studied (unripe heads, green leaves, and upper halves of stems).

Fairbairn and Williamson (30) have reported that the alkaloid pattern of seedlings of *Papaver bracteatum* is similar to those in seedlings of *Papaver orientale* and *Papaver pseudo-orientale.* Only traces of thebaine and about 5 other alkaloids (among these oripavine and isothebaine) were detected in tissue. The *Arya II* variety alone had a predominance of thebaine in the seedlings.

Baytop and Sariyar (7) reported the presence of salutaridine (0.225%) and thebaine (0.3%) (91) as major alkaloids in *Papaver bracteatum* collected near Tunceli in Turkey and the presence of salutaridine and orientalidine as the principal alkaloids in *Papaver lasiothrix* collected near Gümüşhane in Turkey. Although reference was made to the work of Goldblatt (36), these investigators failed to make a reliable plant identification, while reporting dissident alkaloid profiles. In 1978, Sariyar and Baytop (112) reported salutaridine and mecambridine as major alkaloids and orientalidine and thebaine as minor alkaloids for *Papaver lasiothrix*. Another unusual alkaloid profile, reported by Baytop (6), was discovered in a Turkish review by Kaymakçalan (60). Thebaine and oripavine were observed in equal quantities in *Papaver bracteatum*. A collection of plants from Tunceli, identified as *Papaver bracteatum*, yielded salutaridine and thebaine as major alkaloids (111), and this is probably the same plant material reported by Baytop and Sariyar (7) and later recognized as *Papaver pseudo-orientale*, having a diploid chromosome number 2n = 14 (sample "P3") by Phillipson *et al.* (98). These investigators feel that *Papaver bracteatum* does not grow in Turkey (98). Further data on Turkish *Papaver lasiothrix* are presented in the section on the alkaloids from *Papaver pseudo-orientale*.

Hodges *et al.* (49) could detect no codeine, morphine, or northebaine in 5- to 7-month-old *Papaver bracteatum* plants but did report a trace of oripavine (0.0003% fresh weight) along with thebaine (0.06% fresh weight). Theuns *et al.* (136) have reported the occurrence of 2 morphinan alkaloids—14β-hydroxycodeine and 14β-hydroxycodeinone (0.025 and 0.005% of dry weight, respectively) (Figure 8)—in capsules of *Papaver bracteatum*, var. *Arya I*. The presence of the isoquinolone alkaloid *N*-methylcorydaldine (0.044%) was determined by gas chromatography/mass spectrometry. In addition, alpinigenine (0.12%) was isolated, but oripavine and salutaridine could not be detected in the plant material.

Although epialpinine (Figure 9) was mentioned as a constituent of *Papaver bracteatum* in a review by Nyman and Bruhn (91), these authors only referred to a paper by Shamma *et al.* (126) and gave no evidence that this alkaloid was obtained from *Papaver bracteatum* plant material. An even more obscure indication of morphine and codeine in *Papaver bracteatum* was reported in a paper by Duke (26). The occurrence of codeine in this species has been mentioned (18), and the occurrence of morphine was erroneously included in an extensive alkaloid review (154) that referred to a paper by Böhm (11) on interspecific hybrids of *Papaver bracteatum* and *Papaver somniferum*.

In a quantitative determination of thebaine in *Papaver bracteatum*, Wu and Dobberstein (156) report the presence of 2 peaks in a gas chromatography analysis of an extract of the plant, but in high pressure liquid chromatography analysis (HPLC), only 1 major constituent was observed. No positive identification is presented, and the impression is

Figure 8. Structure of Northebaine and *Papaver bracteatum* Alkaloids

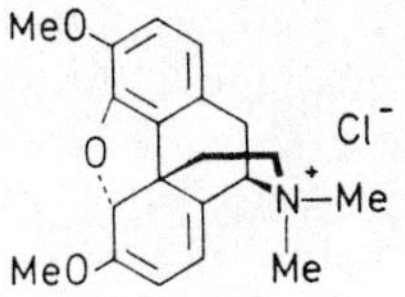

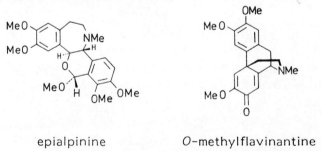

thebaine methochloride 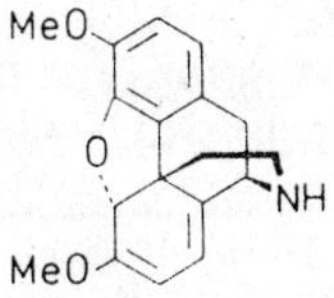   northebaine

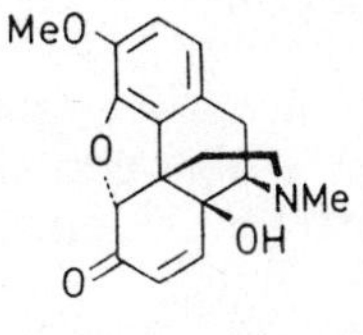

14β-hydroxycodeinone 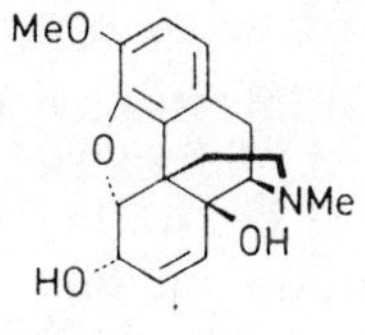   14β-hydroxycodeine 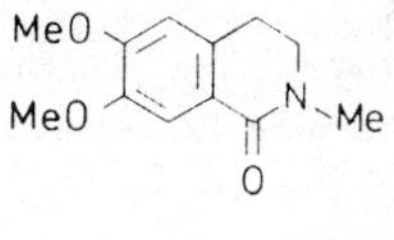   *N*-methylcorydaldine

Figure 9. *Papaver bracteatum* Alkaloids

epialpinine   *O*-methylflavinantine

justified that both gas chromatography peaks resulted only from thebaine with the evidence of 2 different phytoconstituents due only to poor control of the gas chromatography analytical technique.

No marked differences in thebaine content were reported in an examination of capsules and roots from selections of 'Arya I' and 'Arya II' populations (76). 'Arya I' was considered to be more promising for breeding purposes because of the greater variation of horticultural characters, thebaine content, and flowering rate. The high thebaine contents often recorded for capsules (4% to 5%) are applicable only to a few plants in these varieties in which other plants have less than 0.5 percent thebaine (76).

In 1980, the latex of *Papaver bracteatum* was investigated by Novák (90). Thebaine was the dominant alkaloid accompanied by alpinigenine and occasionally also by oripavine. In the same year, Meshulam and Lavie (80) isolated thebaine (2.3%) and 6 other alkaloids from *Papaver bracteatum* var. *Arya II* using large-scale extraction on 3.1 tons of capsules. The alkaloids were 14β-hydroxycodeine, codeine, neopine, alpinigenine, and protopine, plus a yet unknown alkaloid for this species, *O*-methylflavinantine. No 14β-hydroxycodeinone was observed, and this was explained by the known instability of codeinone and similar structural compounds, especially when in solution. 14β-hydroxycodeine was predominant after thebaine. In a previous review, Salemink (108), in error, referred to detection of salutaridine and oripavine in the *Papaver bracteatum* material used by his group.

In 1981, Lavie *et al.* (75) investigated *Papaver bracteatum* capsules collected in the Polour region of Iran and reported a high content of alpinigenine (approximately 15% in the crude extract of capsules). Theuns *et al.* (147), in a report on the search for precursors of the isoquinolone alkaloid *N*-methylcorydaldine in *Papaver bracteatum*, demonstrated the presence of corypalline and *O*-methylcorypalline in *Papaver bracteatum* (Figure 10). For identification of bractamine, an alkaloid of unknown structure (64), the physical data were compared, without success, to the physical data for corypalline and the isomeric tetrahydroisoquinolines I, II, and III.

Figure 10. Tetrahydroisoquinoline Alkaloids

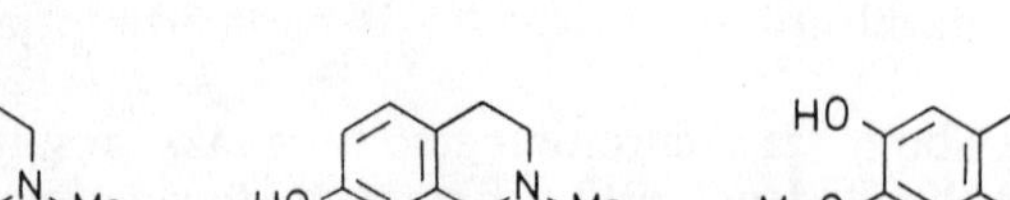

O-methylcorypalline   corypalline

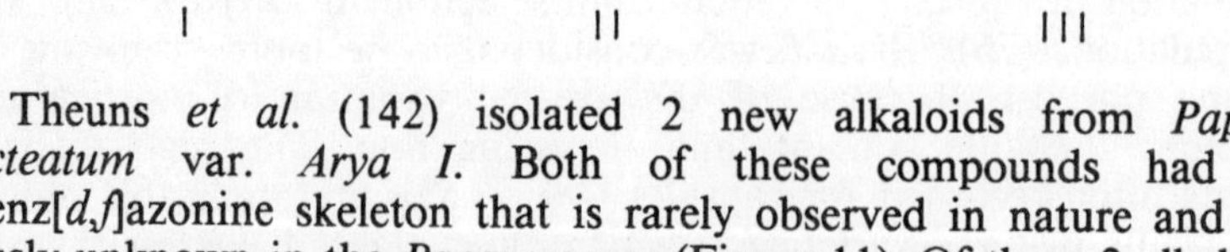

I   II   III

Theuns *et al.* (142) isolated 2 new alkaloids from *Papaver bracteatum* var. *Arya I.* Both of these compounds had the dibenz[*d,f*]azonine skeleton that is rarely observed in nature and previously unknown in the *Papaveraceae* (Figure 11). Of these 2 alkaloids, 1 was eventually identified as neodihydrothebaine and the other as an isomer bractazonine. Syntheses of both of these natural alkaloids (144) and of a number of isomeric substances (143) have been reported. A biomimetic synthesis of neodihydrothebaine and bractazonine from thebaine has also been reported (141). In '*Arya I*' capsules, concentrations of thebaine and the sum of the dibenz[*d,f*]azonine alkaloids were approximately 1.72 percent and 0.036 percent of dry weight, respectively. In '*Arya II*', the concentrations of thebaine and the sum of the dibenz[*d,f*]azonine alkaloids were 2.66 percent and 0.11 percent of dry weight, respectively.

Figure 11. Dibenz[*d,f*]azonine Alkaloids from *Papaver bracteatum*

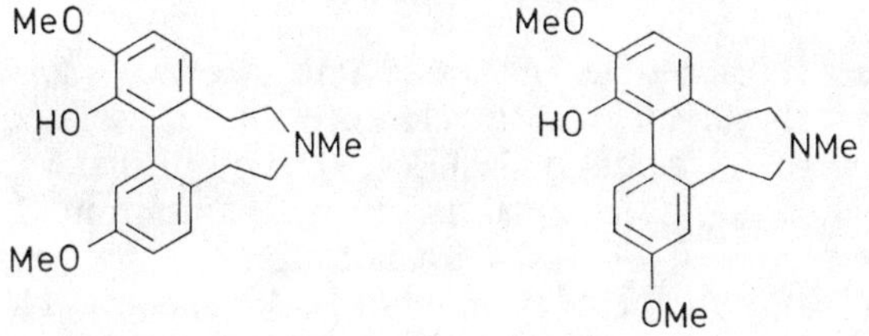

neodihydrothebaine   bractazonine

An alkaloid having unusual characteristics has been isolated from *Papaver bracteatum* var. *Arya I* (142). This alkaloid, named 6,7,8,9,10,14-hexadehydro-4,5-epoxy-3,6-dimethoxy-17-methylthebinan (in agreement with the newly proposed nomenclature system for such rearranged morphinan derivates), is a yellow compound that turns a strong red color in acidic solution. The compound, however, can be recovered unchanged from acidic solutions. The color and chemical behavior of the alkaloid in acid solution are explained by a reversible opening of the 4,5-epoxy ring that results in carbokation IV (Figure 12). The alkaloid can be formed *in vitro* by decomposition of the major isomer of thebaine *N*-oxides. On the basis of this observation, further examination of the structure of the *N*-oxides from *Papaver bracteatum* has resulted in a reversal of the structural assignments for thebaine *N*-oxides, codeine *N*-oxides, and morphine *N*-oxides. A ^{13}C nuclear magnetic resonance (NMR) study on the minor isomer of the thebaine *N*-oxides and other quaternary morphinans (138) supports the reassigned structures.

Theuns (135) has reported that the hemiketale alkaloid alpinigenine decomposes during gas chromatography, causing a number of decomposition peaks to appear in the chromatogram. All decomposition peaks indicate a virtual molecular weight of 355 instead of 401. Presumably the elements of CO and H_2O, the equivalent of 46 mass units, are removed from the molecule under chromatography conditions.

Figure 12. Origin of Acid-Induced Red Color in the Thebinan Alkaloid of
Papaver bracteatum

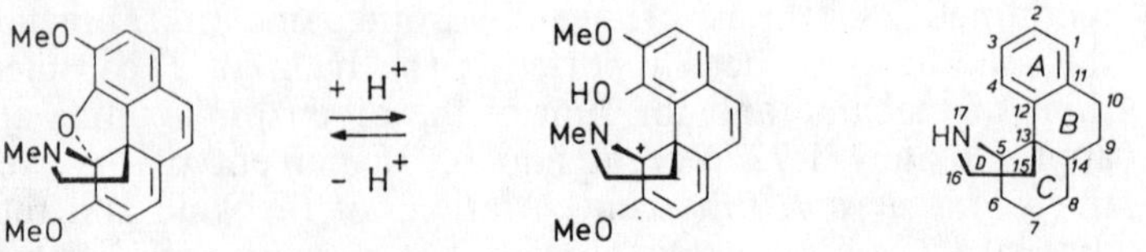

6,7,8,9,10,14–hexadehydro-   IV   thebinan

4,5–epoxy–3,6–dimethoxy–17–methylthebinan

The presence of a trace of isothebaine in *Papaver bracteatum* was
confirmed by comparison with a reference sample isolated from Turkish *Papaver pseudo-orientale* in 1985 (139). Also in that year, Theuns *et
al.* (146) isolated alpinine, epialpinine, and muramine from *Papaver
bracteatum* var. *Arya I.* The structures of alpinine and epialpinine were
assessed by a study of their ^{1}H and ^{13}C NMR spectra. The "alpinine,"
reported earlier by Küppers *et al.* (70), was demonstrated to actually be
the C-14 epimer of alpinine. The spectra of codeine and neopine,
whose presence was reported earlier (70), were definitive for their
configuration. These data strongly support an enzyme-mediated reduction step in the formation of codeine and neopine from neopinone
(possibly nonenzymatic derived). Also a trace of protopine but no
O-methylflavinantine was found.

Slavnik and Slavníková (130) reported in 1985 on the isolation of a
substantial number of alkaloids from *Papaver bracteatum* var. *Halle III*
and Demavend (Iran) population. The *Halle III* variety yielded, along
with thebaine, the significant alkaloids thebain metho salt and
corytuberine. It also yielded the minor alkaloids isothebaine,
scoulerine, protopine, epialpinine, isothebaine metho salt, isoboldine,
corydine, rhoeadine, magnoflorine, a mixture of coptisine and
palmatine, and an alkaloid of yet unknown structure, PB 1, which
possibly is related to the morphinan alkaloids. [The latter alkaloid was
also detected in some extracts of the plants studied by Küppers *et al.*
(70), but its concentration was too low for full characterization.]
Chromatographically, the papaverrubines C, D, E, and G, and
bracteoline were also detected (Figure 13). The Demavend population
from Iran yielded, along with thebaine, the alkaloids thebaine metho
salt, epialpinine, alpinigenine, corytuberine, and a mixture of coptisine
and palmatine. The presence of salutaridine and the papaverrubines C,
D, and G was detected.

Figure 13. New Alkaloids Reported for *Papaver bracteatum* (130)

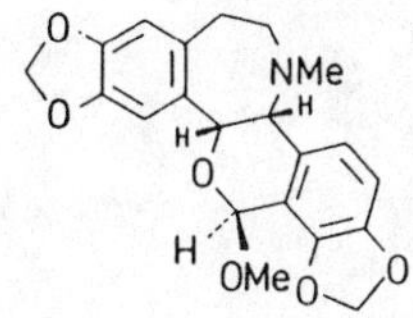

rhoeadine 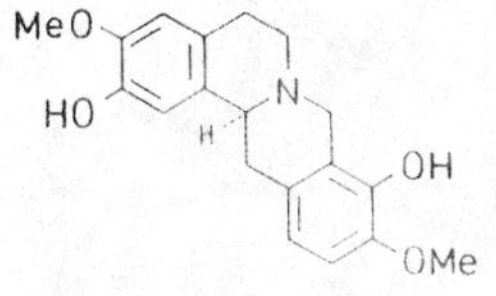 · scoulerine

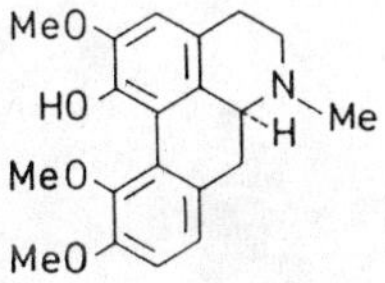

corydine 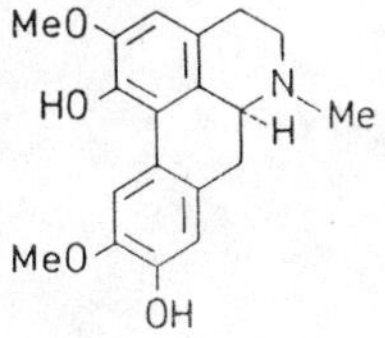 · isoboldine 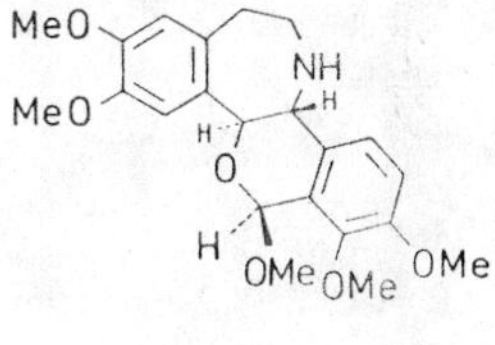 · papaverrubine G

2. Cultures

In callus tissues of *Papaver bracteatum*, Ikuta *et al.* (53) reported the presence of norsanguinarine, sanguinarine, oxysanguinarine, dihydrosanguinarine, chelirubine, protopine, magnoflorine, and 2 unidentified alkaloids (CS and QS) (Figure 14). No thebaine was detected. Kamimura and Nishikawa (59) reported that the 7 common Japanese strains of *Papaver bracteatum* contained isothebaine but no thebaine. The cultured strain used in the research, however, yielded abundant thebaine as the major alkaloid in whole plants (0.14% in leaves and 0.3% to 0.35% in roots) (58). The main alkaloids produced by the callus cells, derived from seedlings and maintained on agar media for over 2 years, were L-stylopine (0.015% to 0.02%) and protopine (0.01% to 0.015%). At an early stage of growth soon after induction of callus cells, formation of thebaine was observed. The concentration of thebaine in the cells was reduced to trace amounts at a later stage of growth, but its production was recovered (highest thebaine yield was 0.013%) when the cells were subcultured in media without 2,4-D. In cultures without 2,4-D, L-stylopine and protopine were present only in trace amounts. In a patent application, Kamimura (57) describes production of callus tissues from *Papaver bracteatum* in a plant hormone-free medium with subsequent culture in a medium containing kinetin and/or coconut milk plus 2,4-D in order to produce thebaine.

Figure 14. Alkaloids Reported for Callus Cultures of *Papaver bracteatum*

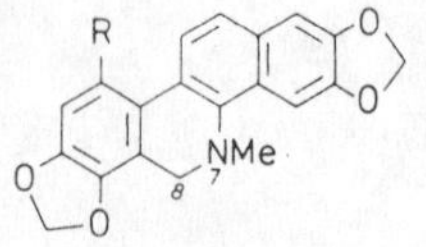

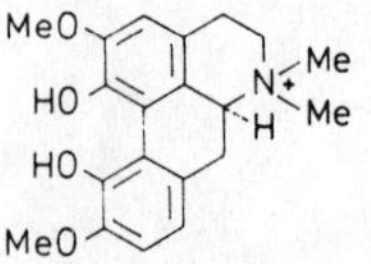

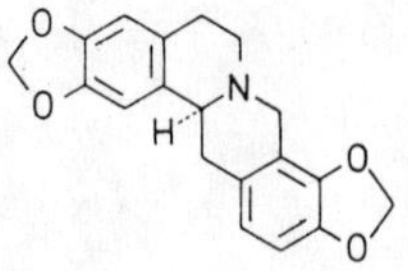

dihydrosanguinarine

  R = H

sanguinarine

  R = H; C^8=N$\overset{+}{\underset{}{<}}$

norsanguinarine

  R = H; *N*-demethyl; C^8=N-

chelirubine

  R = OMe; C^8=N$\overset{+}{\underset{}{<}}$

(+)-magnoflorine   (−)-stylopine

Shafiee *et al.* (122, 123) report the presence of thebaine in tissue cultures of *Papaver bracteatum* var. *Arya II* maintained for only a few transfers but present no information on thebaine yield. Lockwood (77) has reported that callus cultures of *Papaver bracteatum* var. *Arya II* yield orientalidine, isothebaine, and sanguinarine and that the derived suspension cultures yield orientalidine and sanguinarine.

Root cultures derived from cell suspension cultures of *Papaver bracteatum* var. *Arya II* produced thebaine (yield 0.03%) (157). Cell suspension cultures of *Papaver bracteatum* var. *Arya II* containing shoots produced thebaine (0.007% total yield). Codeine was detected in the cell cultures by TLC and HPLC (though identification cannot be regarded as unequivocal; compare the detection of "codeine" in *Papaver somniferum* cell suspension cultures, reported in the same paper) (132).

B. Reports on *Papaver orientale* L.

1. Whole Plants

The species *Papaver orientale* was investigated as early as 1827 by Petit (93), who believed he had isolated morphine and a small quantity of narcotine. In 1911, Gadamer and Klee (34) reported a total alkaloid content of 0.5% for *Papaver orientale* with the major alkaloid being phenolic. Protopine was either absent or present in such a small concentration that it could not be isolated. Klee (65) could not detect morphine or narcotine in *Papaver orientale* but did report the presence of thebaine and isothebaine. While only thebaine was observed during the rapid vegetative growth of the plant, at capsule ripeness the main alkaloid was isothebaine. Gadamer (33), in 1914, reported the presence of at least 3 nonphenolic and 3 phenolic alkaloids, in addition to thebaine and isothebaine. One of the nonphenolic alkaloids was identified as protopine, and one of the phenolic alkaloids, glaucidine, resembled glaucine (Figure 15).

Figure 15. Structures of Narcotine and Glaucine

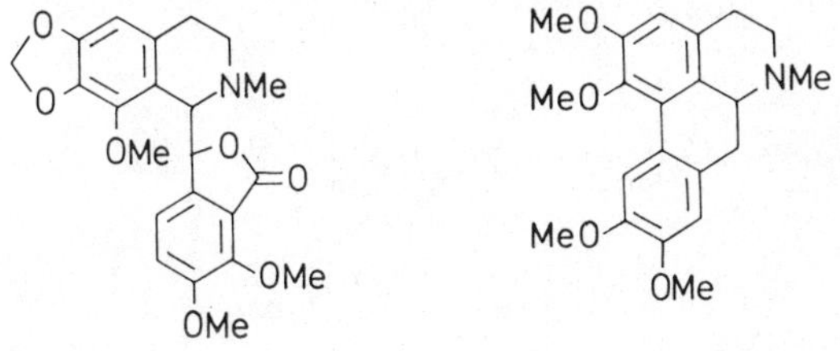

narcotine   glaucine

No isothebaine was detected in *Papaver orientale* collected in 1935 in the Transcaucasus in West-Georgia near Bakuryany, but thebaine (0.02%) and oripavine (0.03%) were isolated (67, 68). The total alkaloid content of the plant was 0.16 percent.

A total alkaloid content for *Papaver orientale* L. of 0.59 percent was reported in 1944 by Fulton (32) with the principal alkaloid being isothebaine (0.22%). No thebaine was detected, but another alkaloid (0.035%), believed to be glaucidine, was obtained. The presence of several other noncharacterized alkaloids was also reported by Fulton (32). Isothebaine (0.11%) has been isolated from roots of *Papaver orientale* (117).

In a population of 297 plants of *Papaver orientale*, Dawson and James (23) observed 102 plants containing both thebaine and isothebaine (the dominant alkaloid), 192 plants containing only isothebaine, and 3 plants containing little or no alkaloids. No indications of opposing seasonal trends in thebaine and isothebaine concentrations were observed in these plants. In another population of 468 plants, all plants contained isothebaine as the major alkaloid, and all but one plant contained thebaine. The differences in observation of alkaloids between the 2 surveys probably result from the use of a more sensitive analytical technique in the latter study (23). In 2 plants of the second population, a third alkaloid was detected. Another group of plants, obtained from a single commercial source, contained, in addition to isothebaine and thebaine, 2 other alkaloids when grown under unfavorable conditions (excessive root binding in the clay pots). One of these latter alkaloids was also observed to occur in a substantial number of other *Papaver orientale* plants.

Bentley and Dyke (10) referred to Hesse (43, 44, 45) on the occurrence of (–)-laudanidine and laudanine [(–)-laudanidine] in *Papaver orientale* (Figure 16). These references, however, describe work performed on opium (the dried latex of *Papaver somniferum*). Apparently confusion was caused by speculations of Bentley and Cardwell (9) on the biosynthesis of thebaine and isothebaine in *Papaver orientale*.

Figure 16. The Structure of (–)-Laudanidine

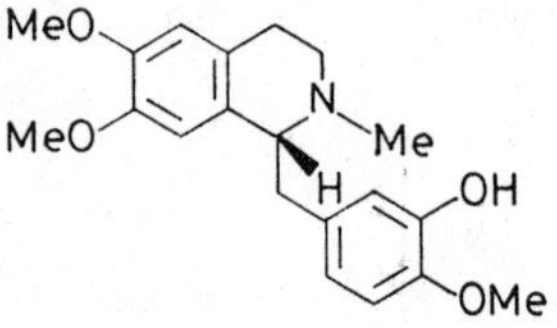

(–)-laudanidine

Kleinschmidt (66), in 1961, studied alkaloid distribution in various parts of *Papaver orientale* during plant development. In all stages of growth, isothebaine was the major alkaloid, with thebaine and protopine present in traces. Three unidentified minor alkaloids were observed, 2 of them being phenolic (possibly oripavine and glaucidine). In a test of 340 individual plants of different origins for alkaloid profiles, Neubauer and Mothes (86) reported that, in general, isothebaine was the major alkaloid with no change in thebaine/isothebaine levels observed throughout the year. Of 12 alkaloids separated and identified by TLC, only 2 were phenolic with 1 of them being isothebaine. The other phenolic alkaloid was neither morphine nor oripavine but was possibly identical to bracteoline and glaucidine (69). The nonphenolic alkaloids included thebaine, protopine, and another that was thought to be orientalidine (100). Some plants were free from isothebaine, and one of these had thebaine as the major alkaloid. Although isothebaine and thebaine occurred together as major alkaloids in some plants, in one plant neither thebaine nor isothebaine was detected. A commercially obtained variety contained thebaine as the sole alkaloid in most individual plants until the plants were 5 months old.

Stermitz and Rapoport (133) observed thebaine, isothebaine, and 5 other phenolic alkaloids in *Papaver orientale* L. Of the phenolic alkaloids, 3 were major components with one conditionally identified as oripavine and a second appearing to resemble the morphine-type alkaloids as well. In a screening for berberine, coptisine, chelerythrine, and sanguinarine (Figure 17), Hakim *et al.* (42) detected the presence of coptisine and sanguinarine independently in 2 separate plants of *Papaver orientale*; no berberine or chelerythrine was detected.

Figure 17. Alkaloids for Which a Screening Test Was Made in *Papaver orientale*

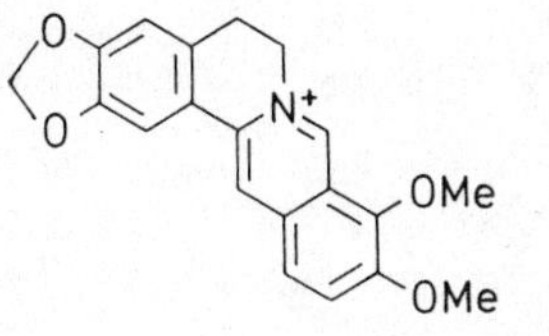

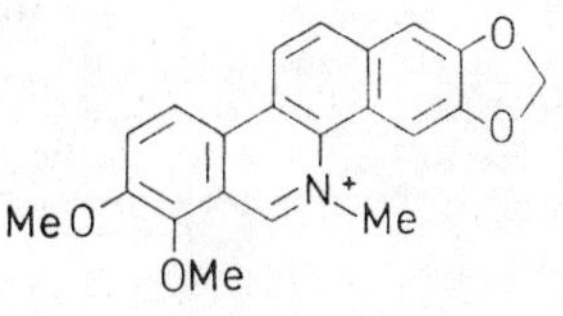

berberine   chelerythrine

Tétényi *et al.* (134) reported isothebaine and an unidentified compound as major alkaloids in *Papaver orientale*. A similar composition with the addition of 10 minor alkaloids was later reported by Lörincz and Tétényi (78). A total alkaloid content of 0.35% was mentioned by Mnatsakanyan and Yunusov (81) for wild-growing *Papaver orientale*. Using paper chromatography, Pfeifer (94) detected papaverrubine D (porphyroxine) as the only alkaloid of this type in *Papaver orientale*. Later Pfeifer and Banerjee (95) reported traces of papaverrubines B and E in addition to D. The presence of papaverrubine F could not be confirmed.

Gross and Dawson (40) reported the presence of isothebaine and oripavine in seedlings of *Papaver orientale* following a few days of growth and, if the seedlings were grown for 1 or 2 weeks, the presence of thebaine as well. In 1965, Heydenreich and Pfeifer (46) mentioned the presence of bractavine (orientalidine) in *Papaver orientale*. Battersby and Brown (5) reported the isolation of 3 alkaloids identified as (–)-orientalinone, (+)-salutaridine, and (+)-dihydro-orientalinone, in addition to the 4 previously isolated from this plant (isothebaine, thebaine, protopine, and oripavine). Preininger and Šantavý (100) isolated isothebaine as the major alkaloid (0.055%) and orientalidine (0.002%); salutaridine (0.0016%); mecambridine (0.0008%); nuciferine (0.0006%); PO-3, PO-4, and PO-5; oxysanguinarine; and thebaine as minor alkaloids (Figure 18). Traces of coptisine were also demonstrated by TLC, but no protopine, glaucidine, or oripavine was detected. The total alkaloid content was 0.53 percent (83).

Délenk-Heydenreich and Pfeifer (24) described in 1969 the isolation of 9 minor alkaloids—bractavine (0.024%), mecambridine (0.012%), (–)-orientalinone (0.002%), OR-1 (0.003%), OR-2 (0.002%), bracteoline (0.002%), salutaridine (0.005%), and the papaverrubines C and D—in addition to isothebaine (0.17%) as the major alkaloid. Thebaine could not be detected, and several other minor alkaloids were present in concentrations too low for characterization. Judging from data presented and a later report by Shafiee *et al.* (121), alkaloid OR-2

Figure 18. Some Alkaloids Reported for *Papaver orientale*

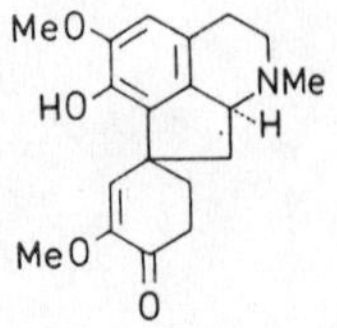

(+)-dihydro-orientalinone 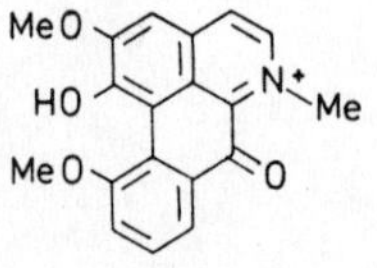   alkaloid PO-3

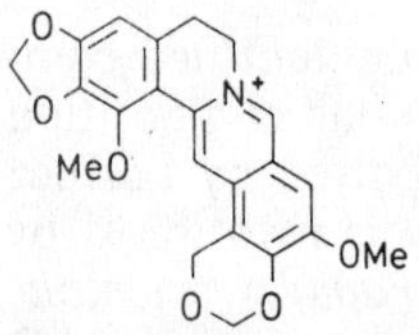

alkaloid PO-4 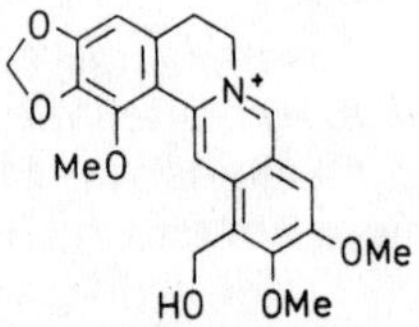   alkaloid PO-5 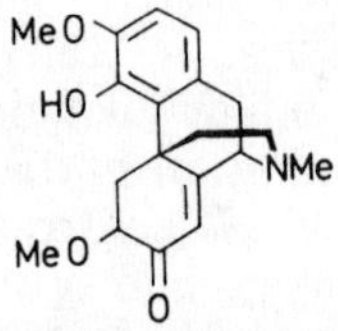   (+)-5,6-dihydrosalutaridine

is most probably a tetrahydro-orientalinol, and although the evidence for a definitive structural assignment is insufficient, alkaloid OR-1 is possibly (+)-5,6-dihydrosalutaridine (24).

Vágújfalvi (151) presented some analytical data in 1970 on the distribution of the alkaloids in various parts of the *Papaver orientale* plant. The major alkaloid was isothebaine with 3 unidentified alkaloids also present. An investigation of 30 individual plants for daily changes in alkaloids indicated that the total alkaloid content had 2 maxima: one at 9 a.m. and another between 9 p.m. and 3 a.m. local time (152). At the minima, the total alkaloid content was 25 percent to 50 percent of the maxima. In some plants, isothebaine was the major alkaloid with a small amount of protopine and 3 unidentified alkaloids. In other plants, all alkaloids were present in nearly equal quantities.

The occurrence of oripavine as the major alkaloid in capsules and roots of *Papaver orientale* has been reported by Böhm (13). Often no thebaine was detected at capsule ripeness, but this alkaloid was clearly recognizable and sometimes even dominating in earlier stages of development. In mature plants, the capsules yielded 0.2 percent oripavine and the roots 0.16 percent oripavine. The presence of another unidentified alkaloid was detected by TLC. In 1972, Cheng (21) isolated isothebaine, orientalidine (bractavine), and an incompletely identified alkaloid that could be identical to oreophiline (mecambridine) from *Papaver orientale* roots.

In 1975, Shafiee *et al.* (121) reported that the latex from *Papaver orientale* collected in northwest Iran contained oripavine (20%) (Figure 19) and thebaine (9%). Trace amounts of isothebaine were also detected in one case. In a later investigation on the alkaloid profiles of Iranian *Papaver orientale* having a diploid chromosome number of 2n = 28 (119), the plants could be classified into 5 different chemotypes based on the occurrences of other alkaloids in addition to the major alkaloid oripavine (120). These chemotypes occur within the same populations of north and northwest Iran. The alkaloid contents are listed in Table 3.

Figure 19. Structures of Isothebaidine and Oripavidine

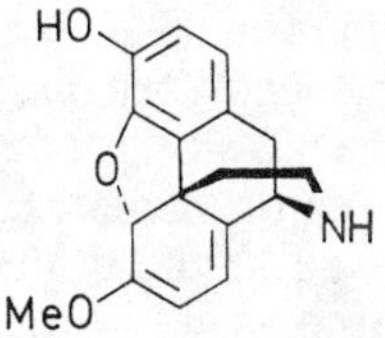

oripavidine 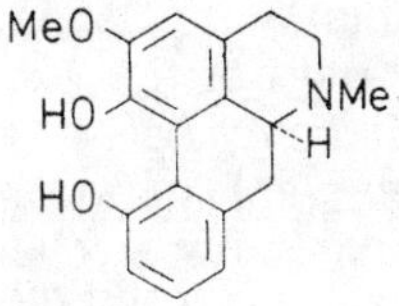   isothebaidine

TABLE 3. Alkaloid Contents of Iranian *Papaver orientale* Chemotypes

Chemotype	oripavine	thebaine	isothebaine	alpinigenine
A	1.0-1.15	-	-	-
B	0.8-0.88	0.1-0.4	-	-
C	0.5	-	0.3	-
D	0.5	-	-	0.3
E	0.8-1.2	0.3-0.35	-	0.05

In 1977, Lalezari and Shafiee (72) reported that plants collected from several regions had a diploid chromosome number of 2n = 28 and contained oripavine as the major alkaloid (1% in dried capsules). During the same year, Israilov *et al.* (56) presented the structure of a phenolic alkaloid, named oripavidine isolated from *Papaver orientale*, collected in Nakhichevan (Azerbaidshan SSR) that proved identical to *N*-demethyloripavine. In a later investigation on the alkaloids of

Papaver orientale, Israilov *et al.* (54) reported that the aerial parts of flowering plants contained 0.49 percent total alkaloids, including isothebaine (0.2%), oripavine (0.15%), thebaine (0.9%), bracteoline (0.02%), mecambridine (0.01%), orientalidine (0.007%), alpinigenine (0.005%), protopine (0.002%), oripavidine (0.0008%), and isothebaidine (0.0001%).

Baytop and Sariyar (7) reported the collection of a chemovar [chromosome number 2n = 28 of Turkish *Papaver orientale* near Agri that contained oripavine (98)] and thebaine. Another chemovar having the same chromosome number (97) and collected near Kars in Turkey (7) had oripavine and isothebaine as major alkaloids. Oripavine was the major alkaloid of *Papaver orientale*, collected from Erzurum in Turkey (112).

Fairbairn and Williamson (30) mentioned in 1978 that the alkaloid patterns in seedlings of the 3 species of the sect. *Oxytona* were similar. A prominent diversity was observed in the alkaloids of mature leaves in *Papaver orientale*. Proportions of the 3 major alkaloids are presented in Table 4. Oripavine was reported by Novák as the dominant alkaloid of *Papaver orientale* in 1980 (90). Isothebaine was also found.

TABLE 4. The Proportion of Major Alkaloids in Leaves of *Papaver orientale**

Plant	thebaine	isothebaine	oripavine
2n = 28	-	++	tr
	+	+	tr
	+	tr	++
2n = 42	-	++	-
	-	++	tr

* Data of Fairbairn and Williamson (30)

In an investigation of 5 different collections of wild *Papaver orientale* from Turkey, Phillipson *et al.* (98) reported in 1981 that oripavine was the major alkaloid in 4 samples, and mecambridine was the major alkaloid in the fifth sample. An analysis of 2 of the oripavine-producing plants indicated a chromosome number of 2n = 28. The differing minor alkaloid patterns are presented in Table 5.

In a screening of ornamental poppies named "*Papaver orientale*" or "oriental poppy," the presence of thebaine was detected in 7 cultivars by Corrigan and Martyn (22). From *Papaver orientale* var. *Goliath* (a plant that according to the report is closely related to

TABLE 5. The Relative Concentration of the Alkaloids of *Papaver orientale* of Turkey*

	Sample				
	01	02§	03	04	05
Diploid Number	28			28	
Compound					
salutaridine				+	+
oripavine	+++	+++		+++	+++
thebaine				+	+
isothebaine	+	+		+	+
mecambridine	+	+	+++		
orientalidine	+	+	+		
alpinigenine	+	+		+	+

* Data of Phillipson et al. (98).
§ The presence of isothebaine in Sample 02 was not otherwise presented in the paper.

Papaver bracteatum), the 2 known thebaine *N*-oxides were isolated, along with thebaine (3% in capsules).

2. Cultures

The alkaloids norsanguinarine, oxysanguinarine, dihydro-sanguinarine, sanguinarine, protopine, magnoflorine, and 2 unknown (CS and QS) alkaloids have been reported in callus tissues of *Papaver orientale* by Ikuta *et al.* (53).

C. Reports on *Papaver pseudo-orientale* (Fedde) Medw.

1. Whole Plants

In a 1975 report on *Papaver pseudo-orientale* growing in Iran, Shafiee *et. al.* (121) described the isolation of 9 alkaloids from the dried latex. The major alkaloids of these plants were isothebaine (11.7%) and orientalidine (0.5%), and the minor alkaloids were bracteoline, salutaridine, OR-1, OR-2, PO-4, alborine (PO-5), and aryapavine (11-demethylmecambridine). In 1977, Lalezari and Shafiee (72) also mentioned caaverine as a minor alkaloid (Figure 20). The chromosome number of the plants, collected from several regions in Iran, was 2n = 42.

Figure 20. Some Alkaloids Reported for *Papaver pseudo-orientale*

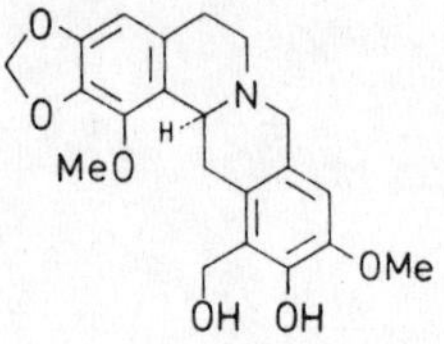

aryapavine 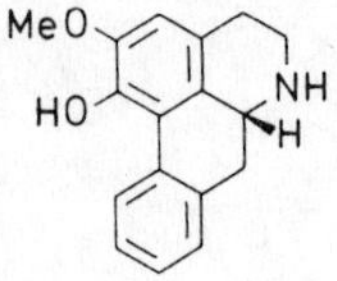   caaverine 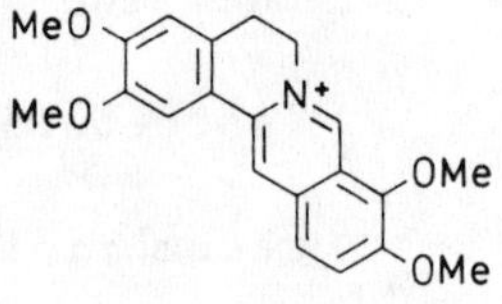   palmatine

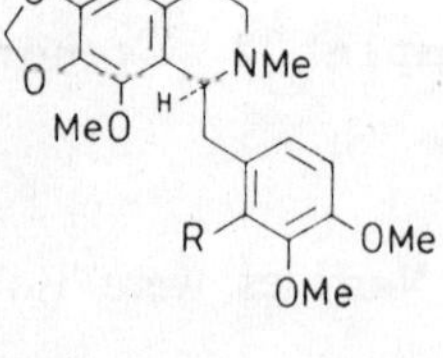

macrantaline   R = CH$_2$OH   isothebaine methohydroxide
macrantoridine   R = COOH

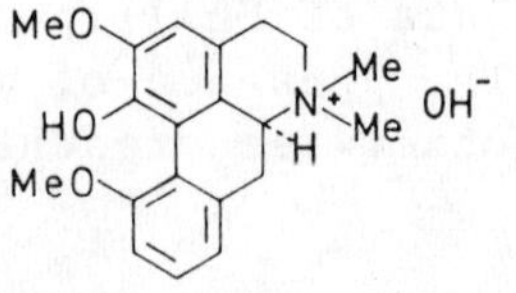

In contrast, Sariyar (109, 110, 114, 115) reported a different alkaloid profile for a Turkish sample of *Papaver pseudo-orientale* plants [chromosome number 2n = 14 (98)] collected at Yildizdag near Sivas. The major alkaloids were salutaridine (0.12%) and macrantaline (0.08%), and the minor alkaloid was macrantoridine with the total alkaloid content being 0.59 percent. A sample of *Papaver pseudo-*

orientale from Artvin in Turkey contained isothebaine as the major alkaloid with orientalidine (0.025%) later thought to be a second major alkaloid (112), mecambridine (0.0025%), and bracteoline (0.030%) as minor alkaloids (98, 111). Baytop and Sariyar (7) reported that a sample of *Papaver pseudo-orientale* collected at Kars in Turkey contained isothebaine and orientalidine as major alkaloids.

The alkaloid patterns of 1-month-old seedlings of the 3 *Papaver* species sect. *Oxytona* were examined by Fairbairn and Williamson (30) in 1978 and reported to be similar. The proportions of the major alkaloids in the leaves of *Papaver pseudo-orientale* are listed in Table 6.

TABLE 6. The Proportion of Major Alkaloids in Leaves of *Papaver pseudo-orientale**

Plant	Sample	thebaine	isothebaine	oripavine
2n = 42	1	-	++	tr
	2	-	++	tr
	3	+	++	tr
2n = 28	1	tr	+	++

* Data of Fairbairn and Williamson (30)

In 1980, Slavnik *et al.* (129) isolated the new alkaloid isothebaine methohydroxide (0.04% in capsules, 0.068% in roots) from *Papaver pseudo-orientale* (Fedde) Medw. The dominant alkaloid was isothebaine (0.93% in capsules, 1.16% in roots); other significant alkaloids were orientalidine, mecambridine, and salutaridine. Traces of coptisine, PO-5 (alborine), and palmatine were also identified. In 1980, Novák (90) reported the dominant alkaloid of *Papaver pseudo-orientale* to be isothebaine with also orientalidine and oripavine.

The isolation of salutaridine (0.07%), mecambridine (0.016%), and orientalidine (0.009%) as major alkaloids and thebaine (0.003%) as a minor alkaloid from a Turkish *Papaver* sample (dried aerial parts bearing capsules) was described by Sariyar and Baytop (113). The plant sample morphologically resembled *Papaver lasiothrix* Fedde [*Papaver bracteatum* according to Goldblatt (36)]. A comparison of the alkaloid profile of the plant material with those of Turkish "*Papaver bracteatum*" and "*Papaver pseudo-orientale*" identified the plants resembling *Papaver lasiothrix* as *Papaver pseudo-orientale*. This indicates that such would be in agreement with Goldblatt's (36) revision of the section *Oxytona* (Table 7). Phillipson *et al.* (98), in an analysis of the same sample ("P2"), indicated a diploid chromosome number of 2n = 28 and listed isothebaine instead of thebaine as a minor alkaloid.

TABLE 7. A Comparison of the Relative Alkaloid Content in *Papaver lasiothrix* with other *Papaver* Species from Turkey*

	lasiothrix	bracteatum	pseudo-orientale var. I	var. II
bracteoline	-	-	+	-
isothebaine	-	-	+++	-
macrantaline	-	-	-	+++
macrantoridine	-	-	-	+
mecambridine	++	-	+	-
orientalidine	++	-	++	-
salutaridine	+++	+++	-	+++
thebaine	+	+++	-	-

* Data of Sariyar and Baytop (113)

An analysis of the alkaloids in 16 different collections of wild *Papaver pseudo-orientale* plants from Turkey indicated 13 contained isothebaine, mecambridine, and orientalidine as their major alkaloids and thebaine and salutaridine as minor alkaloids (Table 8). Alpinigenine was detected in 3 samples, and alpinine was identified in 1 sample ("P16"). However, since spectral data of the alpinine were not presented, this latter identification cannot be positive (140). In a check of chromosome numbers, 4 had a diploid chromosome of number 2n = 42. Two samples contained salutaridine and thebaine as the major alkaloids, and 1 of these samples had a diploid chromosome number of 2n = 14. Another sample had a diploid chromosome number of 2n = 28 and yielded salutaridine as the major alkaloid and isothebaine, mecambridine, and orientalidine as minor alkaloids.

IV. BIOSYNTHESIS OF THE ALKALOIDS

In order to determine the biogenetic relations between *Papaver* sect. *Oxytona* alkaloids, much use has been made of accepted biosynthetic pathways (124, 125). Earlier steps in *Papaver* alkaloid biosynthesis (the intermediacy of norlaudanosoline carboxylic acid) have been studied on *Papaver orientale* seedlings and latex (153).

Most alkaloids of the *Papaver* sect. *Oxytona* are derived from (–)-reticuline (morphinans), (+)-reticuline, and (+)-orientaline

TABLE 8. The Relative Concentrations of Alkaloids in a Collection of *Papaver pseudo-orientale* from Turkey*

	Sample															
	P1	P2*	P3#	P4	P5	P6	P7	P8	P9	P10	P11	P12	P13	P14	P15	P16§
Diploid Number		28	14							42		42	42			42
Compound																
salutaridine	+++	+++	+++	+	+	+	+	+	+	+	+	+	+	+	+	+
thebaine	+++		+++	+	+	+	+	+	+	+	+	+	+	+	+	+
isothebaine		+		+++	+++	+++	+++	+++	+++	+++	+++	+++	+++	+++	+++	+++
mecambridine		+		+++	+++	+++	+++	+++	+++	+++	+++	+++	+++	+++	+++	+
orientalidine		+		+++	+++	+++	+++	+++	+++	+++	+++	+++	+++	+++	+++	+
alpinigenine											+	+				+

* Sample P2 was previously described by Sariyar and Baytop (113).
\# Sample P3 was previously identified as <u>Papaver</u> <u>bracteatum</u> by Sariyar (111).
§ Alpinine was also isolated as a minor alkaloid. The isolation of thebaine, mentioned in the experimental section, was missing from the table presented by Phillipson <u>et al</u>. (98).

[isothebaine-related (pro)aporphines]. The enantiomeric reticulines and (+)-orientaline result from coupling of dopamine and 3,4-dihydroxyphenylpyruvic acid through intermediacy of the norlaudanosoline carboxylic acid (Schemes 1 and 2). A few alkaloids are derived via a biogenetic pathway that starts with dopamine and *p*-hydroxyphenylpyruvic acid (Scheme 3). The alkaloid caaverine is included in the same stereochemical series as (–)-nuciferine and floripavidine, although the propriety of this inclusion cannot be confirmed because, unfortunately, the original paper was unavailable and could not be obtained from Iran.

The simple tetrahydroisoquinolines and the isoquinolone alkaloid *N*-methylcorydaldine involve biosynthesis through another pathway. Generally, isoquinolone alkaloids are thought to originate from oxidation of accompanying 1-benzylisoquinolines (35), but enzymatic oxidation of simple tetrahydroisoquinolines cannot, however, be excluded (135). A study on the low molecular weight alkaloids of *Papaver bracteatum* reveals the presence of traces of both corypalline and *O*-methylcorypalline accompanying the *N*-methylcorydaldine. These findings strongly support the biosynthetic pathway outlined in Scheme 4. The biosynthesis of isothebaine in *Papaver orientale* was studied by Battersby *et al.* (3, 4, 5), who established the biosynthetic pathway from (+)-orientaline to (+)-isothebaine (Scheme 5). Interconversion of

SCHEME 2. The Role of the Reticuline Enantiomers and (+)-Orientaline in the Biosynthesis of *Papaver* section *Oxytona* Alkaloids

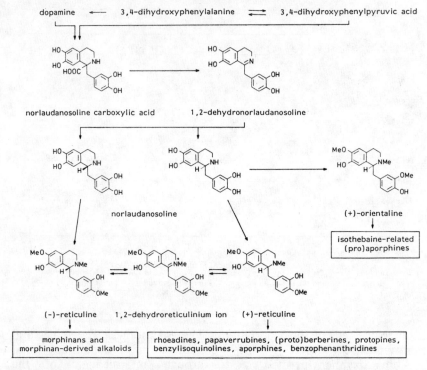

thebaine and isothebaine, as proposed by Gross and Dawson (40), was completely eliminated (4, 133).

The isolation of macrantaline, macrantoridine (109, 110, 114, 115), and aryapavine (121) provides strong support for a mecambridine/orientalidine alkaloid series biosynthetic pathway as proposed in Scheme 6.

Though the stereochemistry of macrantoridine and aryapavine cannot be ensured from the literature, it is nevertheless highly probable that these alkaloids belong to the same stereochemical series as macrantaline, mecambridine, and orientalidine. In contrast to other proposals (102, 128), the aromatization of the alkaloids mecambridine and orientalidine most probably is a secondary process, following initial ring closure of the iminium ion formed from macrantaline that would produce mecambridine and orientalidine as primary products. The alkaloid (+)- magnoflorine is apparently derived from (+)-reticuline through (+)-corytuberine (Scheme 7).

The biosynthesis of alpinigenine has been studied by Böhm (14, 17) and Rönsch (103, 104, 106), who report that in thebaine-type *Papaver bracteatum* plants the biosynthesis of tetrahydropalmatine is

SCHEME 3. *Papaver* section *Oxytona* Alkaloids Derived from Dopamine and *p*-Hydroxyphenylpyruvic Acid

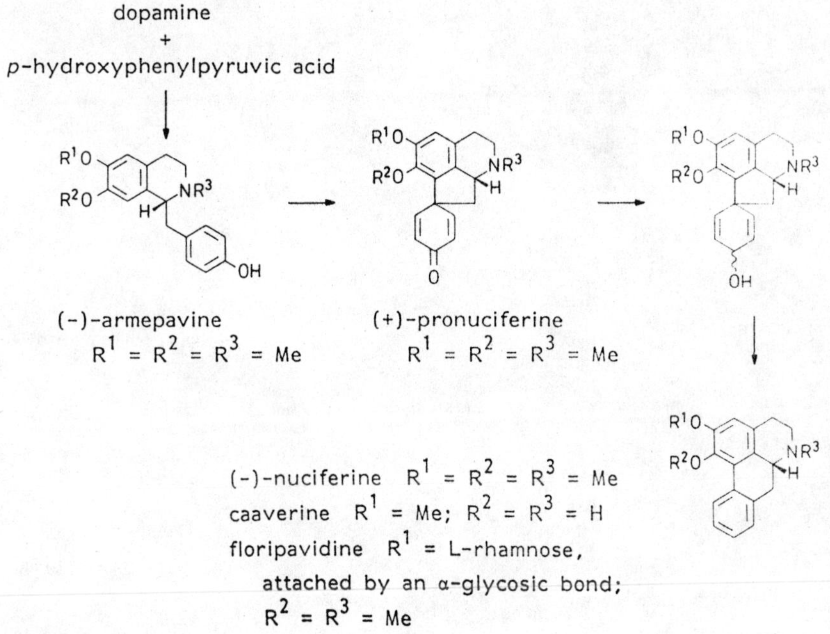

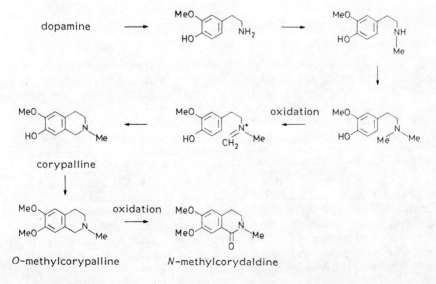

(−)-armepavine
$R^1 = R^2 = R^3 = Me$

(+)-pronuciferine
$R^1 = R^2 = R^3 = Me$

(−)-nuciferine $R^1 = R^2 = R^3 = Me$
caaverine $R^1 = Me$; $R^2 = R^3 = H$
floripavidine $R^1 = L$-rhamnose,
  attached by an α-glycosic bond;
  $R^2 = R^3 = Me$

SCHEME 4. Proposed Biosynthesis of Low Molecular Weight *Papaver bracteatum* Alkaloids

dopamine

corypalline

O-methylcorypalline   *N*-methylcorydaldine

SCHEME 5. Biosynthesis of (+)-Isothebaine and Related Alkaloids

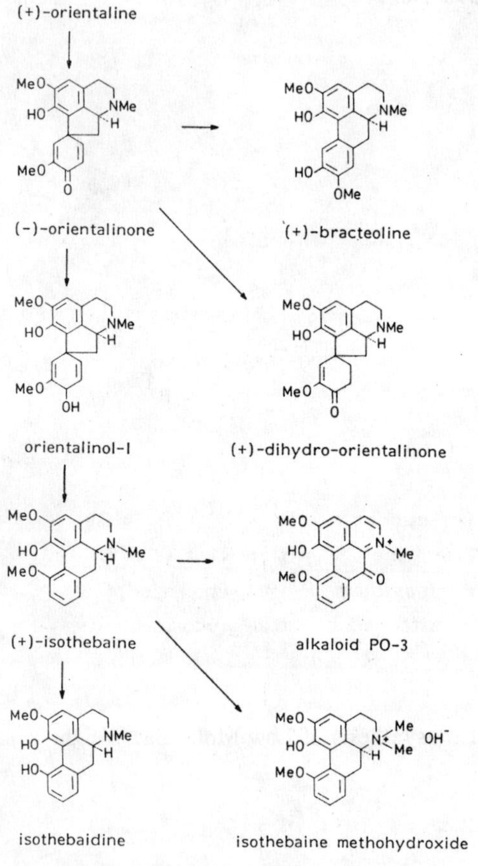

(+)-orientaline

(-)-orientalinone

(+)-bracteoline

orientalinol-I

(+)-dihydro-orientalinone

(+)-isothebaine

alkaloid PO-3

isothebaidine

isothebaine methohydroxide

blocked as this variety of plant can transform exogenous tetrahydropalmatine into alpinigenine (14). There is still, however, a considerable gap in knowledge on the transformations between muramine and alpinigenine and even more so in the biosynthesis of the papaverrubines and the benzophenanthridines (Scheme 8).

The general scheme for the biosynthesis of thebaine in *Papaver bracteatum* and *Papaver orientale* was documented to be quite similar to the biosynthesis scheme operating in *Papaver somniferum* (19, 20, 49, 84, 85, 88). The indication by Nordal *et al.* (88, 89) and Paulsen *et al.* (92) that urea is a precursor of thebaine is incorrect. Stermitz and Rapoport (133) reported that in *Papaver orientale*, thebaine was metabolized into 2 phenolic compounds, one of which presumably was oripavine and the other which may have been oripavidine (135). Oripavine was shown to be derived from thebaine in *Papaver orientale* by Brochmann-Hanssen and Cheng (19).

SCHEME 6. Biosynthesis of Orientalidine and Related Alkaloids

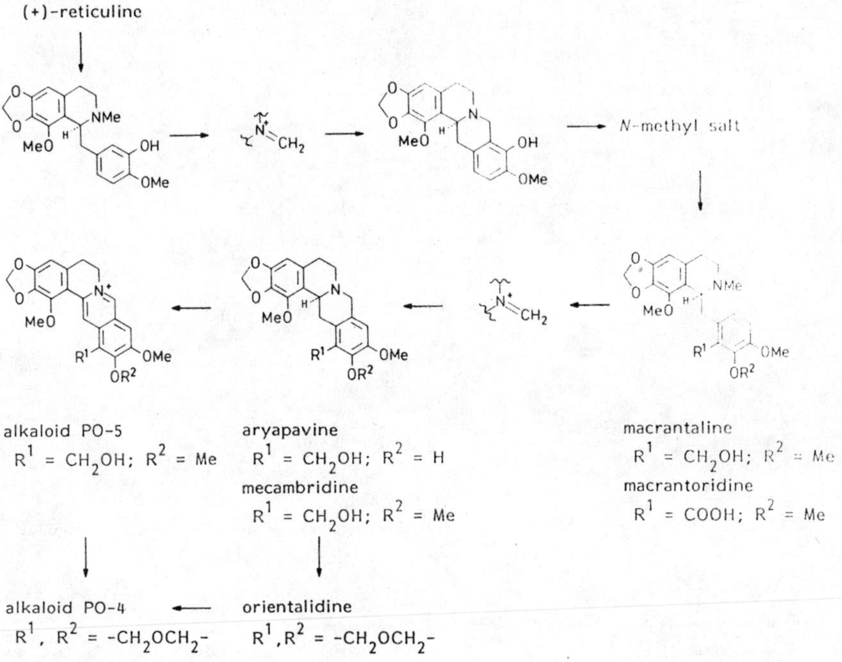

(+)-reticuline

→ *N*-methyl salt

alkaloid PO-5
$R^1 = CH_2OH$; $R^2 = Me$

aryapavine
$R^1 = CH_2OH$; $R^2 = H$
mecambridine
$R^1 = CH_2OH$; $R^2 = Me$

macrantaline
$R^1 = CH_2OH$; $R^2 = Me$
macrantoridine
$R^1 = COOH$; $R^2 = Me$

alkaloid PO-4   ←   orientalidine
R^1, $R^2 = -CH_2OCH_2-$ R^1,$R^2 = -CH_2OCH_2-$

SCHEME 7. Biosynthesis of Magnoflorine

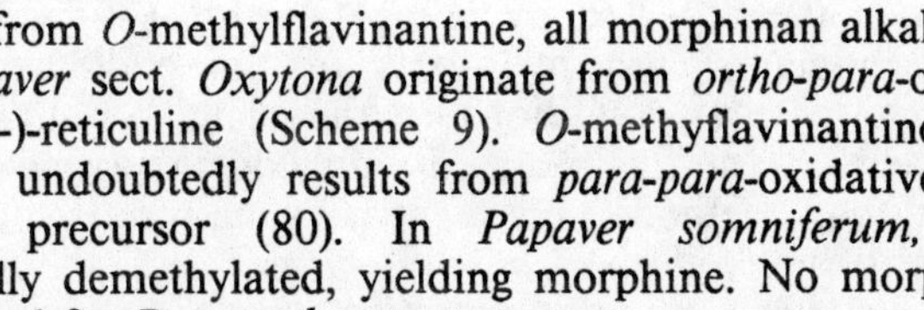

(+)-reticuline →

(+)-corytuberine   (+)-magnoflorine

Apart from *O*-methylflavinantine, all morphinan alkaloids reported in the *Papaver* sect. *Oxytona* originate from *ortho-para*-oxidative coupling of (–)-reticuline (Scheme 9). *O*-methylflavinantine in *Papaver bracteatum* undoubtedly results from *para-para*-oxidative coupling of the same precursor (80). In *Papaver somniferum,* codeine is enzymatically demethylated, yielding morphine. No morphine has yet been reported for *Papaver bracteatum*.

The demethylation of the enol ether group of thebaine to neopinone suffers blockage in *Papaver bracteatum* (20, 49). Brochmann-

SCHEME 8. Biosynthesis of Rhoeadine Alkaloids, Papaverrubines, Protopines, Tetrahydroprotoberberines, Berberines, and Benzophenanthridines

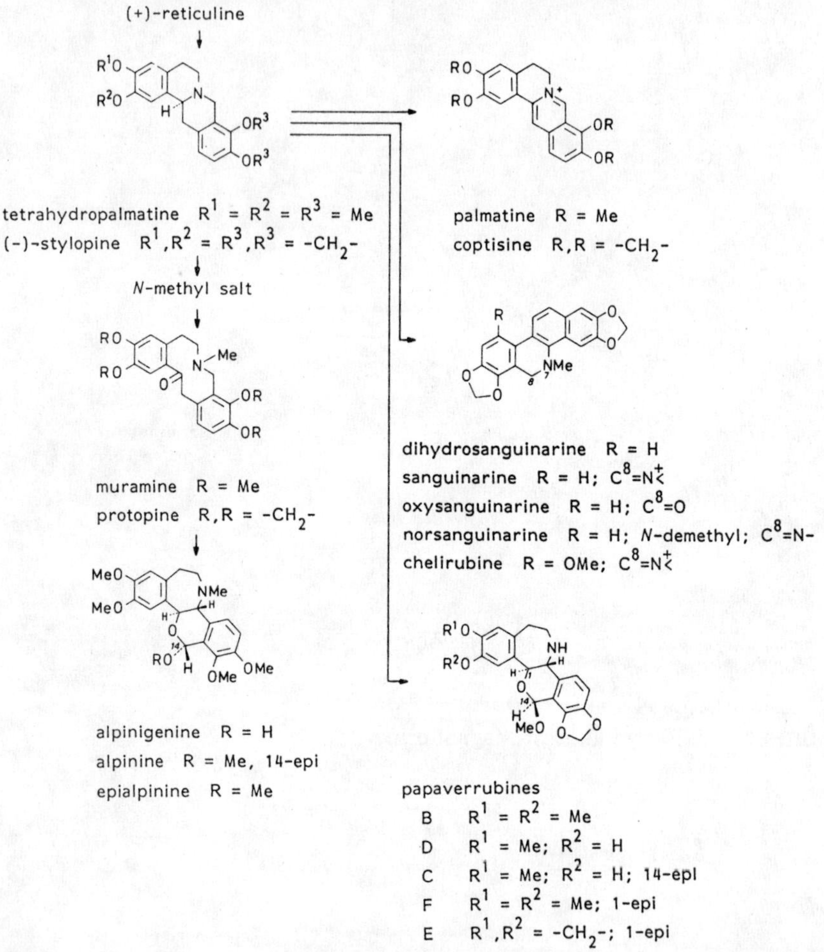

(+)-reticuline

tetrahydropalmatine $R^1 = R^2 = R^3 = Me$
(-)-stylopine $R^1, R^2 = R^3, R^3 = -CH_2-$

N-methyl salt

muramine   R = Me
protopine   R,R = $-CH_2-$

alpinigenine   R = H
alpinine   R = Me, 14-epi
epialpinine   R = Me

palmatine   R = Me
coptisine   R,R = $-CH_2-$

dihydrosanguinarine   R = H
sanguinarine   R = H; $C^8 = N\overset{+}{<}$
oxysanguinarine   R = H; $C^8 = O$
norsanguinarine   R = H; *N*-demethyl; $C^8 = N-$
chelirubine   R = OMe; $C^8 = N\overset{+}{<}$

papaverrubines
B $R^1 = R^2 = Me$
D $R^1 = Me$; $R^2 = H$
C $R^1 = Me$; $R^2 = H$; 14-epi
F $R^1 = R^2 = Me$; 1-epi
E $R^1, R^2 = -CH_2-$; 1-epi

Hanssen and Wunderly (20) supposed that the minute quantities of codeine and neopine reported by Küppers *et al.* (70) were best explained by a nonenzymatic hydrolysis of the enolether group of thebaine caused by acid conditions in the plant. Small amounts of radioactive tracers were incorporated into codeine (isolated through cold carrier dilution method), consistent with the results of Küppers *et al.* (70). In contrast, Hodges *et al.* (49) have detected no codeine in their plant material at a reported detection limit for codeine of 1 ppm per unit of thebaine using gas chromatography. This sensitivity of gas chromatography may be an overstatement as such proportional

SCHEME 9. Biosynthesis of Morphinan Alkaloids

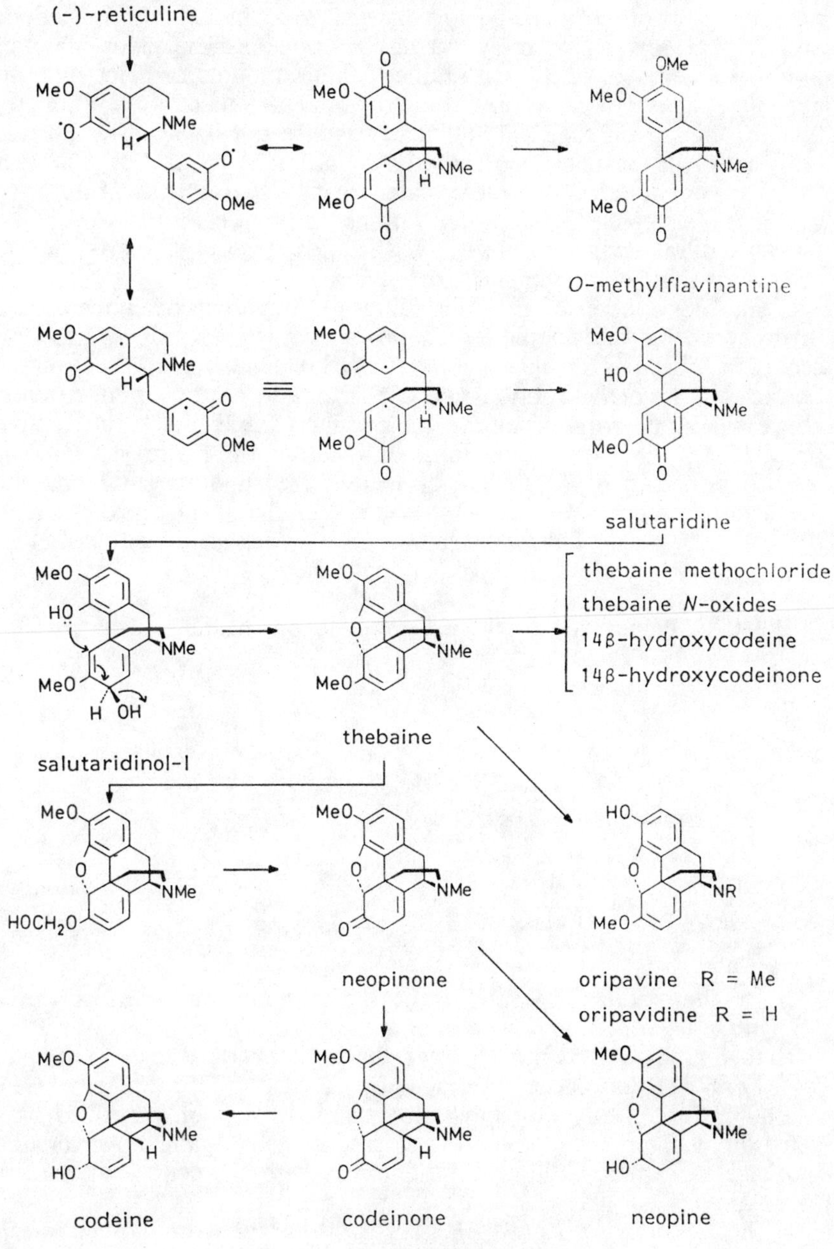

(-)-reticuline

O-methylflavinantine

salutaridine

salutaridinol-I

thebaine

thebaine methochloride
thebaine *N*-oxides
14β-hydroxycodeine
14β-hydroxycodeinone

neopinone

oripavine   R = Me
oripavidine   R = H

codeine

codeinone

neopine

amounts generally cannot be analyzed in a mixture using conventional gas chromatography methods. However, differences in plant strain, age, nutrition, and other factors may very well account for differing minor alkaloid patterns reported by various researchers. The plant material used by Hodges *et al.* (49) contained small amounts of oripavine, an alkaloid that is not mentioned by Brochmann-Hanssen and Wunderly (20) for their plant material and that was also not detected by Theuns *et al.* (136) in the plant sources used by Küppers *et al.* (70). The fact that the codeine and neopine isolated from *Papaver bracteatum* have the same stereochemical configurations around carbon C-6 as the known natural *Papaver somniferum* alkaloids strongly supports natural origins for these compounds (140).

The biosynthesis of the morphinans 14β-hydroxycodeinone and β-hydroxycodeine in *Papaver bracteatum* was originally proposed to proceed from thebaine through neopinone (136). However, in view of the blockage of the demethylation step of thebaine to neopinone, mentioned above, the proposed pathway may be considered unlikely. An alternative proposal for the biosynthetic formation of the 14β-hydroxylated compounds presented by Meshulam and Lavie (80) is quite similar to the mechanism proposed by Iijima *et al.* (52) for the acidic epoxidation of the C-8/C-14 bond of thebaine followed by a then-facilitated enol ether cleavage, yielding 14β-hydroxycodeinone (Scheme 10).

SCHEME 10. Proposed Biosynthesis Pathway for 14β-hydroxycodeinone (80)

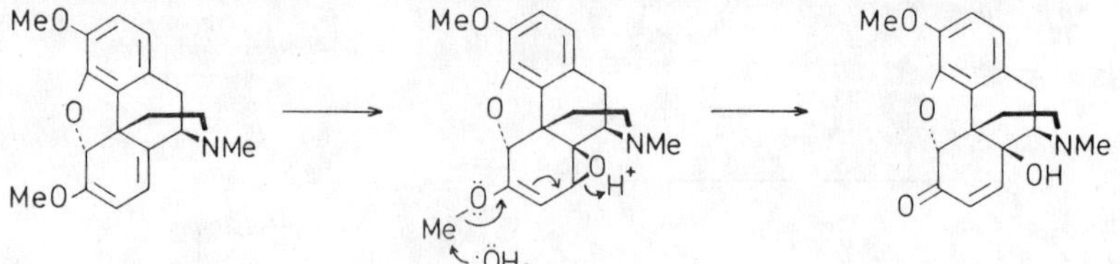

thebaine

hypothetical 8,14β-epoxide
intermediate

14β-hydroxycodeinone

An alternative proposal for the biosynthetic formation of the 14β-hydroxylated compounds similar to biosynthetic pathways operating in the microbial transformation of thebaine by the fungus *Trametes sanguinea* (1) has been outlined by Theuns (135) (Scheme 11). Meshulam and Lavie (80) have also suggested a photosensitized oxygenation of neopinone, involving singlet oxygen. Again, however, the blockage in demethylation of the enol ether group mentioned renders this hypothesis unlikely.

The thebinan alkaloid, 6,7,8,9,10,14-hexadehydro-4,5-epoxy-3,6-dimethoxy-17-methylthebinan, is formed *in vitro* by decomposition of

SCHEME 11. Proposed Pathway for the Biosynthesis of
14β-hydroxycodeinone (135)

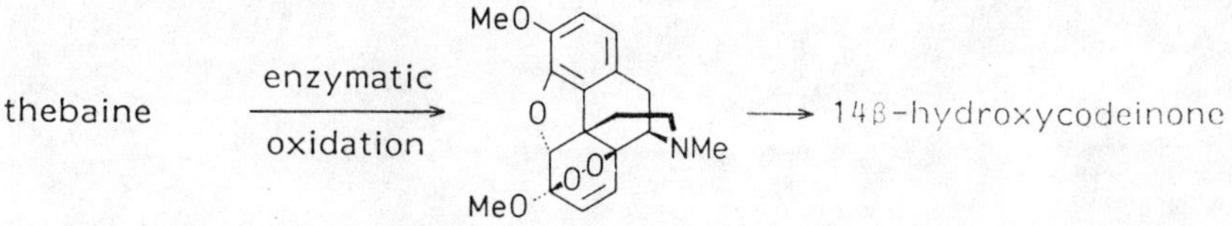

thebaine $\xrightarrow[\text{oxidation}]{\text{enzymatic}}$ [structure] $\longrightarrow$ 14β-hydroxycodeinone

the major isomer of the thebaine *N*-oxides. The natural origin of this
compound would presumably be similar (137) (Scheme 12).

SCHEME 12. Proposed Origin of
6,7,8,9,10,14-hexadehydro-4,5-epoxy-3,6-dimethoxy-17-methylthebinan

thebaine *N*-oxide major isomer

6,7,8,9,10,14-hexadehydro-
4,5-epoxy-3,6-dimethoxy-17-methylthebinan

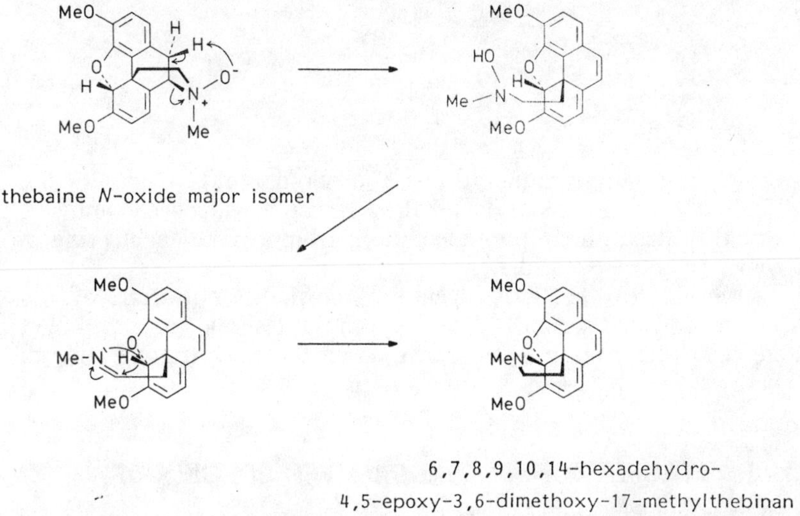

   The   dibenz[*d,f*]azonine   alkaloids   neodihydrothebaine   and
bractazonine are biosynthesized from thebaine (or equally possible
from salutaridinol) through alkyl and aryl migrations, respectively,
followed by a subsequent reduction of the resulting imine (142). A
photochemical biomimetic synthesis of these alkaloids from thebaine
has been reported (141). Probably, the quaternary aziridinium ion V
plays an important part in favoring aryl migration, ultimately resulting
in bractazonine (141, 142) (Scheme 13).
   In the alkaloid production by plant tissue cultures, the growth
conditions appear to exert considerable influences on the nature of the
compounds produced. The alkaloids often differ from those naturally
belonging to the species. Pronounced enzymatic changes occurring in
plant tissue leading to different biosyntheses of alkaloids in culture are
exemplified by the reported production of morphine and other *Papaver
somniferum* alkaloids in plant tissue cultures of *Papaver rhoeas*, a

SCHEME 13. Proposed Pathway for the Biosynthesis of Dibenz[*d,f*]azonines in *Papaver bracteatum*

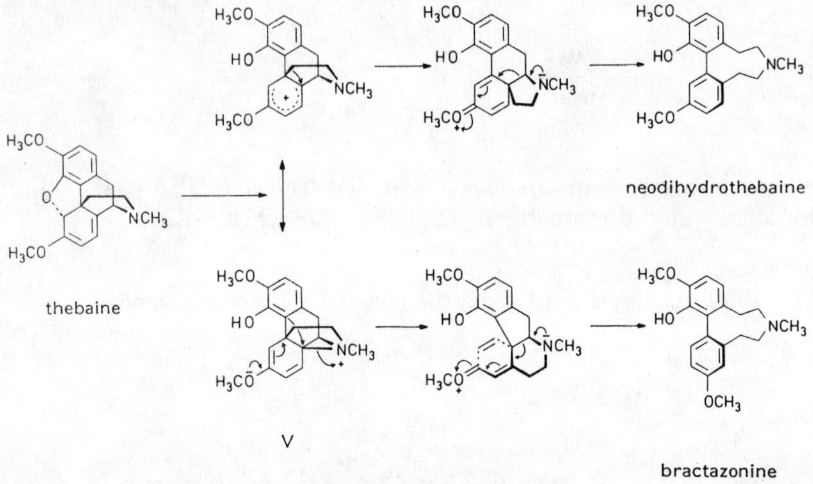

neodihydrothebaine

thebaine

V

bractazonine

species not normally producing these alkaloids (63). Undoubtedly, some dramatic developments in alkaloid research will be encountered in this field in the future. Our expectations from genetic engineering in the *Papaver* field are even higher.

In contrast to the fairly accurate knowledge on some of the biosynthetic transformations, especially those leading to morphinan alkaloids, comparatively little is known about the enzymes operating in these pathways (8, 50, 51, 82).

V. CHARACTERIZATION OF THE *PAPAVER* SPECIES OF SECTION *OXYTONA*

A. Identification

The literature reports on *Papaver* sect. *Oxytona* may be divided into major groups. The first group of reports is comprised of plants for which a reliable identification is possible and includes:

1. Plants having an identified ploidy level and an alkaloid profile that agree with the characteristics of one of the 3 species
   as presented by Goldblatt (36):

   Papaver bracteatum
   2n = 14; thebaine dominant, sometimes accompanied by
   alpinigenine.

Papaver orientale
    2n = 28; oripavine dominant, sometimes accompanied by traces of thebaine and/or isothebaine, as well as several unidentified alkaloids.
Papaver pseudo-orientale
    2n = 42; isothebaine dominant, sometimes accompanied by oripavine, thebaine, or alpinigenine, and traces of other alkaloids.

2. Plants having a ploidy level in accordance with one of the 3 species mentioned which should be identified in agreement with their ploidy levels. Here "chemical races" will be observed.
3. Plants for which the ploidy level is unknown but which have alkaloid profiles in good agreement with one of the 3 species and may be reliably identified by their chemical characteristics.

The second group of reports is comprised of plants for which a positive identification is not possible because of insufficient data and includes:

1. Plants for which the ploidy level is unknown and for which the alkaloid profiles substantially differ from the profiles of identified plants.
2. Plants for which neither the chromosome number nor the major alkaloid(s) is known.

In addition, there is a small third group of reports comprised of obscure references which quote the presence of certain alkaloids that have never been isolated from the identified plants. These reports of alkaloids must not be accepted as belonging to the species.

B. Literature Accommodations

Correct plant identification of plant material can be made for some research reports through an objective comparison of the described plants and alkaloid profiles with known characteristics of plants of the *Papaver* species. A proposed rearrangement of literature reports according to a corrected plant identification would include:

1. *Papaver bracteatum*—Among the plants, identified in the literature as *Papaver bracteatum*, those investigated by Heydenreich and Pfeifer (46, 47, 48), Kiselev and Konovalova (64), Pfeifer (94, 95), and Preininger and Šantavý (101) should be reassigned as *Papaver pseudo-orientale*. The plants investigated by Baytop (7), Sariyar

(111), and Sariyar and Baytop (112) should be reassigned to have "*Papaver lasiothrix*" regarded as *Papaver orientale*, leaving *Papaver bracteatum* correctly identified and not regarded as *Papaver pseudo-orientale* (98).

No positive identification is possible for the plants investigated by Baytop (6), Denisenko *et al.* (25), Ikuta *et al.* (53), Israilov *et al.* (55), and Smith *et al.* (131), and for some of the plants investigated by Cheng (21) and Šarkaný *et al.* (116). Therefore, the results mentioned in the cited articles need further confirmation on correctly identified plant samples. Moreover, the presence of morphine (26, 154) reported in *Papaver bracteatum* must be specifically denied. The nomenclature, proposed by Sárkány *et al.* (116), is highly confusing and should not be used.

    2. *Papaver orientale*—Among the plants identified in the literature as *Papaver orientale*, those investigated by Battersby and Brown (5), Cheng (21), Dawson and James (23), Délenk-Heydenreich and Pfeifer (24), Fulton (32), Kleinschmidt (66), Lörincz and Tétényi (78), Nemecková *et al.* (83), Neubauer and Mothes (86) (except for some plants lacking the dominant alkaloid isothebaine), Preininger and Šantavý (100), Schlittler and Müller (117), Tétényi *et al.* (134), and Vágújfalvi (151, 152), as well as the plants having 2n = 42 investigated by Fairbairn and Williamson (30) should be reassigned as *Papaver pseudo-orientale*.

    The plants named *Papaver orientale* var. *Goliath* investigated by Corrigan and Martyn (22) should be regarded as *Papaver bracteatum*. No positive identification is possible for the plants investigated by Gadamer (33), Gadamer and Klee (34), Gross and Dawson (40), Hakim *et al.* (42), Ikuta *et al.* (53), Israilov *et al.* (54, 56), Klee (65), Mnatsakanyan and Yunusov (81), Heidenreich and Pfeifer (46), Pfeifer (94), Pfeifer and Banerjee (95) [although the latter 3 references (46, 94, 95) probably concern the same plant material reassigned above as *Papaver pseudo-orientale*], Phillipson *et al.* (98) (only for sample "03"), Stermitz and Rapoport (133), for some of the plants studied by Neubauer and Mothes (86) that lack isothebaine as the dominant alkaloid, and for most of the plants studied by Corrigan and Martyn (22). Therefore, the results mentioned in the cited articles need further confirmation on correctly identified plant samples. Moreover, the presence of morphine and narcotine (93), laudanine, and (−)-laudanidine (10) reported in *Papaver orientale* must be specifically denied.

    Strikingly, only a few authors have investigated genuine *Papaver orientale*. They include Konowalowa *et al.* (68) in 1935 and, since 1970, Baytop and Sariyar (7), Böhm (13), Lalezari and Shafiee (72), Novák (90), Phillipson (98) (except for sample "03"), Sariyar and Baytop (112), and Shafiee *et al.* (119, 121).

3. *Papaver pseudo-orientale*—Among the plants identified in the literature as *Papaver pseudo-orientale*, those having a diploid chromosome number of 2n = 14 and reported by Sariyar (109, 110) and Sariyar and Phillipson (114, 115) to yield salutaridine and macrantaline as major alkaloids and macrantoridine as a minor one, and the plants having a diploid chromosome number of 2n = 14 and reported by Phillipson *et al.* (98) to yield salutaridine and thebaine (sample "P3") as major alkaloids [in agreement with the original identification (111) and presumably including sample "P1"], should be reassigned as chemical races of *Papaver bracteatum.*

The plants having a diploid chromosome number of 2n = 28 and reported by Sariyar and Baytop (113) and by Phillipson *et al.* (98) to yield salutaridine (sample "P2") as the major alkaloid along with mecambridine, orientalidine plus thebaine and/or isothebaine as minor alkaloids should be reassigned as a "chemical race" of *Papaver orientale.* Moreover, the plant having 2n = 28 and investigated by Fairbairn and Williamson (30) should be regarded as *Papaver orientale.*

C. The Alkaloids

Identified with each of the *Papaver* species sect. *Oxytona* are both major and minor components including for:

1. *Papaver bracteatum*—The major alkaloids of *Papaver bracteatum* are thebaine (dominant), alpinigenine (sometimes prominent), 14β-hydroxycodeine (in one case predominant after thebaine), salutaridine (in a chemical race dominant next to thebaine), and macrantaline (with salutaridine as the major alkaloids in a chemical race).

The minor alkaloids are protopine, isothebaine, corypalline, both thebaine *N*-oxides, orientalidine, codeine, neopine, alpinine, epialpinine, muramine, tetrahydropalmatine and its metho salt, thebaine methochloride, bractazonine, 6,7,8,9,10,14-hexadehydro-4,5-epoxy-3,6-dimethoxy-17-methycorydaldine, *O*-methylcorypalline, oripavine, macrantoridine, *N*-methycorydaldine, neodihydrothebaine, 1 4β-hydroxycodeinone, *O*-methylflavinantine, corytuberine, isothebaine metho salt, coptisine, scoulerine, isoboldine, the papaverrubines C, D, E, and G, magnoflorine, palmatine, bracteoline, corydine, rhoeadine, the alkaloid PB 1 of yet unknown structure, and any of the major alkaloids.

2. *Papaver orientale*—The major alkaloids of *Papaver orientale* are oripavine (always dominant), sometimes accompanied by

1 or 2 of either thebaine, isothebaine, or alpinigenine. Salutaridine was the dominant alkaloid in a chemical race.

The minor alkaloids are mecambridine, orientalidine, and any of the major alkaloids.

The data of Fairbairn and Williamson (30) for the alkaloids of leaves of *Papaver orientale* (after the rearrangement according to the corrected plant identification, presented above) would indicate a high degree of diversity in alkaloid profiles. These data need further confirmation, as well as the alkaloid profiles of capsules and roots of the plants.

3. *Papaver pseudo-orientale*—The major alkaloids of *Papaver pseudo-orientale* are isothebaine (dominant) and occasionally along with mecambridine and orientalidine.

The minor alkaloids are isothebaine methohydroxide, bracteoline, OR-1, OR-2, PO-3, PO-4, PO-5, aryapavine, salutaridine, thebaine, caaverine, coptisine, palmatine, oripavine, alpinine (structural assessment not certified as no NMR data are available) alpinigenine, protopine, bracteine (structure unknown), bractamine (structure unknown), oxysanguinarine, (−)-orientalinone, (+)-dihydro-orientalinone, nuciferine, papaverrubines B, C, D, and E, and any of the major alkaloids.

Some alkaloids belonging to 1 of the 3 species of the sect. *Oxytona* may also be found in other species than the ones for which they are quoted. Floripavidine, glaucidine (structure unknown), sanguinarine, oripavidine, and isothebaidine cannot be assigned to a specific species because of insufficient data.

Papaver bracteatum and *Papaver orientale* are characterized by high contents of the morphinan alkaloids thebaine and oripavine, respectively. If the biosynthesis of these alkaloids is blocked, chemical races having salutaridine as a dominant or major alkaloid are formed. *Papaver pseudo-orientale* always has isothebaine as a dominant alkaloid, with morphinan alkaloids present in traces only. *Papaver orientale* is clearly intermediate in chemical characteristics having thebaine and/or isothebaine as major alkaloids in addition to oripavine. To know what extent natural hybridization of *Papaver bracteatum* (2n = 14) and *Papaver pseudo-orientale* (2n = 42) is responsible for the chemical characteristics of *Papaver orientale* (2n = 28) would be interesting because such hybrids would expectedly have the same chromosome number and would presumably be genetically compatible with *Papaver orientale*.

Different minor alkaloid patterns reflect natural variabilities and should not be confused with chemical races. In this connection, Lalezari's (73) observations on plants of this section are very intriguing. In the Rahmat-Abad Heights of northern Iran, groups of the 3 species coexist in the same area and flower simultaneously. Chemical studies indicate that for each of the 3 species thebaine, isothebaine, and oripavine were present in the plants in all cases. In localities where the species existed solely, the species-related alkaloid was dominant, agreeing with the "independency of the alkaloid profile for each species." These observations, however, suggest a high incidence of natural hybridization. Unfortunately, chromosome countings have not been reported for the above plants. If hybridization did take place in an early ancestor, the result would be a difference in minor alkaloid patterns.

Plants growing in isolated, remote locations are more likely to develop chemical races. Therefore, not surprisingly, plants like the Turkish *Papaver bracteatum* have developed into selected chemical races. Because some *Papaver bracteatum* plants are known to possess enzymes capable of demethylating the C-3 methyl ether of thebaine and other plants to yield small amounts of codeine, a trace of morphine will likely be observed in some *Papaver bracteatum* plants in the future.

Classifying plants to represent a chemical race of a species requires special care. The concept of a chemical race is only applicable if the dominant biosynthetic pathways characteristic for the species in question are blocked or if another pathway becomes dominant, leading to a major difference in the pattern of the major constituents of the plants. First, one must ascertain the correct identification of the plant. Second, a reliable (and perhaps overall standard) procedure for the analysis of the constituents is necessary. Small variations in the patterns of the natural constituents usually are due to different geographical and climatological conditions or reflect the natural variability of the species. These differences do not represent the existence of chemical races.

A variety of *Papaver bracteatum* studied by Cheng (21) yielded mainly orientalidine in the very young stages of plant development. The concentration of this alkaloid was reduced to traces before the plants reached the age of 4 months, whereas the thebaine content steadily increased. The "*Papaver pseudo-orientale*" (reclassified here as *Papaver bracteatum*) plants yielding salutaridine and macrantaline, studied by Sariyar (109, 110) and Sariyar and Phillipson (114, 115), obviously represent a chemical race. In this chemical race, the biosynthesis of thebaine is blocked in young plants at the salutaridine stage, while in older plants, the orientalidine pathway is maintained but blocked at the macrantaline stage. The preservation of the ability to synthesize substantial amounts of alkaloids representing pathways other than the morphinan route is somewhat similar to the situation described by Böhm (15) for the varieties of *Papaver bracteatum* yielding alpinigenine as well as thebaine. In this latter case there appears to exist a full scale of possibilities with regard to the appearance of alpinigenine, indicating that this is merely a result of natural variability and not a consequence of the existence of chemical races.

As may be seen from this review on alkaloids of the *Papaver* species sect. *Oxytona* Bernh., only a few chemical races can be distinguished, indicating that chemical races are presumably less common than is sometimes suggested (96).

Acknowledgements

Thanks are due to Dr. A. Simay, Chinoin, Budapest, Hungary, for the translation of otherwise inaccessible literature and to Dr. S. D. Cook for linguistic corrections of the manuscript.

VI. REFERENCES

1. Aida, K., K. Uchida, K. Iizuka, S. Okuda, K. Tsuda, and T. Uemura. 1966. Incorporation of molecular oxygen into a morphine alkaloid, 14-hydroxycodeinone by *Trametes sanguinea*. Biochem. Biophys. Res. Commun. 22:13–16.

2. Anonymous. 1980. The peculiar politics of the safer poppy. Chemical Week 127:33–34.

3. Battersby, A.R., T.J. Brocksom, and R. Ramage. 1969. Further studies on the synthesis and biosynthesis of isothebaine. J. Chem. Soc. (D):464–465.

4. Battersby, A.R., R.T. Brown, J.H. Clements, and G.G. Iverach. 1965. On the biosynthesis of isothebaine. J. Chem. Soc. Chem. Commun.: 230–232.

5. Battersby, A.R. and T.H. Brown. 1966. Orientalinone, dihydro-orientalinone, and salutaridine from *Papaver orientale*: Related tracer experiments. J. Chem. Soc. Chem. Commun.: 170–171.

6. Baytop, T. 1974. Türkiyede yetişen çeşitli papaver türleri. Ankara Eczacilik Fakultesinde konferans, 15.5.1974 (through Kaymakçalan, 1976).

7. Baytop, T. and G. Sariyar. 1977. Les alcaloïdes des espèces de *Papaver*, section *Macrantha*. J. Fac. Pharm. Istanbul (Istanbul Ecz. Fak. Mec.) 13:7–9.

8. Benešová, M., P. Kovács, M. Pšenák, A. Barth, and S. Sárkány. 1982. Amino-peptidases in poppy seedlings, *Papaver bracteatum*, Lindl. Biológia (Bratislava) 37:855–862.

9. Bentley, K.W. and H.M.E. Cardwell. 1955. The morphine-thebaine group of alkaloids. Part V. The absolute stereochemistry of the morphine, benzyl-*iso*quinoline, aporphine and tetrahydroberberine alkaloids. J. Chem. Soc.:3252–3260.

10. Bentley, K.W. and S.F. Dyke. 1957. Structure of isothebaine. J. Org. Chem. 22:429–433.

11. Böhm, H. 1965. Über *Papaver bracteatum* Lindl. II. Mitteilung: Die Alkaloide des Reifen Bastards aus der reziproken Kreuzung dieser Art mit *Papaver somniferum* L. Pl. Med. 13:234–240.

12. Böhm, H. 1967. Über *Papaver bracteatum* Lindl. III. Mitteilung: Charakteristische Veränderung des Alkaloidspektrums während der Pflanzenentwicklung. Pl. Med. 15:215–220.

13. Böhm, H. 1970. Ergebnisse und Möglichkeiten der Arbeit an einem Arzneimohn. Pl. Med. 19:93–109.

14. Böhm, H. 1971. Über *Papaver bracteatum* Lindl. 8. Mitteilung: Erneutes Auftreten von Alpinigenin in Thebain-Typen nach Verf Ütterung von Tetrahydropalmatin. Biochem. Physiol. Pflanzen 162:474–477.

15. Böhm, H. 1973. Dissertation. (Dr. Sc.) (Akademie der Wissenschaften der D. D. R., Berlin); through Gröger, 1975.

16. Böhm, H. 1981. *Papaver bracteatum* Lindl.—Results and problems of the research on a potential medical plant. Pharmazie 36:660–667.

17. Böhm, H. and H. Rönsch. 1968. Über *Papaver bracteatum* Lindl. V. Mitteilung: Zur Biosynthese der Alkaloide vom Rhoeadin-Typ. Z. Naturforsch.23b:1552–1553.

18. Braenden, O.J. 1972. Research on poppy species. Report on Mission. United Nations Division of Narcotic Drugs. G XVIII 17/2/17 (46890)-2, d. d. 16 May 1972.

19. Brochmann-Hanssen, E. and C.Y. Cheng. 1982. Biosynthesis of hydrophenanthrene alkaloids in *Papaver orientale*. J. Nat. Prod. 45:434–436.

20. Brochmann-Hanssen, E. and S.W. Wunderly. 1978. Biosynthesis of morphine alkaloids in *Papaver bracteatum* Lindl. J. Pharm. Sci. 67:103–106.

21. Cheng, P.C. 1972. Cultivation and analysis of *Papaver bracteatum* Lindley (M.Sc. Thesis, University of Mississippi). 61 p.

22. Corrigan, D. and E.M. Martyn. 1981. The thebaine content of ornamental poppies belonging to the *Papaver* section *Oxytona*. Pl. Med. 42:45–49.

23. Dawson, R.F. and C. James. 1956. Alkaloids of *Papaver orientale* L. I. Qualitative detection and occurrence. Lloydia 19:59–64.

24. Délenk-Heydenreich, K. and S. Pfeifer, 1969. Über Alkaloide der Gattung *Papaver*. 32. Mitteilung: *Papaver orientale* L. Pharmazie 24:635–645.

25. Denisenko, O.N., I.A. Israilov, D.A. Moerajeva, and M.S. Yunusov. 1977. Alkaloids of *Papaver bracteatum*. Khim. Prir. Soedin. 547–549.

26. Duke, J.A. 1973. Utilization of *Papaver*. Econ. Bot. 27:390–400.

27. Fairbairn, J.W. and F. Hakim. 1973. *Papaver bracteatum* Lindl.—A new plant source of opiates. J. Pharm. Pharmac. 25:353–358.

28. Fairbairn, J.W. and K. Helliwell. 1975. The determination of thebaine in *Papaver bracteatum* Lindl. by gas-liquid chromatography. J. Pharm. Pharmac. 27:217–221.

29. Fairbairn, J.W. and K. Helliwell. 1977. *Papaver bracteatum* Lindley: Thebaine content in relation to plant development. J. Pharm. Pharmac. 29: 65–69.

30. Fairbairn, J.W. and E.M. Williamson. 1978. *Papaver bracteatum* (Lindley) seedling characters as a rapid aid to identification. Pl. Med. 33:365–370.

31. Fedde, F. 1909. *Papaveraceae. In* Das Pflanzenreich IV. 104 A. Engler, ed. Verlag W. Engelmann, Leipzig, Germany: 288–386.

32. Fulton, C.C. 1944. The opium poppy and other poppies. U.S. Treasury Dept., Bureau of Narcotics, U.S. Gov. Printing Office, Washington, D.C. 85 p.

33. Gadamer, J. 1914. 44. Ueber die Nebenalkaloide von *Papaver orientale*. Archiv Pharm. 252:274–280.

34. Gadamer, J. and W. Klee. 1911. 25. Notiz uber die Alkaloide perennierrender Papaveraceen (*Papaver orientale, P. lateritium*). Archiv. Pharm. 249:39–42.

35. Gharbo, S.A., J.L. Beal, R.H. Schlessinger, M.P. Cava, and G.H. Svoboda. 1965. A phytochemical study of *Doryphora sassafras*. I. Isolation of eight crystalline alkaloids from the leaves. Lloydia 28:237–244.

36. Goldblatt, P. 1974. Biosystematic studies in *Papaver* section *Oxytona*. Ann. Missouri Bot. Gard. 61:264–296.

37. Greentree, L.B. 1974. No opium for pain—A threatening medical crisis. N. England J. Med. 291:1411–1412.

38. Greentree, L.B. 1978. No opium for pain. J. Amer. Med. Assoc. 239:1610.

39. Gröger, D. 1975. Chemische Rassen bei Alkaloidpflanzen. Chemical polymorphism and chemical polytypism in alkaloid producing plant species. Pl. Med. 28:269–288.

40. Gross, S. and R.F. Dawson. 1963. The biochemical transformation of the morphothebaine to the morphine ring system. Biochemistry 2:186–188.

41. Guggisberg, A., M. Hesse, H. Schmid, H. Böhm, H. Rönsch, and K. Mothes. 1967. Über *Papaver bracteatum* Lindl. IV. Mitteilung: Zur Struktur des Alkaloids E. Helv. Chim. Acta 50:621–624.

42. Hakim, S.A.E., V. Mijović, and J. Walker. 1961. Distribution of certain *Poppy-Fumaria* alkaloids and a possible link with the incidence of glaucoma. Nature (London) 189:198–201.

43. Hesse, O. 1870. Beitrag zur Kenntniss der Opiumbasen. Liebigs Ann. Chem. 153:47–83.

44. Hesse, O. 1871. Chemische Studien uber die Alkaloide des Opiums. Ber. Deutsch. Chem. Ges. 4:693–697.

45. Hesse, O. 1894. Beitrag zur Kenntniss der Opiumalkaloide. Liebigs Ann. Chem. 282:208–214.

46. Heydenreich, K. and S. Pfeifer. 1965. Bractavin, ein neues *Papaver* alkaloid. Pharmazie 20:521.

47. Heydenreich, K. and S. Pfeifer. 1966. Über Alkaloide der Gattung *Papaver*. 11. Mitteilung: Isolierung von (–)-Orientalinon, Salutaridin und Oreophilin aus *Papaver bracteatum* Lindl. Pharmazie 21:121–122.

48. Heydenreich, K. and S. Pfeifer. 1967. Bracteolin, ein neues Aporphinalkaloid. 21. Mitteilung: Uber Alkaloide der Gattung *Papaver*. Pharmazie 22:124–125.

49. Hodges, C.C., J.S. Horn, and H. Rapoport. 1977. Morphinan alkaloids in *Papaver bracteatum*: Biosynthesis and fate. Phytochemistry 16:1939–1942.

50. Hodges, C.C. and H. Rapoport. 1980. Enzymatic reduction of codeinone *in vitro* cell-free systems from *Papaver somniferum* and *P.bracteatum*. Phytochemistry 19:1681–1684.

51. Hodges, C.C. and H. Rapoport. 1982. Enzymatic conversion of reticuline to salutaridine by cell-free systems from *Papaver somniferum*. Biochemistry 21:3729–3734.

52. Iijima, I., K.C. Rice, and A. Brossi. 1977. The oxidation of thebaine with *m*-chloroperbenzoic acid. Studies in the (+)-morphinan series. III.Helv. Chim. Acta 60:2135–2137.

53. Ikuta, K., K. Syōno, and T. Furuya. 1974. Alkaloids of callus tissues and redifferentiated plantlets in the *Papaveraceae.* Phytochemistry 13:2175–2179.

54. Israilov, I.A., O.N. Denisenko, M.S. Yunusov, D. A. Murav'eva, and S. Yu. Yunusov. 1978. Alkaloids of *Papaver orientale.* Khim. Prir. Soedin. 474–475. Translated in Chemistry of Natural Compounds:14:402–403 (1979).

55. Israilov, I.A., O.N. Denisenko, M.S. Yunusov, and S. Yu. Yunusov. 1976. The structure of floripavidine. Khim. Prir. Soedin. 799-801. Translated in Chemistry of Natural Compounds. 12:716–717 (1977).

56. Israilov, I.A., O.N. Denisenko, M.S. Yunusov, S. Yu. Yunusov, and D.A. Murav'eva. 1977. Oripavidine—A new alkaloid from *Papaver orientale.* Khim. Prir. Soedin. (5), 714. Translated in Chemistry of Natural Compounds. 13:600 (1978).

57. Kamimura, S. 1976. Thebaine from *Papaver.* Japan. Kokai 76,151,316. (4 p.).

58. Kamimura, S., M. Akutsa, and M. Nishikawa. 1976. Formation of thebaine in the suspension culture of *Papaver bracteatum.* Agr. Biol. Chem. 40:913–919.

59. Kamimura, S. and N. Nishikawa. 1976. Growth and alkaloid production of the cultured cells of *Papaver bracteatum.* Agr. Biol. Chem. 40:907–911.

60. Kaymakçalan, S. 1976. The importance of *Papaver bracteatum* in obtaining opium alkaloids. A.ü.Tip Fak.Mec.Cilt, XXIX, Sayi: I - II, 443–452.

61. Kettenes-Van den Bosch, J.J., C.A. Salemink, and I. Khan. 1979. Biological activity of the alkaloids of *Papaver bracteatum* Lindl. WHO-Document MNH/79.31. Geneva.

62. Kettenes-Van den Bosch, J.J., C.A. Salemink and I. Khan. 1981. Biological activity of the alkaloids of *Papaver bracteatum* Lindl. J. Ethnopharmacol. 3:21–38.

63. Khanna P. and G.L. Sharma. 1977. Production of opium alkaloids from *in vitro* tissue culture of *Papaver rhoeas* Linn. Indian J. Exp. Biol. 15:951–952.

64. Kiselev, V.V. and R.A. Konovalova. 1948. On the alkaloids of wild-growing *Papaver* species. VIII. Alkaloids of *Papaver bracteatum.* Zhurn. Obshch. Khim. 18:142–150.

65. Klee, W. 1914. 43. Ueber die Alkaloide von *Papaver orientale.* Archiv Pharm. 252:211–273.

66. Kleinschmidt, G. 1961. Untersuchungen über die Alkaloidverteilung in den Organen von *Papaver orientale* L. im laufe der Vegetationsperiode. Archiv Pharm. 294:254–258.

67. Konovalova, R.A., S. Yunusov, and A.P. Orechov. 1937. On the alkaloids of wild-growing *Papaver* species. 1. Alkaloids of *Papaver orientale* and *Papaver armeniacum.* Zhurn. Obshch. Khim. 7:1791–1796.

68. Konowalowa, R., S. Yunussoff, and A. Orechoff. 1935. Über Alkaloide der *Papaver*-Arten, I. Mitteil.: Alkaloide von *Papaver armeniacum* und *Papaver orientale.* Ber. Deutsch. Chem. Ges. 68:2158–2163.

69. Kühn, L., D. Thomas, and S. Pfeifer. 1970. Die Alkaloide der Gattung *Papaver.* Wiss. Z. Humboldt-Univ. Berlin, Math.-Naturwiss. R. 19:81–119.

70. Küppers, F.J.E.M., C.A. Salemink, M. Bastart, and M. Paris. 1976. Alkaloids of *Papaver bracteatum*: Presence of codeine, neopine and alpinine. Phytochemistry 15:444–445.

71. Lalezari, I., P. Nasseri, and R. Ashgarian. 1974. *Papaver bracteatum* Lindl.: Population *Arya II*. J. Pharm. Sci. 63:1331.

72. Lalezari, I. and A. Shafiee. 1977. Alkaloids of the *Papaver* genus, *Papaver orientale* and *Papaver pseudo-orientale* (*Papaveraceae*). Pazhoohandeh (Tehran) 13:50–56.

73. Lalezari, I. and A. Shafiee. 1978. Thebaine producing plants of Iran. Acta Horticulturae 73:249–253.

74. Lalezari, I., A. Shafiee, and P. Nasseri-Nouri. 1973. Isolation of alpinigenine from *Papaver bracteatum*. J. Pharm. Sci. 62:1718.

75. Lavie, D., H. Berger-Josephs, T. Yehezkel, H.E. Gottlieb, and E.C. Levy. 1981. Alpinigenine from *Papaver bracteatum* Lindl. Restricted rotation in an unusual oxidation product. J. Chem. Soc., Perkin Trans. I:1019–1022.

76. Levy, A., D. Palevitch, and D. Lavie. 1979. Thebaine yield components in selections of *Arya I* and *Arya II* populations of *Papaver bracteatum*. Pl. Med. 36:362–368.

77. Lockwood, G.B. 1981. Orientalidine and isothebaine from cell cultures of *Papaver bracteatum*. Phytochemistry 20:1463–1464.

78. Lörincz, G. and P. Tétényi. 1966. Entfernte Kreuzungen bei *Papaver somniferum* (*Papaver somniferum* L. x *Papaver orientale* L.). Herba Hung. 5:95–105.

79. Maturová, M., H. Potěšilova, F. Šantavý, A.D. Cross, V. Hanǔs, and L. Dolejš. 1967. Isolation and chemistry of the alkaloids from some plants of the genus *Papaver*. XXXVI. The structure of the alkaloids alpinine and alpinigenine isolated from *Papaver alpinum* L. Collect. Czech. Chem. Commun. 32:419–425.

80. Meshulam, H. and D. Lavie. 1980. The alkaloidal constituents of *Papaver bracteatum Arya II*. Phytochemistry 19:2633–2635.

81. Mnatsakanyan, V.A. and S. Yu. Yunusov. 1961. Alkaloids of wild-growing species of *Papaver* and *Roemeria*. Dokl. Akad. Nauk. Uz. SSR. (3):34–36.

82. Mouranche, A. and C. Costes. 1978. Mecanismes et enzymes dans la biosynthèse de la morphine. Ann. Technol. Agric. 27:715–737.

83. Nemecková, A., V. Preininger, and F. Šantavý. 1966. Isolierung und Identifizierung der Alkaloide aus *Papaver orientale* L., *Papaverrhoeas* L. und anderen *Papaver* arten. Abh. Deutsch. Akad. Wiss. (Berlin), Kl. Chem. Geol. Biol.:319–323.

84. Neubauer, D. 1965. Zur Biosynthese des Thebains aus Tyrosin in *Papaver bracteatum*. Archiv Pharm. 298:737–741.

85. Neubauer, D. 1966. Zur Biosynthese von Thebain aus Tyrosin in *Papaver bracteatum*. Abh. Deutsch. Akad. Wiss. (Berlin), K1. Chem. Geol. Biol.: 341–343.

86. Neubauer, D. and K. Mothes. 1961. Zur Dunnschichtchromatographie der Mohnalkaloide. Pl. Med. 9:466–470.

87. Neubauer, D. and K. Mothes. 1963. Über *Papaver bracteatum*. I. Mitteilung. Ein neuer Weg zur Gewinnung von Morphinanen auf pflanzlicher Rohstoffbasis. Pl. Med. 11:387–391.

88. Nordal, A., B.S. Paulsen, and J.K. Wold. 1976. Precursor incorporation experiments in *Papaver* alkaloid biosynthesis. I. *Papaver bracteatum* Lindl. United Nations Document ST/SOA/Ser. J/22. 8 p.

89. Nordal, A., B.S. Paulsen, and J.K. Wold. 1977. Precursor incorporation experiments in *Papaver* alkaloid biosynthesis. I. *Papaver bracteatum* Lindl. Acta Pharm. Suec. 14:37–42.

90. Novák, J. 1980. Chemotaxonomy of the section *Macrantha* Elk. of the genus *Papaver*. Sb. Vys. Sk. Zemed. Praze, Fak. Agron., Rada A 32:3–15.

91. Nyman, U. and J.G. Bruhn. 1979. *Papaver bracteatum*—a summary of current knowledge. Pl. Med. 35:97–117.

92. Paulsen, B.S., J.K. Wold, and A. Nordal. 1979. Precursor incorporation experiments in *Papaver* alkaloid biosynthesis. III. The influence on thebain biosynthesis in *P. bracteatum* Lindl. by repeated surface application of urea or urine. Acta Pharm. Suec. 16:263–266.

93. Petit, P.-H. 1827. Mémoire sur le pavot d'Orient ou de Tournefort, et analyse chimique de cette plante. Journal de Pharmacie et de Sciences Accessoires, Ser. II. 13:170–184.

94. Pfeifer, S. 1962. Uber Rotfärbungs-Alkaloide der Gattung *Papaver*. Pharmazie 17:298–301.

95. Pfeifer, S. and S.K. Banerjee. 1964. Uber Rotfärbungsalkaloide der Gattung *Papaver*. 3. Mitteilung Pharmazie 19:286–289.

96. Phillipson, J.D. 1983. Infraspecific variation and alkaloids of *Papaver* species. Pl. Med. 48:187–192.

97. Phillipson, J.D., S.S. Handa, and S.W. El-Dabbas. 1976. *N*-Oxides of morphine, codeine and thebaine and their occurrence in *Papaver* species. Phytochemistry 15:1297–1301.

98. Phillipson, J.D., A. Scutt, A. Baytop, N. Özhatay, and G. Sariyar. 1981. Alkaloids from Turkish samples of *Papaver orientale* and *P. pseudo-orientale*. Pl. Med. 43:261–271.

99. Preininger, V., J. Novák, and F. Šantavý. 1981. Isolierung und Chemie der Alkaloide aus Pflanzen der *Papaveraceae*, LXXXI. *Glauca*—eine neue Sektion der Gattung *Papaver*. Pl. Med. 41:119–123.

100. Preininger, V. and F. Šantavý. 1966. Isolierung weiterer Alkaloide aus *Papaver orientale* L. Isolierung und Chemie der Alkaloide einiger *Papaver* arten. XXXII. Acta Univ. Palacki. Olomuc., Fac. Med. 43:5–14.

101. Preininger, V. and F. Šantavý. 1970. Isolierung und Chemie der Alkaloide der Gattung *Papaver*. 51. Mitteilung: Isolierung der Alkaloide aus *Papaver bracteatum* Lindl, *P. fugax* Poir. und *P. triniaefolium* Boiss. und Identifizierung einiger fruher isolierter Alkaloide aus Pflanzen der Sektionen *Orthorhoeades*, *Mecones* und *Pilosa*. Pharmazie 25:356–360.

102. Preininger, V., V. Šimanék, and F. Šantavý. 1969. The position of substituents in ring D of the alkaloids mecambridine, orientalidine, and of the alkaloids PO-4, and PO-5. Tetrahedron Lett. 26:2109–2112.

103. Rönsch, H. 1972. Zur Biosynthese der Alkaloide vom Rhoeadin-Typ. Bildung von Alpinigenin aus einer Tetrahydroberberin-Vorstufe und Tetrahydropalmatin-methosalz. Eur. J. Biochem 28:123–126.

104. Rönsch, H. 1977. Biosynthesis of alpinigenine by way of tetrahydroprotoberberine and protopine intermediates. Phytochemistry 16: 691–698.

105. Rönsch, H. and H. Böhm. 1971. Zur Biosynthese des Alpinigenins (Alkaloid E) in *Papaver bracteatum* Lindl. Abh. Deutsch. Akad. Wiss. (Berlin), Kl. Chem. Geol. Biol.:287–291.

106. Rönsch, H., A. Guggisberg, M. Hesse, and H. Schmid. 1977. Konstitution und absolute Konfiguration der Rhoeadin-Alkaloide (+)-Alpinigenin und (+)-*cis*-Alpinigenin. Helv. Chim. Acta 60:2402–2424.

107. Rönsch, H. and W. Schade. 1979. Thebaine methochloride from *Papaver bracteatum*. Phytochemistry 18:1089–1090.

108. Salemink, C.A. 1980. Problems involved in structure determination of active principles of plants used in traditional medicine: Extraction, separation, and determination of characteristics of active principles. J. Ethnopharmacol. 2:135–143.

109. Sariyar, G. 1975. Dissertation (University of Istanbul, Faculty of Pharmacy). Through Sariyar and Phillipson, Ref. 115.

110. Sariyar, G. 1976. Alkaloids from *Papaver pseudo-orientale* (Fedde) Medw. J. Fac. Pharm. Istanbul 12:171–173.

111. Sariyar, G. 1977. Alkaloids from *Papaver bracteatum* Lindl. and *P. pseudo-orientale* (Fedde) Medw. of Turkish origin. J. Fac. Pharm. Istanbul 13:171–177.

112. Sariyar, G. and T. Baytop. 1978. Symp.Pap.—IUPAC Int. Symp. Chem. Nat. Prod., 11th. 2:387–389.

113. Sariyar, G. and T. Baytop. 1980. Alkaloids from *Papaver pseudo-orientale* (*P. lasiothrix*) of Turkish origin. Pl. Med. 38:378–380.

114. Sariyar, G. and J.D. Phillipson. 1977. Alkaloids from a Turkish Sampleof *Papaver pseudo-orientale*. J. Pharm. Pharmacol. 29 Suppl.:14P.

115. Sariyar, G. and J.D. Phillipson. 1977. Macrantaline and macrantoridine, new alkaloids from a Turkish sample of *Papaver pseudo-orientale*. Phytochemistry 16:2009–2013.

116. Sárkány, S., K.M. Nyomárkay, and I.S. Kiss. 1977. Pharmakobotanische Untersuchung und Auswertung von einzelnen Individuen der *Papaver bracteatum* Lindl.—Bestände verschiedener Herkunft und verschiedenen Alters.Pl. Med. 32A:60–61.

117. Schlittler, E. and J. Müller. 1948. Über die Konstitution des Isothebains. Helv. Chim. Acta 31:1119–1132.

118. Seddigh, M., G.D. Jolliff, W. Calhoun, and J.M. Crane. 1982. *Papaver bracteatum*, potential commercial source of codeine. Econ. Bot. 36:432–441.

119. Shafiee, A., I. Lalezari, and F. Assadi. 1977. Studies on Iranian orpiavin producing plants. Pazhoohandeh (Tehran) 16: 9–15.

120. Shafiee, A., I. Lalezari, F. Assadi, and F. Khalafi. 1977. Alkaloids of *Papaver orientale* L. J. Pharm. Sci. 66:1050–1052.

121. Shafiee, A., I. Lalezari, P. Nasseri-Nouri, and R. Ashgarian. 1975. Alkaloids of *Papaver orientale* and *Papaver pseudo-orientale*. J. Pharm. Sci. 64:1570–1572.

122. Shafiee, A., I. Lalezari, and N. Yassa. 1976. Thebaine in tissue culture of *Papaver bracteatum* Lindl., population *Arya II*. Lloydia 39:380–381.

123. Shafiee, A., I. Lalezari, and N. Yassa. 1978. Process for the production of thebaine. U. S. Patent 4,114,314. 5 p.

124. Shamma, M. 1972. The Isoquinoline Alkaloids, Chemistry and Pharmacology (Academic Press, New York, NY). 594 pp.

125. Shamma, M. and J.L. Moniot. 1978. *Isoquinoline Alkaloids Research, 1972-1977.* (Plenum Press, New York, NY). 425 pp.

126. Shamma, M., J.A. Weiss, S. Pfeifer, and H. Döhnert. 1968. The stereochemistry at C-14 for the rhoeadine-type alkaloids. J. Chem. Soc., Chem. Commun. (4):212–214.

127. Sharghi, N. and I. Lalezari. 1967. *Papaver bracteatum* Lindl., a highly rich source of thebaine. Nature 213:1244.

128. Šimánek, V., V. Preininger, P. Sedmera, and F. Šantavý. 1970. Isolation and chemistry of the alkaloids from some plants of the genus *Papaver.* XLVIII. Studies in exhaustive methylation of tetrahydroprotoberberine alkaloids and the structure of the alkaloids PO-4, PO-5, orientalidine and mecambridine. Collect. Czech. Chem. Commun. 35:1440–1455.

129. Slavík, J., K. Picka, L. Slavíková, E. Táborská, and F. Vežlík. 1980. Quaternary alkaloids of some species of the *Papaveraceae* family. Collect. Czech. Chem. Commun. 45:914–920.

130. Slavík, J., and L. Slavíková. 1985. Alkaloids from *Papaver bracteatum* Lindl. Collection Czechslov. Chem. Commun. 50:1216–1226.

131. Smith, D.W., T.H. Beasley, R.L. Charles, and H.W. Ziegler. 1973. Quantitative determination of thebaine in poppy plants using high speed liquid chromatography. J. Pharm. Sci. 62:1691–1694.

132. Staba, E.J., S. Zito, and M. Amin. 1982. Alkaloid production from *Papaver* tissue cultures. J. Nat. Prod. 45:256–262.

133. Stermitz, F.R. and H. Rapoport. 1961. The biosynthesis of opium alkaloids. Alkaloid interconversions in *Papaver somniferum* and *P. orientale.* J. Amer. Chem. Soc. 83:4045–4050.

134. Tétényi, P., C. Lörincz, and E. Szabó. 1961. Untersuchung der infraspezifischen chemischen Differenzen bei Mohn. Beiträge zur Charakterisierung der Hybriden von *Papaver somniferum* L. x *Papaver orientale* L. Pharmazie 16:426–433.

135. Theuns, H.G. 1984. Constituents of *Papaver bracteatum* Lindl. Dissertation. State University of Utrecht, Utrecht, The Netherlands. 141 p.

136. Theuns, H.G., J.E.G. van Dam, J.M. Luteijn, and C.A. Salemink. 1977. Alkaloids of *Papaver bracteatum*: 14β-Hydroxycodeinone, 1 4β-hydroxycodeine and *N*-methylcorydaldine. Phytochemistry 16:753–755.

137. Theuns, H.G., R.H.A.M. Janssen, H.W.A. Biessels, F. Menichini, and C.A. Salemink. 1984. A new rearrangement product of thebaine, isolated from *Papaver bracteatum* Lindl. Structural assignment of thebaine -N--oxides. J. Chem. Soc., Perkin Trans.I:1701–1706.

138. Theuns, H.G., R.H.A.M. Janssen, H.W.A. Biessels, and C.A. Salemink. 1984. Electric field effects in ^{13}C NMR of some quaternary morphinan derivatives. Org. Magn. Res. 22:793–794.

139. Theuns, H.G., R.H.A.M. Janssen, H.W.A. Biessels, and C.A. Salemink. 1985. Constituents of *Papaver bracteatum*: *O*-Methyl-a-thebaol and 10-n-nonacosanol. Lanthanide-induced chemical shifts in ^{1}H and ^{13}C NMR. Phytochemistry 24:163–169.

140. Theuns, H.G., R.H.A.M. Janssen, D. Seykens, and C.A. Salemink. 1985. Alpinine, epialpinine and other alkaloids from *Papaver bracteatum.* Phytochemistry 24:581–584.

141. Theuns, H.G., G.F. La Vos, M.C. ten Noever de Brauw, and C.A. Salemink. 1984. Biomimetic synthesis of neodihydrothebaine and bractazonine from thebaine. Tetrahedron Lett. 25:4161–4162.

142. Theuns, H.G., H.B.M. Lenting, C.A. Salemink, H. Tanaka, M. Shibata, K. Ito, and R.J.J.Ch. Lousberg. 1984. Neodihydrothebaine and bractazonine, two dibenz[d,f]azonine alkaloids of *Papaver bracteatum*. Phytochemistry 23: 1157–1166.

143. Theuns, H.G., H.B.M. Lenting, C.A. Salemink, H. Tanaka, M. Shibata, K. Ito, and R.J.J.Ch. Lousberg. 1984. Synthesis of some neodihydrothebaine and bractazonine isomers. Heterocycles 22:1995–2005.

144. Theuns, H.G., H.B.M. Lenting, C.A. Salemink, H. Tanaka, M. Shibata, K. Ito, and R.J.J.Ch. Lousberg. 1984. Total synthesis of neodihydrothebaine and bractazonine, two dibenz[d,f]azonine alkaloids from *Papaver bracteatum*. Heterocycles 22:2007–2011.

145. Theuns, H.G. and C. A. Salemink. 1980. Alkaloïdes nouveaux, isolés de *Papaver bracteatum* Lindley. J. Pharm. Belge 35:122–132.

146. Theuns, H.G., H.L. Theuns, and R.J.J.Ch. Lousberg. 1985. Search for new natural sources of morphinans. Econ. Bot. In press.

147. Theuns, H.G., E.J. Vlietstra, and C.A. Salemink. 1983. Corypalline and O-methylcorypalline, two alkaloids from *Papaver bracteatum*. Phytochemistry 22:247–250.

148. United Nations Document. 1973. Report of the second working group on *Papaver bracteatum*. Teheran, 13-17 September 1973. ST/SOA/Ser.J/2. 12 p.

149. United Nations Document. 1976. The feasibility of the conversion of thebaine into drugs of abuse and of potential abuse. MNAR/4/1976. Geneva. 9 p.

150. United Nations Document. 1980. Report of the International Narcotics Control Board for 1980, Demand and Supply of Opiates for Medical and Scientific Needs. E/INCB/52/Supp. Vienna. 211 p.

151. Vágújfalvi, D. 1970. Untersuchungen über die Lokalisation der Alkaloide in einigen *Papaveraceae*-Taxa. Bot. Közlem 57:113-120.

152. Vágújfalvi, D. 1973. Changes in the alkaloid pattern of latex during the day. Acta Bot. Acad. Sci. Hung. 18:391–403.

153. WHO-Advisory Group. 1980. The dependence potential of thebaine. Bull. Narc. 32:45–54.

154. Willaman, J.J. and H.-L. Li. 1970. Alkaloid-bearing plants and their contained alkaloids, 1957–1968. Lloydia 33:1–286 +VII p.

155. Wilson, M.L. and C.J. Coscia. 1975. Studies on early stages of *Papaver* alkaloid biogenesis. J. Amer. Chem. Soc. 97:431–432.

156. Wu, F.-F. and R.H. Dobberstein. 1977. Quantitative determination of thebaine in *Papaver bracteatum* by high-pressure liquid chromatography. J. Chromatog. 140:65–70.

157. Zito, S.W. and E.J. Staba. 1982. Thebaine from root cultures of *Papaver bracteatum*. Med. 45:53–54.

Botanical Characteristics of Ginseng

Gary A. Thompson
**Department of Botany and Plant Pathology, Purdue
University, West Lafayette, IN 47906**

CONTENTS

I. INTRODUCTION

Ginseng is the common name for plants in the genus *Panax* that have gained recognition from their use in traditional Oriental medicines. The term "ginseng" is considered by many to refer specifically to a single species, *Panax ginseng* (Oriental ginseng), that is cultivated primarily in China, Korea, and Japan. Other members in the genus *Panax* also synthesize biologically active compounds that are identical or similar to those isolated from *Panax ginseng*. In addition to *Panax ginseng*, plants include American ginseng (*Panax quinquefolium* L.), dwarf American ginseng (*Panax trifolium* L.), Sanchi ginseng (*Panax pseudoginseng* Wallich), Japanese ginseng (*Panax japonicum* C.A. Meyer), and numerous wild Asiatic ginsengs.

Many of the minor Asiatic plants are collected from the wild for use in local folk remedies, and wild American ginseng is collected for export to Hong Kong. Only Oriental ginseng, American ginseng, and Sanchi ginseng are cultivated extensively for medicinal use in the Orient. New markets for ginseng products are being generated by increased health awareness and interest in natural products in Europe and North America.

Active research on agronomic and medicinal aspects of ginseng occurs in Korea, China, Japan, and the Soviet Union. In North America, active investigation was undertaken for a brief period in the early 1900s, coinciding with the initiation of cultivation of American ginseng. A resurgence in research activity with the American species has paralleled the increasing popularity of ginseng production and usage over the past decade.

Research has concentrated on 3 biological areas: (1) the biology and conservation of wild populations, (2) the cultivation of plants, and (3) the medicinal properties and applications of plants and extracts. Information from all of these areas has contributed greatly to our overall understanding of this group of plants. This paper reviews some of the significant aspects of this literature to provide a broad background of the basic botanical features of the plants in the genus *Panax* that are commonly called ginseng.

II. ARALIACEAE—THE GINSENG FAMILY

The Araliaceae or ginseng family is primarily composed of woody species, including shrubs, trees, vines, or perennial herbs with alternate, often compound or decompound, leaves (16). Members of this family have an umbellate inflorescence that generally consists of 5-merous regular flowers with an inferior ovary. Ovules are solitary and pendulous in each locule, and the fruit is a drupe with 2 to 5 or more oblong seeds. Typical characteristics of the ginseng family are secretory canals in the pith, phloem, and cortex that vary according to species.

The family is divided into 3 tribes on the basis of petal shape and arrangement in the bud (aestivation) (16). The tribes Schefflereae and Aralieae have petals with a broad base, the former being valvate in the bud and the latter being somewhat imbricate. The tribe Mackinlayeae has petals that are narrowed at the base and valvate in the bud. Ginseng is included within the tribe Aralieae.

The Araliaceae family is composed of 60 to 70 genera and 700 to 750 species (16, 34, 58). Although the 2 major centers of speciation are tropical America and Indo-Malaya, the family is represented by 3 temperate genera (16, 39). *Aralia*, the type genus for the family, contains approximately 30 species of herbs or deciduous shrubs to trees (39). The distribution of *Aralia* is primarily in warm temperate and tropical regions of Asia, Australia, and North America. Three species of thorny, deciduous shrubs in the genus *Oplo panax* (*Echino panax*) are observed in western North America and northeastern Asia (39). *Panax*, the genus of the true ginsengs, has a bicentric distribution (20). In North America, the genus ranges from 70° to 97° W longitude and 34° to 47° N latitude. The range for plants in eastern Asia extends from 85° to 140° E longitude (Nepal to Japan) and 22° to 48° N latitude (North Vietnam to eastern Siberia).

Phylogenetically, members of the Araliaceae are quite old. Fossils of *Panax* have been reported from the Oligocene of Colorado, and fossil evidence of *Aralia* occurs in the Upper Cretaceous and Palaeocene of Alaska (16). According to Graham (16), the Cretaceous occurrence of Araliaceae places it among the oldest known angiosperm families. Another indication of the evolutionary position of *Panax* is the bicentric generic distribution pattern. Hu (20) stated that genera with this type of disjunct distribution are thought to be of "great antiquity,"and the members of the genus can be viewed as "living fossils."

The lectotype species for the genus *Panax quinquefolium* (American ginseng) was determined by Linnaeus and published in *Species Plantarum* in 1753 (13, 16). The name *Panax*, a conjugation of 2 Greek terms, Pan (all) and akos (cure), is based on the reputed use of the plant in China as a panacea (19, 58). The misconception of the plant's cure-all properties has been perpetuated in the West. However, the use of ginseng in Chinese medical practice appears to be very restricted and specific (19).

Botanical descriptions of the genus are numerous (6, 7, 14, 15, 16, 55). According to Hu (20), *Panax* typified by *Panax quinquefolium* (Figure 1) "...contains only the species with an underground morphogenetic point, an aerial shoot, a whorl of digitately compound leaves, serrate, double serrate, orpinnatifid-serrate leaflets, terminal umbellate inflorescence, small flowers, 5 petals, inferior ovary, and fleshy red or orange fruits containing 2-3 pyrenes." References in the older literature and herbaria may be confusing to those initiating studies with these plants as the 2 Linnaean genera *Aralia* and *Panax* were originally treated as the single genus *Aralia* Tournef. (18). This designation was followed for many years and is evidenced by the original determinations in collections of many of the herbaria from the late 1800s and early 1900s. The Linnaean genera are now universally accepted as correct.

Figure 1. The Ginseng Plant

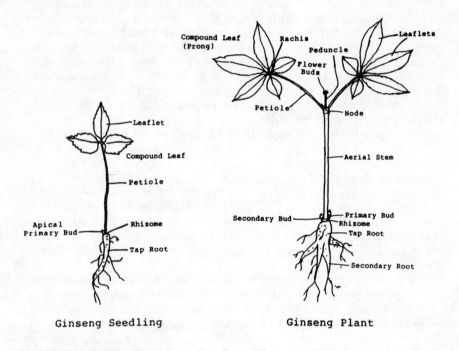

Ginseng Seedling   Ginseng Plant

III. *PANAX* SPECIES

Generally, 5 major species are considered within the genus *Panax* (33, 39). Of these species, *Panax quinquefolium* L. and *Panax trifolium* L. are native to North America; *Panax ginseng* C.A. Meyer, *Panax japonicum* C.A. Meyer, and *Panax pseudoginseng* Wallich *Panax notoginseng* (Burk.) F.H. Chen are native to eastern Asia. The 2 North American species and *Panax ginseng* are well established while the rank of the remaining Asiatic species are often in question. Occasionally, *Panax zingiberensis*, *Panax bipinnatifidum*, *Panax wangianum*, *Panax augustifolium*, *Panax major*, or *Panax elegantior* are included within the major Asiatic species (17, 19, 20, 33). These latter species represent polymorphic races (17) and are usually treated as minor species or reassigned as subspecies or varieties of *Panax pseudoginseng* or *Panax japonicum* (Table 1).

Panax species have also been grouped according to root and rhizome characteristics (20) (Figure 2). The primary root of all species of *Panax* is fleshy, although not all are persistent. The tap root degenerates and adventitious roots form along the rhizome in some species. Species with creeping rhizomes and fibrous root system are

TABLE 1. The Panax species

Scientific Nomenclature	Common Name
Panax augustifolia Harn	
Panax bipinnatifidum	Featherleaf bamboo ginseng
Panax elegantior (Burk.) Hu	Pearl ginseng
Panax ginseng C.A. Meyer	Oriental, Chinese, or Korean ginseng
Panax japonicum C.A. Meyer	Japanese or bamboo ginseng
Panax major Ting	Big leaf bamboo ginseng
Panax notoginseng (Burk.)Chen	
Panax pseudoginseng Wallich	Sanchi or tienchi ginseng
Panax quinquefolium Linnaeus	American or Canadian ginseng
Panax trifolium Linnaeus	Dwarf American ginseng
Panax wangianum Sun	
Panax zingiberensis Wu & Feng	Ginger ginseng

WILD ASIATIC GINSENGS REASSIGNED AS SUBSPECIES AND VARIETIES

Panax japonicum C.A. Meyer	var. major (Burk.) Wu & Feng
Panax pseudoginseng Wall.	subsp. himalaicum (Nees) Hara
	subsp. japonicum (Nees) Hara
	subsp. pseudoginseng
	var. angustifolium
	var. bipinatifidum
	var. elegantior (Burk.) Hoo & Tseng
	var. notoginseng (Burk.)Hoo & Tseng
	var. wangianum (Sun) Hoo & Tseng

References: 7,17,19,20,21,33,39,58.

considered primitive taxa. Those species with a fleshy root and erect rhizomes are derived taxa. Species with a persistent fleshy root and erect rhizome include *Panax quinquefolium, Panax ginseng, Panax trifolium, Panax pseudoginseng, Panax wangianum*, and *Panax zingiberensis*. Root shape and color vary within this group. *Panax quinquefolium* and *Panax ginseng* have thick, light yellow fusiform roots. *Panax pseudoginseng* roots are obconical or short cylindrical and are colored yellowish green to brownish yellow (19). *Panaxtrifolium* has a small, globose root, and *Panax zingiberensis* has numerous fleshy tuberous roots on a short rhizome.

Variation also exists in rhizome characteristics of the primitive ginseng species (20). *Panax japonicum* has a stout horizontal rhizome with short internodes, giving the appearance of bamboo. *Panax elegantior* has a slender rhizome with elongated internodes and enlarged nodes, having the appearance of a string of pearls.

Figure 2. The Ginseng Rhizome

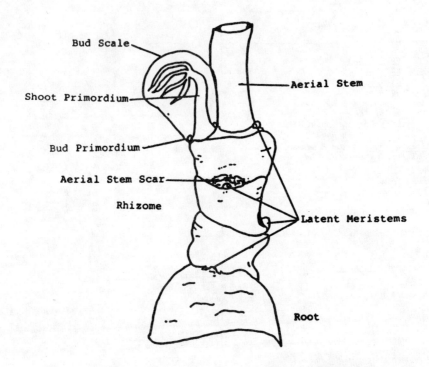

A wild Asiatic race, designated as *Panax pseudoginseng* subsp. *himalaicus* by Hara (17), has variable rhizome characteristics associated with the altitude at which the plants are growing. Thickened nodes and thin internodes are typical of plants located at altitudes near 3900 m. Internodes thicken and rhizomes become less nodulose as elevation decreases and conditions for survival become less severe. Ecological conditions apparently account for the morphological characteristics of rhizomes included in the determination of many of the minor species (17). A Chinese species reported to be identical to *Panax japonicum* is located in southern China at elevations of 1,500 to 2,500 m, while at higher elevations, typical *Panax pseudoginseng* var. *himalaicum* Hara is observed (42).

Cytogenetic characteristics for the 5 major species are presented in Table 2. Blair (5), in a comparison of the karyotypes of 8 populations of *Panax quinquefolium* from the Mountain-Piedmont disjunction in North Carolina, South Carolina, and Virginia, observed little difference among populations that have been separated for 10,000 years, suggesting considerable karyotypic stability. The detailed karyotype of *Panax quinquefolium*, which shows a gradient in chromosome length ranging

TABLE 2. Cytology of Selected Ginseng Species

Species	Somatic Chromosome Number	Ploidy	Authority	Reference
Panax ginseng	2n=44	Tetraploid	Sagiura 1936	21,22
	2n=48		Harn & Wang 1963	21,22
Panax japonicum	2n=48	Tetraploid	Matsuura & Suto 1935	21,22
Panax pseudoginseng	2n=24	Diploid	Kurosawa 1971	17,21
Panax quinquefolium	2n=44	Tetraploid	Taylor 1967	21,60
	2n=48		Blair 1975	5,21
			Rüdenberg 1980	21,22
Panax trifolium	2n=24	Diploid	Rüdenberg 1980	21,22

from 1.8 to 4.0 μm, has been presented by Blair (5). Based on length, the 48 chromosomes are placed into 5 groups.

The relative content and types of saponins have been suggested as useful taxonomic markers for the genus in order to demonstrate botanical relationship among *Panax* species (9, 65, 66). Saponins are considered to be the primary biologically and pharmaceutically active component of *Panax* species, thus, extensive research has been undertaken to isolate and chemically characterize the major and minor saponins. Ginseng saponins are triterpene glycosides that yield an aglycone (sapogenin) and a sugar moiety upon acid hydrolysis. Sugars associated with the aglycone include glucose, glucuronic acid, arabinose, rhamnose, and xylose. The major sapogenins reported in *Panax* species are dammarane triterpenoids and oleanolic acid. The dammarane triterpenoids are further divided into panaxadiol and panaxatriol types (53). A third ocotillol-type aglycone is a minor saponin of *Panax quinquefolium*, *Panax pseudoginseng*, var. *himalaicum* and *Panax pseudoginseng* var. *major* (43, 59).

A major division in sapogenin component occurs between morphological types. Species with a persistent, fleshy, tap root contain saponins largely of the dammarane type, while primitive species with a well-developed rhizome but fibrous root system contain a larger percentage of oleanolic acid type saponins (42, 43, 51, 53). An interesting exception to this separation are the saponins of *Panax trifolium*. The roots of this species have the lowest overall levels of saponins in the genus (32), having low levels of the oleanolic type ginsenoside-Ro typical of a derived species (40). However, the leaves of these plants contain large quantities of ginsenoside-Ro in addition to the dammarane-type ginsenosides-Rb_1, -Rb_2, and Rc (40).

Current ginseng saponin terminology is based on the species name from which a specific compound was isolated. Shibata *et al.* (52) coined the term ginsenoside for the saponins isolated from *Panax ginseng* by thin-layer chromatography. Dammarane-type saponins were designated alphabetically according to the arrangement of spots, from top to bottom, on a chromatograph (52). Minor saponins include: quinquesides from *Panax quinquefolium* (3), notoginsenosides from *Panax pseudoginseng* var. *notoginseng* (66, 67), pseudoginsenosides from *Panax pseudoginseng* var. *himilaicum* (59), and majonosides from *Panax pseudoginseng* var. *major* (43). An exception to this naming procedure are the chikusetsusaponins named after Chikusetsu-Ninjin, the drug derived from the rhizomes of *Panax japonicum* (42, 61, 65). Gypenosides were first isolated from *Gynostemma pentaphyllum* (Cucurbitaceae) and are minor saponins of *Panax quinquefolium* roots (3) as well as the leaves, stems, and seeds of *Panax pseudoginseng* var. *notoginseng* (66). Oleanolic acid saponins include ginsenoside-Ro (chikusetsusaponin V) and chikusetsusaponins Ib, IV, IV$_a$ (42). Ocotillol-type triterpines include majonosides -R2, -R1, and pseudoginsenoside-F11 (42). The chemical nomenclature for many of the dammarane-type saponins is presented in Table 3.

Saponins are reported in all plant parts of *Panax* species at different concentrations (Table 4). The roots of *Panax ginseng* contain high levels of saponins that vary seasonally from the first year of growth (57) with levels of free carbohydrates (24). The major saponins of *Panax ginseng*, *Panaxquinquefolium*, and *Panax pseudoginseng* var. *notoginseng* are similar quantitatively with slightly different patterns (51). Although the roots and rhizomes of ginseng are usually used in medicinal preparations, Yahara (64) has noted that the levels of ginsenosides -Rg_1, -Re, and -Rd in *Panax ginseng* leaves are 10 times the concentrations observed in the root. Buds and flowers of this species yield a high level of ginsenoside-Re (63).

Saponins in the aerial portions of the genus can be used as chemotaxonomic markers to segregate *Panax pseudoginseng* var. *notoginseng* from the remaining species. Yang *et al.* (66) could isolate only panaxadiol-type saponins from *Panax pseudoginseng* var. *notoginseng*, while the remaining species contained both panaxatriol- and panaxadiol-type saponins, the latter in larger amounts than the former. Other taxonomic relationships based on saponin content have been suggested (9), but the significance of these classifications is unclear.

TABLE 3. The Dammarane Type Saponins of Ginseng

Saponin	Chemical Nomenclature

Ginsenosides

-Rb_1 20S-protopanaxadiol-3-[O-β-D-glucopyranosyl(1→2)-β-D-
glucopyranoside)-20-(O-β-D-glucopyranosyl(1→6)-β-D-
glucopyranoside]

-Rb_2 20S-protopanaxadiol-3-[O-β-D-glucopyranosyl(1→2)-β-D-
glucopyranoside]-20-(O-∝-L-arabino-pyranosyl(1→6)-β-D-
glucopyranoside]

-Rc   20S-protopanaxadiol-3-[O-β-D-glucopyranosyl(1→2)-β-D-
glucopyranoside-20-(O-∝-L-arabinofuranosyl(1→6)-β-D-
glucopyranoside]

-Rd   20S-protopanaxadiol-3-[O-β-D-glucopyranosyl(1→2)-β-D-
glucopyranoside]-20-(O-β-D-glucopyranoside]

-Re   20S-protopanaxatriol-6-[O-∝-L-rhamnopyranosyl(1→2)-β-D-
glucopyranoside]-20-O-β-D-glucopyranoside

-Rf   20(S)-protopanaxatriol-6-O-β-D-glucopyranosyl(1→2)-β-D-
glucopyranoside

-Rg_1 6,20-di-O-β-D-glucosyl-20S-protopanaxatriol

-Rg_2 20S-protopanaxatriol-6-O-∝-L-rhamnopyranosyl(1→2)-β-D-
glucopyranoside

-Rh_1 6-O-β-D-glucopyranosyl-20(S)-protopanaxatriol

-F_1 20-O-β-glucopyranosyl-20(S)-protopanaxatriol

-F_2 3,20-di-O-β-glucopyranosyl-20(S)-protopanaxadiol

-F_3 20-O-[∝-arabinopyranosyl-(1→6)-β-glucopyranosyl]-20(S)-
protopanaxatriol

-M_{7cd} 20-O-β-D-glucopyranoside of dammar-25-ene-3β,6,6∝,12β,20(S),
24∝-pentaol

Notoginsenosides

-R_1 20(S)-protopanaxatriol-6-[O-β-D-xylopyranosyl-(1→2)-β-D-
glucopyranosyl]-20-O-β-D-glucopyranoside

-R_2 20(S)-protopanaxatriol-6-O-β-D-xylopyranosyl(1→2)-β-D-
glucopyranoside

-Fa   (20S)-protopanaxadiol 3-O-β-xylopyranosyl-(1→2)-β-
glucopyranosyl-(1→2)-β-glucopyranoside-20-O-β-
glucopyranosyl-(1→6)-β-glucopyranoside

TABLE 3. The Dammarane Type Saponins of Ginseng (cont.)

-Fc   (20S)-protopanaxatriol 3-O-β-xylopyranosyl-(1→2)-β-
         glucopyranosyl-(1→2)-β-glucopyranoside-20-β-xylopyranosyl-
         (1→6)-β-glucopyranoside

-Fe   (20S)-protopanaxadiol 3-O-β-glucopyranoside-α-O-α-
         arabinofuranosyl-(1→6)-β-glucopyranoside

Chikusetsusaponins

-L5   20-O-[β-xylopyranosyl-(1→4)-α-arabinopyranosyl-(1→6)-β-
         glucopyranosyl]-20(S)-protopanaxatriol

-L10   12-O-β-glucopyranosyl-20(S)-protopanaxatriol

-LN4   dammar-24-ene-3β,20S-diol-12-one-3-[O-β-xylopyranosyl(1→6)-β-
         glucopyranoside]-20-[O-α-arabinopyranosyl(1→6)-β-glucopyranoside]

-LT5   dammar-24-ene-3β,20S-diol-3-(O-β-glucopyranoside)-20-[O-β-
         glucopyranosyl(1→6)-β-glucopyranoside)

-LT8   dammar-24-ene-3β,20S-diol-12-one-3,20-di(O-β-glucopyranoside)

Pseudoginsenosides

-F_8 mono-acetyl-3,20-di-O-glycosyl-(20S)-protopanaxadiol

-F_{11} 6-O-α-rhamnopyranosyl(1→2)-β-glucopyranoside of 3β,6α,12β,25
         tetrahydroxy-(20S,24R)-epoxydammarane

Majonosides

-R_1 3β,6α,12β,25-tetrahydroxy-(20S,24S)-epoxydammarane-6-O-β-
         sophoroside

-R_2 3β,6α,12β,25-tetrahydroxy-(20S,24S)-epoxydammarane-6-O-β-
         xylopyranosyl(1→2)-β-glucopyranoside

Quinquesides

-R_1 mono-O-acetyl-ginsenoside-Rb_1

Gypenosides

-XVII   3-O-β-D-glucopyranosyl-20-O-gentiobiosyl-20(S)-protopanaxadiol

---

References: 3,42,43,44,48,49,59,61,62,63,65,66,67.

A. Distribution of the *Panax* Species

Panax quinquefolium is distributed throughout the Eastern temperate forest region of North America, ranging from southern Quebec to Minnesota, and south from Oklahoma to Georgia (1, 36). Populations have been discovered along the eastern borders of South Dakota and in Nebraska and northern Louisiana, although their occurrence is rare.

TABLE 4. Saponins of the *Panax* Species

Plant Material:
1 = Panax ginseng
2 = Panax quinquefolium
3 = Panax pseudoginseng (3a = notoginseng; 3b = himalaicum; 3c = major)
4 = Panax japonicum (4a = Japanese; 4b = Chinese)
5 = Panax trifolium

COMPOUNDS*	ROOTS					LEAVES & STEMS						RHIZOMES				FLOWERS	
	1	2	3a	4	5	1	2	3a	3b	4	5	3b	3c	4a	4b	1	3a
Ginsenoside																	
-Ra$_1$	x																
-Ra$_2$	x																
-Rb$_1$	0.5	x	x	x	x	0.1	x	0.03			x	1.05				0.2	0.001
-Rb$_2$	0.2	x	x	x		0.4					x					0.2	
-Rb$_3$		0.03					0.1	0.71	0.9		x						1.2
-Rc	0.3	x	x	x		0.2	x	0.39			x					0.2	0.42
-Rd	0.15	x	x	x		1.5	x		0.1		x		0.67			0.5	0.067
-Re	0.15	x	x	x	0.0005	1.5	x		0.1		x				0.12	2.8	
-Rf	0.05				0.0008												
-Rg$_1$	0.2	0.15	x	x	x	1.5	0.1								0.15	0.3	
-Rg$_2$		0.008	0.03		0.0008		x							x	0.05		
-Rh$_1$	0.0015		0.06														
-Ro	x	x	x	x	0.0004		x				x	7.25	0.95	5.35	3.1		
20-glc-Rf	x												0.01				
-F$_1$						0.4				0.01							
-F$_2$		0.018				0.2											
-F$_3$						0.2											0.03
-M$_7$																	0.03
Notoginsenoside																	
-R$_1$			0.16														
-R$_2$			0.04														
-Fa								0.01					0.03	x			0.087
-Fe								0.005		x				x			
-Fc								0.05									0.15
Pseudoginsenoside																	
-F$_8$								0.1									
-F$_{11}$		0.04	x			x		0.4							0.24		
Quinqueside																	
-R$_1$		0.01															
Majonoside																	
-R$_1$													0.07				
-R$_2$													0.11				
Gypenoside																	
XVII		0.03															
IX									0.03								0.014
Chikusetsusaponin																	
-Lg$_a$										0.2							
-Lg$_{bc}$										x							
-L$_{10}$										0.1							
-L$_5$										0.2							
-LT$_5$										2.0/0.5							
-LT$_8$										0.1							
-LN$_4$										1.4							
-Ia													x	x			
-Ib														x			
-III												x	1.17				
-IVa												0.6	0.19	x	2.8		
-IV												0.3	0.19	0.43	3.4		
-V (Ro)																	
Me ester of V														x			

* As percentage yield from dried material; x = compound reported, but concentration not specified.

References: 3, 4, 9, 12, 25, 32, 40, 42, 43, 44, 45, 48, 49, 53, 56, 59, 61, 62, 63, 64, 65, 66, 67.

American ginseng is limited to forested areas and is absent from the prairie regions within the ecological range (1). In the United States, ginseng has been observed in 33 states and is fairly common in Appalachia, the Midwest, and the Ozark Plateau (33, 41). Ginseng is less common along the Eastern seaboard and is considered extinct in Rhode Island (33,41). Overharvesting and habitat destruction have contributed to the decline of this species in several areas, leaving the plant "threatened" in 16 states and "endangered" in 10 (41). In only 6 states is American ginseng considered "not endangered or threatened."

Dwarf American ginseng, *Panax trifolium*, has a smaller and more northern range than *Panax quinquefolium*. Populations extend from Nova Scotia and Ontario to Minnesota and southward to Kentucky, Tennessee, North Carolina, and northern Georgia (39). This plant grows from April to June and is known for its hardiness, quick growing habit, capacity to withstand wet soils, and tolerance to stronger light conditions than *Panax quinquefolium* (21).

Wild populations of *Panax ginseng*, although extremely rare, still occur in the Long White Mountain area of northeastern China and adjacent Korea (20). In China, wild plants grow in mixed broadleaf and coniferous forests in the provinces of Heilungkiang, Kirin, Liaoning, and northern Hopei (19). The historical range, reduced due to overharvesting, once extended from central China to Korea and Siberia (47).

The range of *Panax japonicum* extends from Japan to the warm temperate and subtropical regions of China, northern India, and Nepal (20). *Panax pseudoginseng* is indigenous to the mountains of the Chinese provinces of Heilungkiang, Kirin, Liaoning, and northern Hopei (19). The ecological range also extends from Nepal eastward into northern India, northern Burma, and southeastern Tibet. The minor Asiatic species of *Panax* are more limited in their distribution (20). *Panax zingiberensis* is restricted to southeastern Yunnan Province, and *Panax wangianum* is located in the high mountains of western Szechuan and southeastern Yunnan. *Panax elegantior* is observed from Yunnan to Szechuan and northward to southern Shensi and Kansu.

B. Growth and Development of *Panax quinquefolium* and *Panax ginseng*

At the time of fruit maturation, ginseng seeds contain copious endosperm and poorly developed immature embryos. Seeds normally require a minimum of 18 to 22 months before they germinate. Lewis (35) observed that seed continued to germinate for 5 years following the destruction by harvesters of all the reproductively mature plants in a wild population of *Panax quinquefolium*. During the first year, approximately 60 percent of the embryos within a given population of seed develop at a rate that will result in germination in the spring of the second year.

Ginseng seeds undergo 3 after-ripening stages to complete the stratification process and germinate (10). The first after-ripening stage occurs after the fruits are mature and involves the development of a rudimentary embryo into a morphologically complete embryo. In the second stage, the embryo (approximately 0.2 to 0.3 mm in length) of seeds under cultivation continues to grow, reaching a length of 4.3 to 5.0 mm during August to September of the year following fruit maturation. At this stage, the leathery endocarp dehisces along the sutures and is referred to by growers as being "cracked." Although the embryo is morphologically mature, the seed fails to germinate due to a poorly understood physiological block (11). The final stage of seed dormancy is satisfied by the cold temperature of the following winter, and completion of this stage allows the seed to germinate.

After-ripening processes can be satisfied by storing moist seed at a temperature of 15°C for 3 to 4 months. The endocarp becomes dehiscent, and embryo development is completed (11). The physiological block can be overcome by a moist chilling of the seed at 2° to 5°C, allowing the seed to germinate (11). The response is identical in both *Panax ginseng* and *Panax quinquefolium* (11, 30).

Germination is initiated by the eruption of the radicle through the membranous seed coat that is exposed due to the dehiscence of the endocarp. As the radicle elongates, the cotyledonary node emerges through the combined enlargement of the cotyledons and epicotyl. The seedling shoot, a single trifoliate leaf differentiated during the elongation phase of embryo development, emerges in a characteristic epicotyl hook during late April or early May. The leaf, pulled between cotyledons that have continued to enlarge in the seed below the ground surface during germination, continues to grow until fully expanded (26, 54). The cotyledons later abscise (54).

The petiole of a seedling plant joining the primary root at the cotyledonary node ranges from 4 to 10 cm but can be much longer if the mulch is very thick or the leaf litter is difficult to penetrate. A single bud at the base of the leaf petiole differentiates into shoot and bud primordia for the next season's vegetative growth. Seedlings also have meristems in the axils of the cotyledons that remain quiescent (1).

Growth of the aerial shoot of ginseng plants is determinant. A single shoot primordium, differentiated the year prior to expression, is so completely developed that the number of leaves and leaflets can be counted and the inflorescence, if present, can be seen by mid to late summer (1). Growth of the aerial shoot in any year is limited to the expansion of the preformed primordium. This annual determinant shoot growth continues throughout the life of the plant.

The majority of seedling plants are senescent by late August to mid October, and the subterranean portions of the ginseng plant (root, rhizome, and developing bud) remain dormant during the late fall and winter until growth can resume in the following spring. Little is known about the chilling requirements needed to break dormancy in the field. Konsler (27) has reported that one-year-old American ginseng roots require 75 to 90 days in temperatures ranging from 0° to 9°C to obtain 100 percent emergence. The total dormancy period averaged 126.5 days under his experimental conditions with the days to emergence inversely proportional to the days of the cold treatment. Lee *et al.* (32)

have indicated that the dormancy requirement of American ginseng could be met by temperatures ranging from 0° to 10°C for 100 days (32). Within this temperature range, maximum plant growth occurred with 3-year-old roots stored at 5°C for 100 days and subsequently grown at 15°C.

Following the seedling year, ginseng plants grow from the apical bud on the rhizome (26). Compound leaves composed of 3 to 5 leaflets, commonly called prongs, join at the terminus of an elongated internode (aerial stem). Because shoot primordia are differentiated the year prior to emergence, the status of the storage root and environmental factors during the year the root was formed have a strong morphological effect upon shoot characteristics. Root mass determines the phenotype of the aerial shoot with stem height, the number of prongs and leaflets, and the leaf area being good indicators of root mass (1).

Under cultivation, there is an enhanced linear accumulation of root mass, and the number of prongs often directly corresponds to the age of the plant (2 prongs = 2 years; 3 prongs = 3 years) (1, 37). Ginseng plants, however, rarely obtain 5 or more prongs even under extended cultivation. Growth in the wild is slow and is reflected by the development of the aerial shoot. Lewis and Zenger (37) have reported a positive correlation between age and prong development of American ginseng that was linear although not annual. Normally, cultivated ginseng flowers the third and subsequent years, but vigorously growing plants will flower the second year (26). The umbellate inflorescence is borne on a single elongated peduncle that joins the stem at the junction of the whorl of compound leaves. For American ginseng growing in the northern part of the ecological range, immature flower buds can be observed as the plant emerges in the spring. In southern areas, the immature inflorescence is not visible until elongation of the shoot occurs (28).

Peduncle elongation and floral maturation take place after the plant has attained full size. The American ginseng plant flowers over a period of 3 to 8 weeks from late May to early August, depending on the plant location (1, 8, 38). Fruit set is from late June through early August, and ripening of the bright red drupe occurs from late August into October (8, 38). Oriental ginseng flowers from June through July, and the fruit ripens from July through September (19). The entire aerial portion of the cultivated plant becomes senescent, although the stem often persists at the rhizome, only rotting away with time. In wild plants, the fruit is often persistent during senescence (37).

C. The Morphology and Anatomy of Ginseng

1. *Panax quinquefolium* and *Panax ginseng*

Panax quinquefolium and *Panax ginseng* have a thick, fleshy, persistent, fusiform primary root that is often irregularly branched. The root ranges from cream-colored to yellow and has numerous, irregular, transverse wrinkles that become more evident with age. The wrinkling of roots has been attributed to contractile activity within the root, a mechanism to counterbalance the lengthening rhizome and ensure placement of the dormant bud at the soil surface (1, 2). Root shape is strongly determined by the soil environment (21) with light sandy soils producing a long, straight, carrot-like, tap root with little secondary branching. Heavy or rocky soils produce a short, thickened, primary root with many thickened secondary roots. Adventitious roots can form from the rhizome and also become thick and fleshy (1).

The primary structure of the *Panax quinquefolium* root is 4 thin-walled, compact layers of cortex surrounded by an epidermis and a distinct endodermis with readily visible Casparian strips (18). Inside the endodermis is a 2-layered pericycle. In the primary roots of 2-layered *Panax ginseng* a triarch vascular cylinder with 3 oil ducts formed from the pericycle and located outside the protoxylem vessels is most commonly observed (54). Specimens of American ginseng have been reported to have a diarch vascular cylinder with 2 broad strands of phloem and 2 oil ducts (6). During secondary growth, cell layers from the epidermis to the endodermis are sloughed and subsequently replaced by athin-walled periderm originating from the pericycle. The new cortex is composed of thin-walled parenchyma containing starch and 4 oil ducts located just inside the periderm. Several layers of cambium develop outside the old vascular cylinder, and 4 secondary xylem rays and 4 strands of secondary phloem are formed. Kubo *et al.* (29) determined that ginsenosides are localized outside of the cambium in the periderm and cortex of *Panax ginseng*. As the roots become tuberous, a starch containing pith develops in the center of the old vascular cylinder, and 2 additional bands of oil ducts develop in the cortex with the innermost ones located near the phloem. The cambium is continuous, producing small strands of phloem and deep rays of xylem with few vessels. Broad rays of parenchyma separate the vascular strands. As the roots continue to age, the width of the cortex increases and oil ducts become more numerous. Secondary vascular elements are produced annually from the cambium, crushing and obliterating the older vascular elements (1).

The ontogeny of oil ducts (secretory canals) in roots of *Panax ginseng* has been described by Slepyan (54) as having primary and secondary schizogenous-type oil ducts formed in separate locations. Primary oil ducts originate from the pericycle in the young root during germination. Cells within the pericycle divide anticlinally and separate at the middle lamella, forming triangular or quadrangular intercellular spaces bordered by 3 or 4 epithelial cells. As the surrounding parenchyma cells are crushed during secondary growth, the primary oil ducts become distorted and often joined together.

Secondary oil ducts are formed in the cambium at the onset of secondary growth. In seedling ginseng plants, secondary oil ducts first occur at the cotyledonary node and later in the lower root. Small groups of 4 to 5 parenchyma cells with dense cytoplasm and no starch can be seen in the cortex close to the cambium. These cells separate, forming cavities lined with 4 to 6 epithelial cells.

The epithelial cells of both types of oil ducts are filled with a dense yellow to light brown cytoplasm. When exposed to ultraviolet light, these cells fluoresce the golden yellow color typical of woody Aralies rather than the blue color seen in herbaceous Aralies. This response, in combination with the characteristic episodic growth of ginseng that is also typical of some woody plants, may have significant implications for the phylogeny of these species.

The rhizome, which remains underground, is the true stem of all ginseng plants. In the wild, rhizomes can become elongated, but under cultivation, most are modified into short, thick, compact, erect structures. Normally unbranched, the rhizome length is extended with each annual growth cycle. A single, actively developing bud, composed of 3 membranous, distichous (2 ranked, 2 rows) bud scales that enclose the shoot primordium, is located at the apex of the rhizome (1). As the bud develops throughout the growing season, the number of leaves, leaflets, and floral primordia can be seen by removing the bud scales.

Bud primordia differentiate in the axils of the 2 superior bud scales. The bud subtending the uppermost scale continues to develop throughout the growing season, enlarging to form the shoot primordium for the following year's aerial growth. Unless the apical bud is damaged or conditions for vigorous growth exist, the second bud remains dormant. This growth results in an annual, sympodial development with compressed internodes and latent meristems on the rhizome. Successive buds and aerial stem scars are located 90° apart due to the distichous nature of the bud scales (1). The conspicuous, annual abscission scars and the latent buds create a rotational pattern on the rhizome and are often used to determine the age of wild ginseng plants (1, 8, 37).

The anatomy of the *Panax quinquefolium* rhizome is similar to other rhizomatous plants (18). Internodes contain several layers of thin-walled phellem that develop inside the epidermis. Several layers of collenchyma inside the periderm provide most of the supportive tissue for the structure.

Numerous oil ducts surrounded by secretory cells are located in a circular band in the cortex close, but not corresponding, to the vascular bundles. Cortical parenchyma cells containing starch and numerous druses extend to the center of the pith without interruption and have a single band of regular collateral vascular bundles. Secondary xylem and phloem, produced annually, crush older vascular tissue, maintaining the discrete collateral vascular bundles (1). Fibrous elements of the xylem and phloem are absent or are parenchymous (1). The xylem has several wide scalariform vessels. The pith is thin-walled, contains starch, and has a single oil duct near the center. There is little increase in diameter of the rhizome due to the crushing of vascular tissue as well as the pith and cortical parenchyma by newly formed tissues (1).

The aerial shoot of a *Panax quinquefolium* and *Panax ginseng* seedlings consist of a single trifoliate leaf. The serrate, elliptic leaflets have small, unbranched trichomes along the midrib on the upper surface (1). Leaflets join at the terminus of a 4 to 10 cm petiole that is channeled along the length on the adaxial side. The petiole arises from the cotyledonary node, and the hypocotyl does not elongate (1).

The aerial vegetative shoot of mature plants is composed of a single, glabrous, erect stem arising from the rhizome and terminating in a whorl of 3 to 5 palmately compound leaves. Juvenile or early maturing plants may have only 1 or 2 compound leaves. Compound leaves, commonly called prongs, have 3 to 7, normally 5, leaflets with short, adaxially, convex petiolules with 2 narrow wings (18). The basal leaflets are ovate to obovate and the center longer leaflets oblong-ovate to obovate. All the leaves are conspicuously serrate with deltoid teeth and accuminate at the apex. The leaf base of *Panax quinquefolium* is rounded and *Panax ginseng* is cuneate, a characteristic that can be used to distinguish the 2 morphologically similar species (16). Stems of 2-year-old cultivated ginseng plants range from 10 to 18 cm and 30 to 60 cm in length in subsequent years (26). Multiple shoots occasionally will arise from dormant buds along the rhizome (37).

In strict botanical terms, the entire aerial vegetative shoot of ginseng plants may be considered to be a leaf (21). This is due to the position of the bud on the rhizome and the lack of vegetative buds in the axils of the compound leaves. However, the terms aerial stem and compound leaves or prongs are in keeping with the vast majority of the literature.

The aerial stem of *Panax quinquefolium* has a thick, smooth cuticle and a thin-walled epidermis (18). Surrounded by 2 hypodermal layers of collenchyma are 6 layers of compact thin-walled cortical parenchyma containing chlorophyll. The vascular bundles are arranged in a single band and are separated by broad rays of thin-walled parenchyma cells which extend from the cortex to the pith. Conspicuous scalariform vessels are present in the xylem and an arch of thin-walled sterome is located on the phloem side of the vascular bundles. Within the cortex are located 2 bands of oil ducts corresponding with the number of vascular bundles. The stem is hollow in the center from 2 wide lacunae.

The stem (or petiole) of seedling plants is similar to more mature plants but has a thicker cuticle and oil ducts between the vascular bundles in addition to those associated with the vascular bundles. An endodermis surrounds each of the vascular bundles.

Petioles of older plants have a small-celled epidermis and 2 to 3 layers of hypodermal collenchyma surrounding the chlorophyll-containing cortex. The vascular bundles are collateral and form an open arch with oil ducts, corresponding to those in the stem, on both faces. A thin-walled central pith also contains a single oil duct. Petiolules have an anatomy similar to the petiole, but with fewer vascular bundles and no oil duct in the pith.

Leaves have a single layer of epidermis on each face that encloses several layers of irregular-shaped spongy mesophyll parenchyma with wide intercellular spaces. Palisade parenchyma are absent. Stomata lack subsidiary cells and are located exclusively on the abaxial side of the leaf lamina. Large multicellular trichomes cover the midrib on the adaxial surface. The midrib, which contains a single arch-shaped vascular bundle and a single oil duct located close to the phloem, projects on both faces but is pronounced on the abaxial side due to the presence of large water storage tissue. On the adaxial side, several layers of collenchyma cover the xylem while only a single layer of collenchyma cells is on the abaxial side. The midrib cuticle is thick and the epidermis thick-walled.

The inflorescence of *Panax quinquefolium* is solitary globose umbel that terminates on a 1 to 25 cm long peduncle that extends from the axis of the whorl of compound leaves. A small involucre of lanceolate-acute bracts subtend short (12 mm) pedicels on which the individual small flowers are borne (18). Flowers are 5-merous with triangular acute calyx teeth and greenish-white petals. All of the flowers are perfect with 5 stamens and an inferior ovary with 1, 2, or rarely 3 styles (50).

Ginseng flowers are protandrous. Soon after the petals are reflexed, the anthers mature and dehisce prior to the stigmatic tips becoming receptive (50). Lewis and Zenger (37) have observed that the degree of protandry varied with the ecological range in which the plants were growing. The interval between maturation of the anthers and stigmas was shorter or occasionally the same in a population of plants in Missouri as compared with New York. The flowers within the inflorescence mature centripetally over a period of 1 to 3 weeks (50). Thus, the inflorescence has in unison functional male and female flowers that are self-compatible (8, 38).

The fruit is a drupe with a bright red exocarp and a lignified leathery endocarp surrounding each of the 1 to 3 subglobose pyrenes (37). The combination of the endocarp and pyrene form a flattened hemispherical seed.

2. *Panax trifolium*

The *Panax trifolium* plant has a globose root that grows to approximately 1 to 2 cm in diameter (18). During secondary growth, the basal portion of the primary root enlarges, forming the rounded tuberous root. The primary xylem has a diarch structure, although this is difficult to recognize after the secondary xylem begins to develop. Thin-walled phellem and 2 to 3 layers of secondary cortex replace the epidermis during root enlargement, and 2 oil ducts of pericyclic origin form just inside the phellem, opposite of the primary xylem.

Secondary vascular growth occurs from a continuous cambium producing small strands of phloem with little parenchyma and deep rays of xylem with few vessels and abundant parenchyma. Starch and druses formed of calcium oxalate accumulate in the cortica l parenchyma. Within the cortex, several concentric bands of secondary oil ducts with 5 to 7 epithelial cells develop. The outer layers of the cortex are composed of collenchyma, and the root is covered with layers of heterogenous phellem with occasional sclerified tangential cell walls. Primary oil ducts are observed on the inner face of the periderm. The center of the root is composed of a broad pith.

The rhizome of *Panax trifolium* is vertical and straight with short internodes and alternate axillary buds that remain latent, similar to other members of the genus (18). During growth, the epidermis is sloughed and replaced by homogenous thin-walled phellem. The cortex, composed of parenchyma that contains druses of calcium oxalate, extends from the phellem to a small solid pith of thin-walled cells. Within the cortical parenchyma, a circular band of oil ducts and collateral vascular bundles develop.

The annual aerial stem (or internode) of *Panax trifolium* has the most unusual anatomy of the *Panax* species (18). The smooth glabrous stem is cylindric in shape at the base and becomes polygonal toward the apex. A thickened cuticle covers a thin-walled epidermis above several hypodermal layersof collenchyma. In the 6 to 8 layers of chlorophyll-containing cortical parenchyma is a circular band of 8 discrete, collateral, vascular bundles, each surrounded by a thin-walled endodermis with a Casparian strip. In the basal portion of the internode, amphicribral (phloem surrounding xylem) vascular bundles can be seen. The pith is thin-walled and hollow at the center.

Oil ducts are more numerous in the upper than lower stem. A total of 32 oil ducts are located in the apical portion of the stem: 2 on each side of the vascular bundles, 1 in the cortex outside of the vascular bundle, and a single oil duct in the periphery of the pith. In contrast, the basal portion of the stem has a single oil duct located outside of each vascular bundle with 2 or more often located on the sides. Each oil duct has 5 epithielial cells.

Palmately compound leaves, typical of the genus, are borne on petioles that join in a whorl at the apex of the stem. A wrinkled cuticle covers a thick-walled epidermis above several layers of collenchyma surrounding the cortex. Cortical parenchyma cells accumulate neither starch nor calcium oxalate. Each of the 5 amphicribral vascular bundles is surrounded by an endodermis and, similar to the stem, is associated with oil ducts.

The *Panax trifolium* plant has a bifacial leaflet with stomata exclusively on the abaxial face and multicellular trichomes sparsely distributed along the midrib on the adaxial side. Although thin-walled on both faces, the comparatively larger cells on the adaxial side emphasize the bifacial nature of the leaflets. A single layer of palisade cells resides above 4 layers of spongymesophyll that have wide intercellular spaces, enabling this species to withstand higher light intensities than *Panax quinquefolium*. The midrib has collateral vascular bundles that form an arch open toward the adaxial face. Of the 4 oil ducts located in the midrib, 3 are on the abaxial face with the remaining duct above the very short xylem rays. The lateral veins are surrounded by parenchyma and embedded in the spongy mesophyll. Connecting the leaf to the petiole is a short petiolule that has a structure similar to the midrib. However, in the cortex on the adaxial face, the cells are elongate similar to the palisade layer of the leaf blade.

The polygamous umbellate inflorescence of *Panax trifolium* is borne on a longitudinally furrowed, elongated peduncle arising from the whorl of leaves. Anatomically, the peduncle is similar to the apical portion of the stem, regarding epidermis, collenchyma, cortex, and amphicribral or collateral vascular bundles (18). The pith is solid, and there is 1 rather than 2 oil ducts on the side of each vascular bundle (18).

Inflorescences of *Panax trifolium* are androdioecious, with either staminate or hermaphroditic flowers on separate plants. All of the flowers have 5 sepals that alternate with the petals and anthers that are opposite of the sepals. Pollen grains from the 2-celled anthers are radially symmetrical, and the surface appears to be reticulate under the light microscope but is striate when examined by scanning electron microscopy (SEM). Staminate plants have a reduced and nonfunctional ovary and single style. Hermaphroditic flowers have 3 functional styles located above a tricarpellate inferior ovary that can produce a single seed in each carpel. According to Philbrick (46), 69 percent of the inflorescences within a population are staminate, 30 percent are hermaphroditic, and the remaining 1 percent is andromonoecious with staminate and hermaphroditic flowers in a single inflorescence.

The secondary sex characteristics of *Panax trifolium* have been studied by Philbrick (46). The staminate inflorescence flowers mature centripetally, extending the period of bloom for 15 days. The inflorescence of hermaphroditic plants has fewer flowers than the staminate inflorescence, and these flowers bloom almost simultaneously for 6 days. Flowers on both types of inflorescences are open for 4 to 5 days, making pollen available over an extended period. The perfect flowers are also protandrous which, combined with simultaneous bloom, favors outcrossing. The entire aerial portion of staminate plants dies several days post-anthesis. The dry, yellow fruit matures approximately 28 days after pollination. Upon maturation, an abscission layer forms at the base of the ovary and the fruits fall to the ground, rotting and exposing the small (2.5 to 3.5 mm x 1.5 to 2.5 mm), white seed. The aerial portion of the hermaphroditic plants also turns yellow and dies soon after the fruit has fallen.

Unlike *Panax quinquefolium* seed, the endocarp of the seed dehisces along the suture in the late fall. Seeds germinate in the spring of the following year. The entire annual period of growth for this species is very short, lasting only from very early spring to about the time that many of the associated tree species have fully leafed out.

3. *Panax japonicum*

Rhizomes of *Panax japonicum* from Japan and a morphologically similar -Panax- species observed at altitudes of 1,500 to 2,500 m in southern China have been compared by Morita *et al.* (42). These rhizomes have a cortex that varies from 2 to 4 layers of elongated to tangential sclerenchymatous cells surroundinga continuous cambium. The periderm of the Japanese and Chinese plants ranges from 5 to 8 layers of thin-walled cells, with the Chinese plants occasionally having secondary growth. Oil ducts with 6 to 8 epithelial cells are located in 2 to 3 circular layers near the phloem, and fiber bundles are occasionally located in the xylem. Tissues contain both starch grains distributed through the various tissue types and druses of calcium oxalate scattered in the cortex, and occasionally, in the xylem.

4. *Panax pseudoginseng*

The floral characteristics of *Panax pseudoginseng* are similar to the polymorphic races of wild Asian *Panax* that Hara (17) classifies as varieties of *Panax pseudoginseng*. Like the American diploid species, flowers are either hermaphroditic or staminate and often androdioecious. However, the occurrence of andromonoecious individuals is more common than seen with *Panax trifolium*. In addition, a secondary staminate umbel will occasionally branch off the peduncle that terminates with an umbel of perfect flowers.

Hermaphroditic flowers have 3 (occasionally 4) styles that can be free or united toward the base. Staminate flowers also have 2 styles that are shorter than those of the hermaphroditic flowers and that can be united in a single column. Anthers are either oblong, elliptic, or oval and produce pollen grains (22 to 24 μm in diameter) that have a very fine reticulation on the surface. Deciduous petals are small (2 to 2.5 mm) and oblong to ovate in shape. Calyx lobes, variable between populations, but generally uniform within a population, may be ovate-triangular to depressed-triangular or, sometimes, rounded-flattened. Glabrous pedicels are subtended by lanceolate or linear bracts that are usually prominent in Japanese plants and inconspicuous in Himalayan plants.

Fruits of *Panax pseudoginseng* are typically bright red with a black spot at the calyx end. These fruits contain 2 to 3 seeds, varying from a slightly flattened coccoon shape to subglobose or ovoid.

IV. SUMMARY

The major division between the primitive and derived taxa within the genus is well documented by morphological and biochemical evidence. The existence of various morphological types of the primitive plants in Asia and their absence in North America is indicative of the center of speciation of this genus. However, classification within the primitive taxa is not consistent throughout the current literature. Hara (17) designated the wild Japanese and Himalayan plants with well-developed rhizomes and fibrous root system as subspecies and varieties of *Panax pseudoginseng* due to the variability of characteristics that often overlap among populations. Within this designation, *Panax japonicum* is reduced to a geographical subspecies of *Panax pseudoginseng*. This interpretation of the wild Asian ginsengs is often followed in the pharmaceutical literature while much of the general botanical literature treats this group of plants as individual species. Additional research into the chemotaxonomy, anatomy, and breeding systems are needed to elucidate relationships within the primitive taxa.

The American diploid species, *Panax trifolium*, has an interesting combination of primitive and derived characteristics. The fleshy persistent root and erect rhizome of these plants are typical of a derived species. However, the floral morphology and the high levels of oleanolic-type saponins isolated from the stems and leaves are primitive characters. The unusual anatomy and short duration of growth are also unique within the genus.

The 3 economically important species, *Panax ginseng* (Oriental ginseng), *Panax quinquefolium* (American ginseng), and *Panax pseudoginseng* (Sanchi ginseng), that are cultivated for their persistent fleshy root are clearly derived species. The Asiatic and American tetraploid species, *Panax ginseng* and *Panax quinquefolium* respectively, are very similar in their ecology, morphology, and anatomy. In addition to minor morphological differences, the 2 species can be differentiated by examining the relative composition and concentration of saponins.

The wild species of *Panax* growing in North America and Asia are irreplaceable sources of genetic diversity from which desirable traits may be incorporated into the cultivated species. While the botanical characteristics of this group of plants are well documented, many basic biological questions prevent researchers from using the available germplasm. Studies on interspecific barriers, generation time, tissue culture, manipulation of ploidy, characterization of populations, identification of selectable genetic markers, and basic genetic studies are all fertile areas for continued research to obtain new varieties of ginseng from this group of ancient plants.

V. REFERENCES

1. Anderson, R.C., J.S. Fralish, J. Armstrong, and P. Benjamin. Biology of ginseng *Panax quinquefolium.* Illinois Dept. of Conservation, Division of Forest Resources and Natural Heritage, Springfield, IL. pp. 1-32.

2. Baronov, A. 1966. Recent advances in our knowledge of the morphology, cultivation and uses of ginseng *Panax ginseng* (C.A. Meyer). Econ. Bot. 20:403-406.

3. Besso, H., R. Kasai, J. Wei, J-F. Wang, Y-I. Saruwatari, T. Fuwa, and O. Tanaka. 1982. Further studies on dammarane-saponins of American ginseng, roots of *Panax quinquefolium* L. Chem. Pharm. Bull. 30(12):4534-4538.

4. Betz, J., A.H. Der Marderosian, and T.M. Lee. 1984. Continuing studies on the ginsenoside content of commercial ginseng products by TLC and HPLC, II. Proc. 6th N. Amer. Ginseng Conf., Univ. of Guelph, Guelph, Ontario. pp. 65-83.

5. Blair, A. 1975. Karyotypes of five plant species with disjunct distributions in Virginia and the Carolinas. Amer. J. Bot. 62(8):833-837.

6. Britton, N.L. 1901. *Manual of the Flora of the North Eastern States and Canada.* Henry Holt and Co., New York. 668 p.

7. Britton, N.L. and A. Brown. 1913. *An Illustrated Flora of the Northeastern U.S., Canada, and the British Possessions.* Charles Scribner and Sons, New York. pp. 618-619.

8. Carpenter, S.G. and G. Cottam. 1982. Growth and reproduction of American ginseng *Panax quinquefolius* in Wisconsin, U.S.A. Canad. J. Bot. 60:2692-2696.

9. Chen, S.E., E.J. Staba, S. Taniyasu, R. Kasai, and O. Tanaka. 1981. Further study on dammarane-saponins of leaves and stems of American ginseng, *Panax quinquefolium.* Planta Medica 42:406-411.

10. Choi, K.G. 1977. Studies of seed germination in *Panax ginseng* C.A. Meyer. 2. The effect of growth regulators on dormancy breaking. Bull. Inst. Agr. Res. Tohoku Univ. 28:159-170.

11. Choi, K.G. and N. Takahashi. 1977. Studies of seed germination in *Panax ginseng* C.A. Meyer 1. The effect of germination inhibitors in fruits on dormancy breaking. Bull. Inst. Agr. Res. Tohoku Univ. 28:145-157.

12. Der Marderosian, A.H., J. Betz, and M. Lee. 1983. Automated HPLC analysis of commercial ginseng (*Panax* spp., Araliaceae) preparations. Proc. 5th Nat'l. Ginseng Conf. Lexington, KY. pp. 48-53.

13. Farr, E.R., J.A. Leussink, F.A. Stafleu, eds. Index Nominum Genericorum (Plantarum) Vol. II, 1978. Bohn, Scheltema and Holkema, Utrecht dr. W. Junk b.v., Publishers, The Hague. p. 1250.

14. Fernald, M.L. 1970. *Gray's Manual of Botany* (8th Ed.), D. Van Nostrand Co., New York. pp. 1077-1078.

15. Gleason, H.A. and A. Cronquist. 1963. in *Manual of Vascular Plants of Northeastern United States and Canada.* D. Van Nostrand Co., New York. p. 499.

16. Graham, S.A. 1966. The genera of Araliaceae in the Southeastern United States. J. of the Arnold Arboretum 47:126-136.

17. Hara, H. 1970. On the Asiatic species of the genus *Panax.* J. Jap. Bot. 45(7):197-211.

18. Holm, T. 1916. Medicinal plants of North America, Merck's Rept. 97. *Aralia* L. and *Panax* L. 25:11-15, 62-65, 126-130, 177-180.

19. Hu, S.Y. 1976. The genus *Panax* (ginseng) in Chinese medicine. Econ. Bot. 30:11-28.

20. Hu, S.Y. 1978. The ecology, phytogeography, and ethnobotany of ginseng. Proc. 2nd Int'l Ginseng Symp., Seoul. pp. 149-157.

21. Hu, S.Y. 1980. Biological and cytological foundation for better ginseng to more people. Proc. 3rd Int'l. Ginseng Symp., Seoul. pp. 171-179.

22. Hu, S.Y., L. Rudenberg, and P. Del Tredici. 1980. Studies of American ginsengs. Rhodora 82:627-636.

23. Kim, J.Y. and E.J. Staba. 1974. Biochemistry of ginseng constituents and plant triterpenes. Kor. Jour. of Pharmacog. 5(2):85-101.

24. Kim, S.K., I. Sakamoto, K. Morimoto, M. Sakata, K. Yamasaki, and O. Tanaka. 1980. Chemical evaluation of ginseng extracts: Seasonal variation of saponins and sucrose in cultivated roots. Proc. 3rd Int'l. Ginseng Symp., Seoul. pp. 5-8.

25. Kondo, N., J. Shoji, and O. Tanaka. 1973. Studies on the constituents of Himalayan ginseng, *Panax pseudoginseng.* I. The structures of the saponins. (1). Chem. Pharm. Bull. 21(12):2702-2711.

26. Konsler, T.R. 1983. Ginseng Production Guide for North Carolina. North Carolina Ag. Ext. Bull. AG 323. pp. 1-15.

27. Konsler, T.R. 1984. Root chilling dormancy requirements for American ginseng (*Panax quinquefolium* L.). Proc. 4th Int'l. Ginseng Symp. Sept. 18-20, 1984, Daljen, South Korea. pp. 49-55.

28. Konsler, T.R. 1986. Some Opportunities in American Ginseng (*Panax quinquefolium* L.). Proc. 7th N. Amer. Ginseng Conf., June 13-15, 1986, Delhi, NY (in press).

29. Kubo, M., T. Tani, T. Katsuki, K. Ishizaki, and S. Arichi. 1980. Histochemistry. I. Ginsenosides in ginseng (*Panax ginseng* C.A. Meyer) root. J. of Nat. Products 43(2):278-284.

30. Lee, J.C., J.S. Byen, and J.T.A. Proctor. 1983. Effect of temperature on embryo growth and germination of ginseng seed. Proc. 5th Nat'l. Ginseng Conf. Lexington, KY. pp. 11-21.

31. Lee, J.C., B.C. Strik, and J.T.A. Proctor. 1985. Dormancy and growth of American ginseng as influenced by temperature. J. Amer. Hort. Sci. 110(3):319-321.

32. Lee, T.M. and A.H. Der Marderosian. 1981. Two-dimensional TLC analysis ginsenosides from root of dwarf ginseng (*Panax trifolius* L.) Araliaceae. J. Pharm. Sci. 70(1):89-91.

33. Lewis, W.H. 1979. Ginseng of Northeastern China. Proc. 1st Nat'l. Ginseng Conf. Lexington, KY. pp. 69-77.

34. Lewis, W.H. 1979. The healing herbs. Well Being Mag. 46:45-47.

35. Lewis, W.H. 1985. Restoration of a population of *Panax quinquefolium* in a Missouri climax forest. (Manuscript in preparation.) Copies available from author on request. Washington Univ., St. Louis, MO.

36. Lewis, W.H. and G.A. Thompson. 1985. *Panax quinquefolium* (Araliaceae) in southeastern Oklahoma. Rhodora 87:131.

37. Lewis, W.H. and V.E. Zenger. 1982. Population dynamics of the American ginseng *Panax quinquefolium* (Araliaceae). Amer. J. Bot. 69(9):1483-1490.

38. Lewis, W.H. and V.E. Zenger. 1983. Breeding systems and fecundity in the American ginseng *Panax quinquefolium* (Araliaceae). Amer. J. Bot. 70(3):466-468.

39. Li, H.L. 1952. Distribution of genera: Dicotyledons. 36. Araliaceae. Floristic Relationships between Eastern Asia and Eastern North America. Vol. 42, Pt. 2. p. 393.

40. Lui, J.H. and E.J. Staba. 1980. The ginsenosides of various ginseng plants and selected products. J. of Nat. Prod. 43(3):340-346.

41. McMahan, L. 1981. A summary of the biology and management of American ginseng. Proc. 3rd Nat'l. Ginseng Conf., Asheville, NC. pp. 3-16.

42. Morita, T., R. Kasai, H. Kohda, O. Tanaka, J. Zhou, and T-R. Yang. 1983. Chemical and morphological study on Chinese *Panax japonicus* C.A. Meyer (Zhujie-Shen). Chem. Pharm. Bull. 31(9):3205-3209.

43. Morita, T., R. Kasai, O. Tanaka, J. Zhou, T.R. Yang, and J. Shoji. 1982. Saponins of Zu-Tzing, rhizomes of *Panax japonicus* C.A. Meyer var. Major (Burk.) C.Y. Wu ex K.M. Feng, collected in Yunnan, China. Chem. Pharm. Bull. 30(12):4341-4346.

44. Nagai, Y., O. Tanaka, and S. Shibata. 1971. Chemical studies on the Oriental plant drugs - XXIV. Structure of ginsenoside-Rg$_1$, neutral saponin of ginseng root. *Tetrahedron* 27:881-892.

45. Nagasawa, T., T. Yokozawa, Y. Nishino, and H. Oura. 1980. Application of high-performance liquid chromatography to the isolation of ginsenoside - Rb$_1$, -Rb$_2$, -Rc, -Rd, -Re, and -Rg$_1$ from ginseng saponins. Chem. Pharm. Bull. 28(7):2059-2064.

46. Philbrick, C.T. 1983. Contributions to the reproductive biology of *Panax trifolium* L. (Araliaceae). Rhodora 85(841):97-113.

47. Polczinski, L.C. 1982. Ginseng (*Panax quinquefolius* L.) culture in Marathon County, Wisconsin: Historical growth, distribution and soils inventory. M.S. Thesis, Univ. of Wisconsin, Stevens Point, WI. p. 16.

48. Sanada, S., N. Kondo, J. Shoji, O. Tanaka, and S. Shibata. 1974. Studies on the saponins of ginseng. I. Structures of ginsenoside -Ro, - Rb$_1$, -Rb$_2$, -Rc, and -Rd. Chem. Pharm. Bull. 22(2):421-428.

49. Sanada, S., N. Kondo, J. Shoji, O. Tanaka, and S. Shibata. 1974. Studies on the saponins of ginseng. II. Structures of ginsenoside-Re,-RF, and -Rg$_2$. Chem. Pharm. Bull. 22(10):2407-2412.

50. Schlessman, M.A. 1985. Floral biology of American ginseng *Panax quinquefolium*. Bull. Torey Bot. Club 112:129-133.

51. Shibata, S. 1974. Some chemical studies on ginseng. Proc. Int'l. Ginseng Symp. Seoul. pp. 69-76.

52. Shibata, S., T. Ando, and O. Tanaka. 1966. Studies on the oriental plant drugs. XVII. The prosapogenin of the ginseng saponins (ginsenosides-Rb$_1$, -Rb$_2$, and -Rc). Chem. Pharm. Bull. 14(10):1157-1161.

53. Shibata, S. and H. Saito. 1977. Some recent studies on ginseng saponins. Proc. Int'l. Geront. Symp. Singapore. pp. 183-195.

54. Slepyan, L.I. 1973. Anato-morphological description of emerged seedlings of *Panax ginseng*. Akad. Nauk SSSR, Rast. Resur. 9(1):18-30.

55. Smith, A.C. 1944. *Panax*. North American Flora. 28B(9):9-10.

56. Soldati, F. 1980. HPLC and quantitative determination of ginsenosides from *Panax ginseng*, *Panax quinquefolium* and from ginseng drug preparations. Proc. 3rd Int'l. Ginseng Symp. Seoul. pp. 59-69.

57. Soldati, F. and O. Tanaka. 1984. *Panax ginseng*. Relation between age of plant and content of ginsenosides. Planta Medica 51:351-352.

58. Staba, E.J. 1979. Ginseng, what is it? Well Being Mag. 48 (December).

59. Tanaka, O. and S. Yahara. 1978. Dammarane saponins of leaves of *Panax pseudo-ginseng* subsp. *himalaicus*. Phytochemistry 17:1353-1358.

60. Taylor, R.L. 1967. I.O.P.B. Chromosome number reports. Taxon 16:566.

61. Yahara, S., K. Kaji, and O. Tanaka. 1979. Further study on dammarane-type saponins of roots, leaves, flower-buds, and fruits of *Panax ginseng* C.A. Meyer. Chem. Pharm. Bull. 27(1):88-92.

62. Yahara, S., R. Kasai, and O. Tanaka. 1977. New dammarane-type saponins of leaves of *Panax japonicus* C.A. Meyer. 1. Chikusetsusaponins -L5, - L$_9$a, and -L$_1$0. Chem. Pharm. Bull. 25(8):2041-2047.

63. Yahara, S., K. Matsuura, R. Kasai, and O. Tanaka. 1976. Saponins of buds and flowers of *Panax ginseng* C.A. Mcyer. (1). Isolation of ginsenosides-Rd$_1$, -Re, and -Rg$_1$. Chem. Pharm. Bull. 24(12):3212-3213.

64. Yahara, S., O. Tanaka, and T. Komori. 1976. Saponins of the leaves of *Panax ginseng* C.A. Meyer. Chem. Pharm. Bull. 24(9):2204-2208.

65. Yahara, S., O. Tanaka, and I. Nishiola. 1978. Dammarane-type saponins of leaves of *Panax japonicus* C.A. Meyer 2. Saponins of the specimens collected in Tottori-ken, Kyoto-shi, and Niigata-ken. Chem. Pharm. Bull. 26(10):3010-3016.

66. Yang, T.-R., R. Kasai, J. Zhou, and O. Tanaka. 1983. Dammarane saponins of leaves and seeds of *Panax notoginseng* Phytochemistry 22(6):1473-1478.

67. Zhou, J., M.-Z. Wu, S. Taniyasu, H. Besso, O. Tanaka, Y. Saruwatari, and T. Fuwa. 1981. Dammarane-saponins of sanchi-ginseng, roots of *Panax notoginseng (Burk.) F.H. Chen (Araliaceae)*. Structures of new saponins, notoginsenosides -R1 and -R2, and identification of ginsenosides -Rg$_2$ and -Rh$_1$. Chem. Pharm. Bull. 29(10):2844-2850.

Synergism and Antagonism in the Pharmacology of Alkaloidal Plants

Mohamed Izaddoost
College of Pharmacy, University of Tehran, Tehran, Iran

Trevor Robinson
Department of Biochemistry, University of Massachusetts, Amherst, MA 01003

CONTENTS

I. Introduction
II. Pharmacology of *Atropa belladonna* L.
   A. Alkaloids
   B. Other Compounds
   C. Interactions
III. Pharmacology of *Cephaelis ipecacuanha* A. Rich
   A. Alkaloids
   B. Other Compounds
   C. Interactions
IV. Pharmacology of *Cinchona* spp.
   A. Alkaloids
   B. Other Compounds
   C. Interactions
V. Pharmacology of *Colchicum autumnale* L.
   A. Alkaloids
   B. Other Compounds
   C. Interactions
VI. Pharmacology of *Ephedra sinica* L.
   A. Alkaloids
   B. Other Compounds
   C. Interactions
VII. Pharmacology of *Papaver somniferum* L.

I. INTRODUCTION

Drug plants, as a first approximation, are generally assumed to owe their efficacy to the high concentration of some constituent that may be isolated and characterized. The administration of this pure constituent should then, theoretically, produce exactly the same pharmacological effects as the original plant.

There may be some cases where the above paradigm fits the facts. However, practitioners of herbal medicine will immediately deny the validity of this statement, and pharmaceutical chemists will be able to think of cases where it is certainly inadequate to explain the facts. In this review, some examples of alkaloid-containing medicinal plants are examined to illustrate the considerable complexity arising from the actions and interactions of the many different constituents that are present.

Pharmacological effects from administration of whole plant extract can be quite different from the effects of administering a single active principle. A commonly recognized fact of drug treatments is that "...the presence of inert substances may modify or prevent the absorbability or potency of the active constituents" (14). Moreover, more than one active constituent may be present in drug plant extracts. At the molecular level, 2 or more active constituents could compete for the same site of action or act at different sites that are both connnected with a larger physiological system. The resultant, overall pharmacological effect on the organism could be synergistic or antagonistic action. Some interactions, such as tannins that form slightly soluble precipitates with alkaloids or the presence of acids or bases that control the ionic form of an active constituent and thereby influence solubility and/or absorbability, can be understood as simple, chemical phenomena. More subtle pharmacological effects of drug plants could result if one constituent stimulates an excitatory receptor while an accompanying constituent stimulates an inhibitory receptor of the same system or if one constituent inhibits an endogenous enzyme that metabolizes a second active constituent.

In theory, a great many such possibilities of interaction among plant constituents can be imagined. The selected examples that follow demonstrate that some of these possibilities are natural occurrences that need to be incorporated into any full understanding of the actions of herbal drugs.

II. PHARMACOLOGY OF *ATROPA BELLADONNA* L.

Various parts of the deadly nightshade plant (*Atropa belladonna* L.) act as a parasympathetic depressant, which accounts for its use as a spasmolytic agent. The juice of the berries placed in the eyes causes dilation of the pupils, giving a striking appearance to the face. The pharmacological effects of this plant are due primarily to the alkaloid content, but the other constituents of the plant agonize or antagonize the effects of the alkaloids.

A. Alkaloids

Alkaloids belonging to a variety of chemical types are present in *Atropa belladonna* (Figure 1). Most important are the tropanes. The naturally occurring tropane alkaloids l-hyoscyamine, l-scopolamine (hyoscine), apoatropine, and belladonnine as well as compounds derived from them (such as atropine and tropine) show, to different degrees, antimuscarinic activity (25, 28, 36, 77, 86, 89). Thus, the plant extracts are used to relieve spasms of the intestinal tract or respiratory tract. The plant extracts also demonstrate different levels of other pharmacological actions. For instance, the tropanes can act as antihistamines (80) and as effectors of the central nervous system (CNS). Low doses of plant extracts may stimulate the CNS, while higher doses depress. Scopolamine has a greater effect than atropine on the CNS (77), and apoatropine has a greater effect than atropine as an antispasmodic (80).

B. Other Compounds

Quercetin, kaempferol, and glucosidic flavones are reported in the herb *Atropa belladonna* (68) (Figures 2 and 3). Some of these compounds exhibit antispasmodic and diuretic activity (9, 10, 65). Chlorogenic acid is a CNS stimulant similar to caffeine (27) and also acts as an antihistaminic (30) and antibacterial agent (20).

C. Interactions

Among themselves, the alkaloids of this plant demonstrate synergistic pharmacological effects in their various activities. However,

Figure 1. Alkaloids of *Atropa belladonna* L.

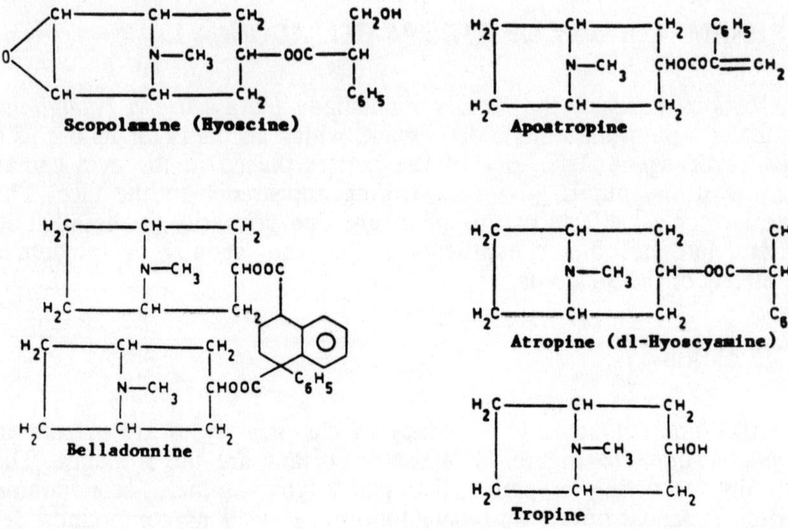

Scopolamine (Hyoscine)

Apoatropine

Belladonnine

Atropine (dl-Hyoscyamine)

Tropine

Figure 2. Quercetin

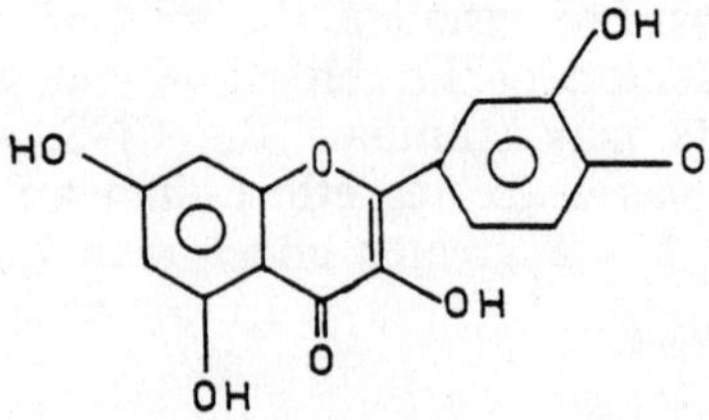

Figure 3. Kaempferol

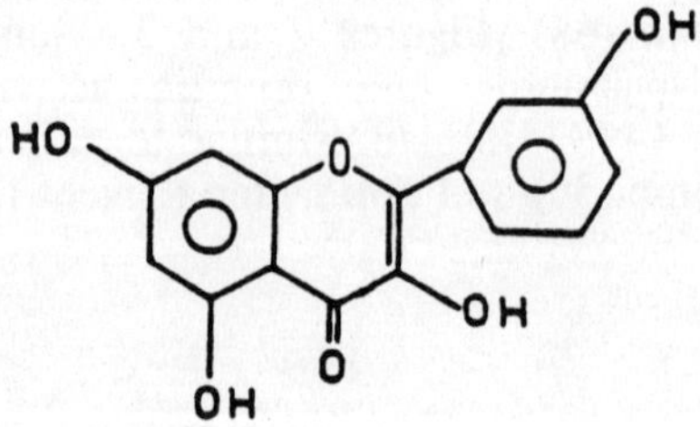

depending on the proportions of different alkaloids present within the plant, different types of response to treatments with plant extracts may be emphasized. Different plant preparations may contain different proportions of these different alkaloids; since standardization is normally only for total alkaloid content, variability in pharmacological effects may be expected from whole plant extracts. Synergism and antagonism among the alkaloids means that spasmolytic activity of a total extract cannot be predicted accurately from knowledge of either the l-hyoscyamine content or the total alkaloid concentration (47).

When plant constituents other than alkaloids are considered, flavonoids appear to be synergistic with the alkaloids in spasmolytic action but antagonistic to the alkaloids in action on urine retention. Chlorogenic acid maybe synergistic with the alkaloids in antihistaminic activity but antagonistic to alkaloids in the CNS. Considering that differences in the amounts of compounds secondary to the alkaloids are observed in different varieties of the plants, widely varying effects would be expected when whole plant extract is administered.

III. PHARMACOLOGY OF *CEPHAELIS IPECACUANHA* A. RICH

Rhizomes and roots of the shrub *Cephaelis ipecacuanha* A. Rich are known as ipecac. From this plant, an emetic-acting syrup can be extracted. The alkaloid constituent, emetine, induces vomiting; the hydrochloride of emetine is an antiamebic when administered intramuscularly or subcutaneously.

A. Alkaloids

Isoquinoline-type alkaloids are reported in the extract of *Cephaelis ipecacuanha* (Figure 4). The expectorant and emetic action of ipecacuanha is due mostly to its content of emetine (11). For patients with amebic dysentery, amebic abscess, or amebic hepatitis, pure emetine is preferable (48). This compound has bacteriostatic potency (46) and a high pharmacological activity against pathogenic amebas (18). The compound is also an adrenergic neuron-blocking agent (57) and is known to produce a histopathological change: hyperplasia in the bone marrow (60). Emetine inhibits multiplication of viruses (61) and exhibits an anti-inflammatory effect (10 mg/kg) (43). The compound is used for the antihelmintic effect against *Oxyuris* and *Taenia* (59). Growth of mouse tumors can be inhibited with emetine (31), and the compound causes a regular reduction of stroke volume of the heart in laboratory animals (8). Cephaeline is also an expectorant agent and acts synergistically with emetine (11).

Figure 4. Alkaloids of *Cephaelis ipecacuanha* A. Rich

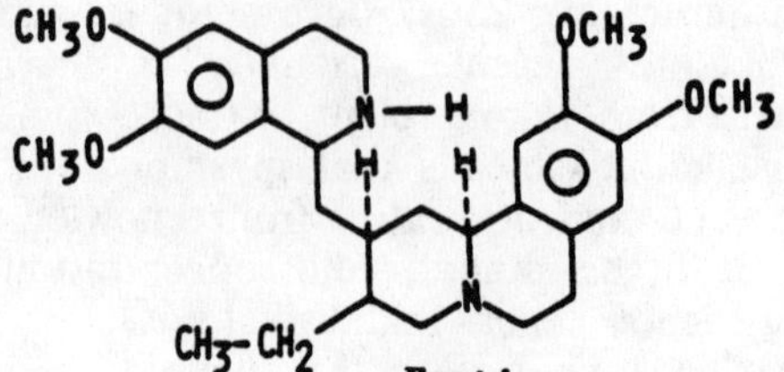

Emetine

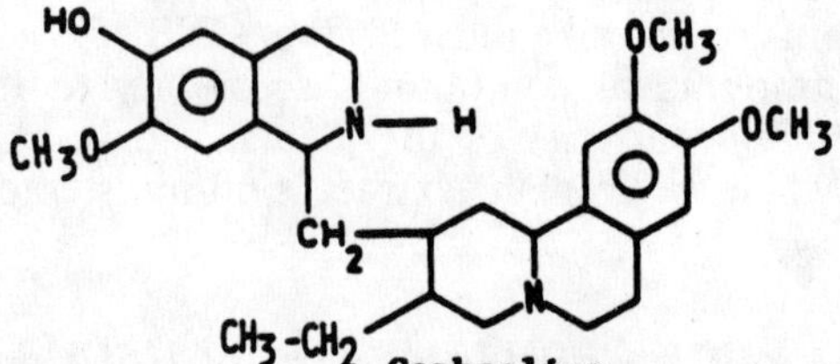

Cephaeline

B. Other Compounds

Tannins and anthraquinone constituents are reported in *Cephaelis ipecacuanha* (17, 45).

C. Interactions

The presence of tannins reduces the absorption of alkaloids from the intestinal tract. The cathartic effects of the anthraquinone compounds are opposite to the astringent effects of tannins but could also decrease the effective activity of alkaloids by decreasing the available time for absorption from the intestinal tract.

IV. PHARMACOLOGY OF *CINCHONA* SPP.

A. Alkaloids

Alkaloids belonging to at least 2 chemical types—quinoline and indole—are reported in the extract of bark of *Cinchona* spp. (Figure 5). These alkaloids share a common precursor, the amino acid tryptophan.

Quinine, the major alkaloid, is best known as an antimalarial agent. In addition, this alkaloid is antimitotic and slows the differentiation of tissues in culture media (66). The compound also acts as a sedative and febrifuge (79), is effective in the prevention of fibrillation (4), and has fungicidal and anti-inflammatory activity (35, 74). Intravenous injection of quinine sulfate reduces gastric secretion (42).

Among the other alkaloids of *Cinchona*, quinidine, a stereoisomer of quinine, is an important antiarrhythmic agent (79) that is effective in the prevention of heart fibrillation (4). The compound also inhibits cholinesterase action (5, 81). Cinchonine and cinchonidine are known antihistaminic agents (30). Cinchonine action resembles that of quinidine (19) in prevention of heart fibrillation. Epiquinine, cinchonine, and quinidine have a negative inotropic action on heart muscles (3).

Figure 5. Alkaloids of *Cinchona* spp.

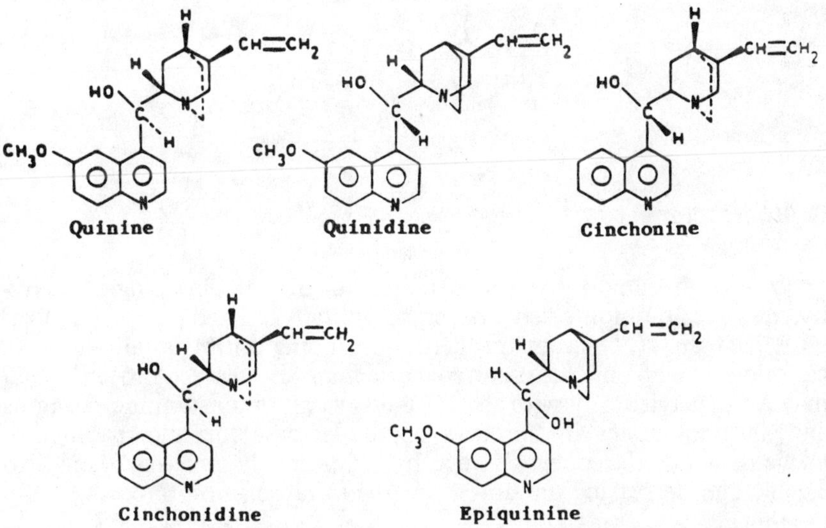

Quinine   Quinidine   Cinchonine

Cinchonidine   Epiquinine

B. Other Compounds

Chlorogenic acid, protocatechuic, and caffeic acid are present in *Cinchona* spp. (Figures 6 and 7). Chlorogenic acid is a CNS stimulant and antihistaminic (30, 81). Tannins (45) and anthraquinones (17) in these plants may influence the absorption of alkaloids from the intestinal tract.

Figure 6. Chlorogenic Acid

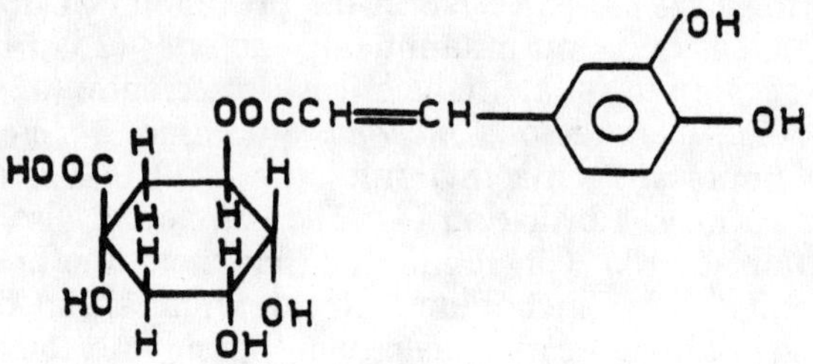

Figure 7. Protocatechuic Acid

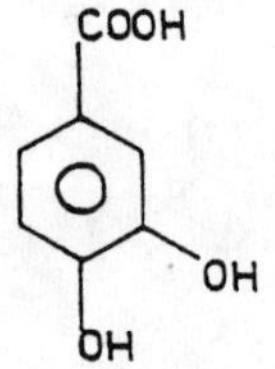

C. Interactions

Although quantitatively different in degree of physiological activity, quinine, quinidine, and other structurally related *Cinchona* alkaloids have many common properties including antimalarial action. A consideration of nonalkaloidal constituents indicates cholorogenic acid may act synergistically with the alkaloids as an antihistaminic. Tannins and anthraquinones in the bark could decrease the absorbability of alkaloids from the internal tract by, respectively, making them less soluble and decreasing the time available for absorption to occur.

V. PHARMACOLOGY OF *COLCHICUM AUTUMNALE* L.

The seed and corm of the autumn crocus are used as an antirheumatic agent and for other remedies.

A. Alkaloids

Of the amine types of alkaloids reported in this plant, colchicine is the preferred compound in the symptomatic treatment of acute attacks of gouty arthritis (25) (Figure 8). Although the mechanism of this pharmacological action is unknown, molecular interaction with tubulin may be the initial step (22). Colchicine is very toxic, and medicinal use should be discontinued at the first evidence of any toxicity, including diarrhea, nausea, vomiting, or abdominal pain. Human platelet aggregation (40) and histamine release from mast cells are inhibited by colchicine (26, 40). Parenteral administration of colchicine causes severe degeneration in the mucosa (85). The compound has analgesic, anti-inflammatory, and teratogenic effects (64, 84).

Figure 8. Alkaloids of *Colchicum autumnale* L.

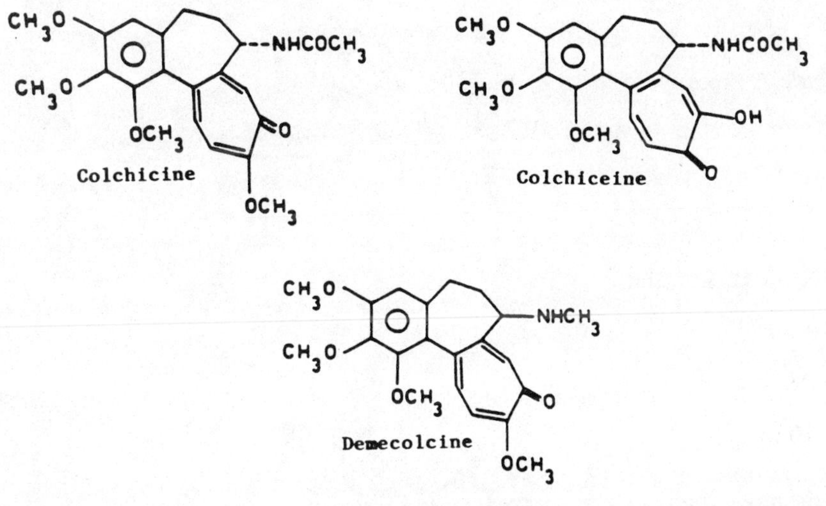

Colchicine

Colchiceine

Demecolcine

Another alkaloid in *Colchicum autumnale*—colchiceine—is not effective against gout (82) but inhibits the aggregation of platelets similar to colchicine (67). Demecolcine, an alkaloid effective in the treatment of gout, causes agranulocytosis (82) and inhibits the release of histamine and the production of agglutinating and hemolysing antibodies (58). Colchicoside is an alkaloid that is mildly effective in the treatment of gout (26) and, like colchicine, has an antimitotic effect (39). The compound also inhibits the production of agglutinating and hemolysing antibodies (58).

B. Other Compounds

Of the flavonoids in *Colchicum autumnale*, apigenin has demonstrated a bronchodilator action that is longer lasting, but 3 to 4 times weaker, than that of papaverine. This compound both antagonizes the pharmacological action of histamine and reduces the

146 Herbs, Spices, and Medicinal Plants, Volume 2

hypotensive action of histamine in cats (32). Significant spasmolytic and anti-inflammatory effects are noted following treatment with apigenin (Figure 9). This flavonoid also decreases the tone and motility of intestine and antagonizes the stimulating effect of carbamoylcholine on the intestine (38). Another flavonoid—luteolin (Figure 10)—reduces the diastolic and, to a lesser extent, the systolic amplitudes. This compound also reduces the heartbeat frequency and cardiac output (56), causing a slight increase of the arterial and lowering of the venous blood pressure (56).

Figure 9. Apigenin

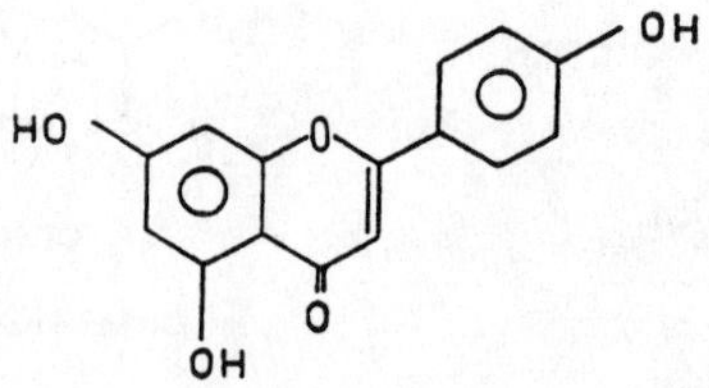

Figure 10. Luteolin

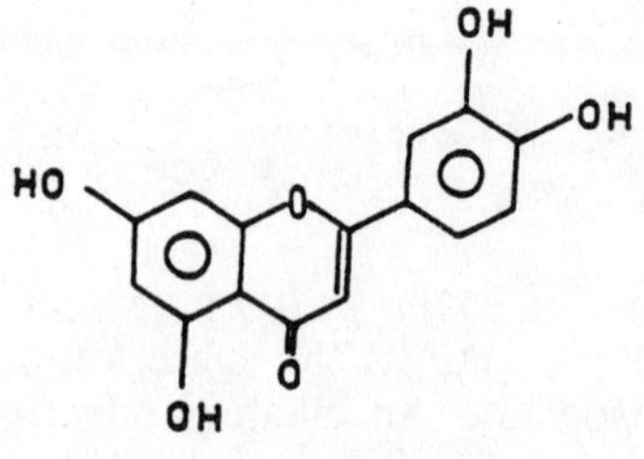

C. Interactions

Several of the alkaloids of *Colchicum autumnale* have similar and thus additive action. Colchicine and demecolcine are effective in the treatment of gout; colchicine and demecolcine cause agranulocytosis; colchicine, demecolcine, and colchicoside have antimitotic and antineoplastic effects; colchicine, colchiceine, and demecolcine inhibit the aggregation of platelets; and demecolcine and colchicoside inhibit the production of agglutinating and hemolysing antibodies. Colchicine, colchicoside, and the flavonoid apigenin are synergists in their anti-inflammatory effect but via different mechanisms. Colchicine and demecolcine reduce the release of histamine while apigenin acts an antagonist of the histamine action in the body.

VI. PHARMACOLOGY OF *EPHEDRA SINICA* L.

The Chinese drug ma huang is the dried aerial part of the herb *Ephedra sinica* L. This plant has been used in China for a variety of medications but primarily for the treatment of pulmonary diseases.

A. Alkaloids

Alkaloids belonging to a variety of chemical structures, especially the phenylpropanoid nucleus, are reported in the plant. The stereoisomers l-ephedrine and d-pseudoephedrine are both present and are about equally effective as bronchodilators. However, pseudoephedrine differs from ephedrine in that its pressor, cardiac, mydriatic, and central stimulant actions are relatively weaker even though there is strong antiinflammatory activity (25, 34). Ephedrine is effective in control and curing of high urinary frequency, whereas pseudoephedrine dilates renal blood vessels and, as a result, increases urine output (25, 34). Use of the total extract from the shoot on the majority or the alkaloids reported in the plant will cause an increase in blood pressure (21). The 3 ephedradines A, B, and C, that are present in the plant, conversely, reduce hypertension (21, 34). Thus, the overall effect of the plant material on the body results from a number of competing pharmacological actions.

B. Other Compounds

Leucoanthocyanidins and other flavonoids are present in *Ephedra sinica* (2, 62, 73).

C. Interactions

The overall physiological effect of the plant material on the body results from a number of competing pharmacological actions of the alkaloids. The nonalkaloidal constituents of *Ephedra* interfere with the absorption of alkaloids from the intestinal tract into the portal vein, making the effects of the alkaloids appear slowly and last longer (29). The nonalkaloidal substances responsible for this effect are not known for sure, but leucoanthocyanidins and other flavonoids could be re-

Figure 11. Alkaloids of *Ephedra sinica* L.

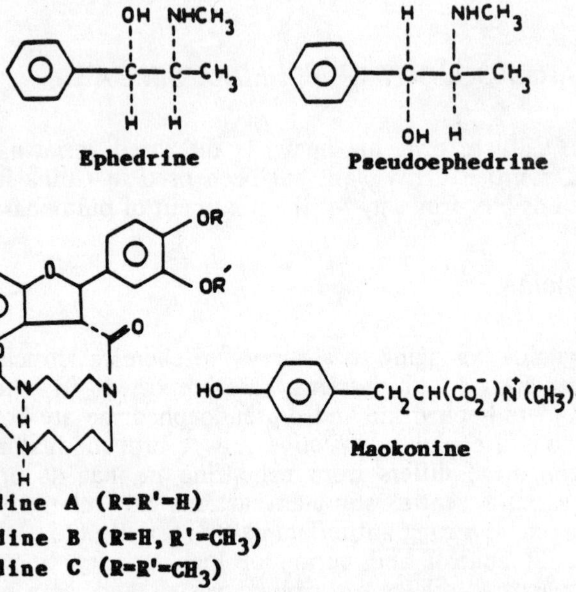

Ephedrine

Pseudoephedrine

Maokonine

Ephedradine A (R=R'=H)
Ephedradine B (R=H, R'=CH₃)
Ephedradine C (R=R'=CH₃)

sponsible (2, 62, 73). In addition, the total extract from the roots is hypotensive but contains the alkaloid maokinine, whose effect is hypertensive (71).

VII. PHARMACOLOGY OF *PAPAVER SOMNIFERUM* L.

The opium poppy *Papaver somniferum* L. is one of the best known of all medicinal plants, with its physiological effects commonly ascribed to only 2 or 3 prominent alkaloids among the dozens of constituents that have been characterized in opium, the dried latex of the capsules.

A. Alkaloids

Alkaloids belonging to a variety of chemical types are reported in *Papaver somniferum* (Figure 12). Most commonly recognized are those alkaloids of the phenanthrene, isoquinoline, and protoberberine nuclei.Morphine, one of the better-known compounds, is used as an analgesic, antitussive, and nonspecific antidiarrheal agent. Morphine increases the activity and tone of the smooth muscles of gastrointestinal, biliary, and urinary tracts, causing constipation, gall bladder spasms,

Figure 12. Alkaloids of *Papaver somniferum* L.

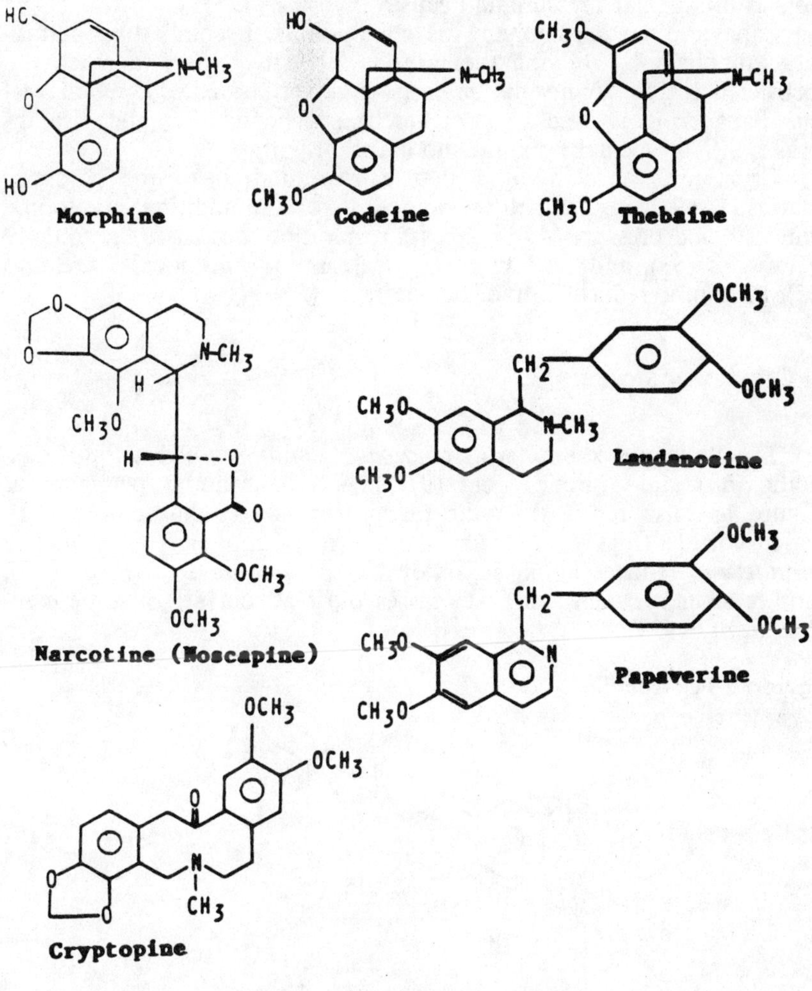

Morphine

Codeine

Thebaine

Narcotine (Noscapine)

Laudanosine

Papaverine

Cryptopine

and urinary retention (25). In addition, morphine also depresses respiration and causes myosis (25). Codeine is used as antitussive, analgesic, sedative, narcotic, and antiperistaltic (25). Thebaine, in low doses, reduces the intraocular pressure (87) but in higher doses causes convulsions (25), releases histamine (37, 88), and initiates vasodilation (54).

Narcotine, used as an anticonvulsant, narcotic, and antitussive, increases the intraocular pressure (76, 86). Laudanosine, which is used as a spasmolytic (76), has a noticeable contradictory effect to phenobarbital and causes convulsions (25). In low doses, this compound reduces intraocular pressure and causes mydriasis (25).

Papaverine is spasmolytic; its chief use is in combatting pulmonary embolism by dilating the arteries, allowing blood to reach the obstructed region. In normal subjects, papaverine dilates cerebral vessels. Papaverine is used to treat cerebral ischemia (86) and also increases the intraocular pressure and causes mydriasis (25).

Cryptopine, a compound that causes dilation of the coronary arteries (1, 49), also has antitussive activity (1). In addition, cryptopine reduces blood pressure (49), increases respiration, decreases the tonicity of muscles (53), and, in low doses, decreases the intraocular pressure (25). Protopine reduces intraocular pressure (25).

B. Other Compounds

The flavonoid kaempferol in *Papaver somniferum* is an antispasmodic (63) and diuretic agent (9). The anthocyanidin pelargonidin (Figure 13) also reported in the plant decreases cardiac output (78). Caffeic acid (Figure 14), an aromatic compound in *Papaver somniferum*, reduces blood sugar levels (13). Ferulic acid (Figure 15), another aromatic compound, depresses the reaction rate of some cerebral enzymes (33).

Figure 13. Pelargonidin

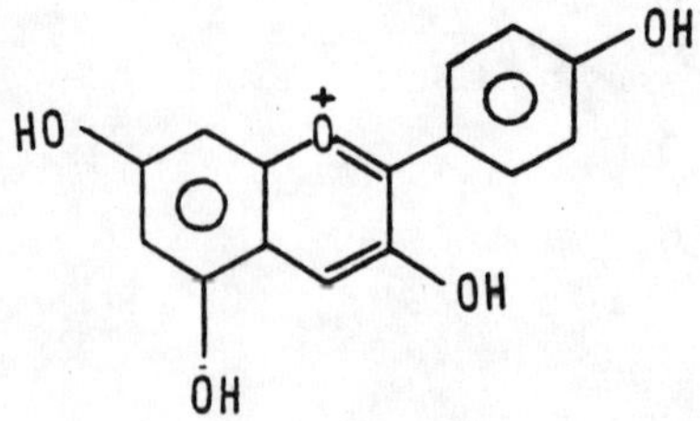

Figure 14. Caffeic Acid

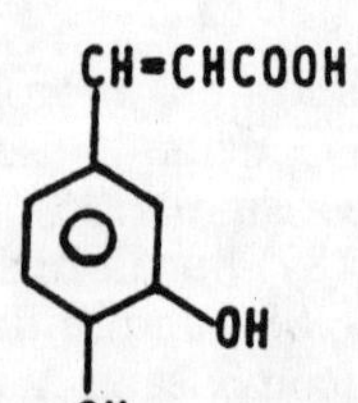

Figure 15. Ferulic Acid

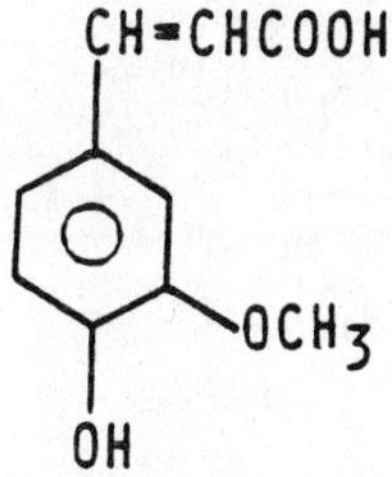

C. Interactions

The alkaloids morphine, codeine, laudanosine, and papaverine, as well as the flavonoid kaempferol, collectively account for sedative and antispasmodic effects of opium from *Papaver somniferum*. The alkaloids thebaine, cryptopine, and protopine reduce the intraocular pressure while narcotine increases the intraocular pressure. Morphine induces myosis in the eye while laudanosine causes mydriasis.

Because of the complementary and opposing physiological effects of the compounds, the expected pharmacological effects following administration of opium are complicated. The numerous interactions indicate unexpected effects can result from the use of a plant exudate.

VIII. PHARMACOLOGY OF *VERATRUM VIRIDE* AIT.

The American hellebore *Veratrum viride* Ait. consists of the dried rhizome and roots of the herb. This drug plant was used by prehistoric American Indians.

A. Alkaloids

Based on chemical structure, 3 classes of alkaloids are observed in this plant (Figure 16). One of the alkaloids—cevadine—causes transient stimulation in isolated intestines with the locus of spasmogenic action appearing to be directly on the intestinal muscle. Tachyphylaxis is also observed (16). Cevadine is extremely irritating, particularly to mucous membranes, and caution must be used in handling the compound (86). Cevadine also has a hypotensive effect and is a cardiac stimulant (15, 50). Sinus tachycardia is a characteristic irregularity with cevadine (6). Intracisternal injection of cevadine and protoveratrine into rabbits causes increased inspiration, motor disorder, and convulsions (41).

Figure 16. Alkaloids of *Veratrum viride* Ait.

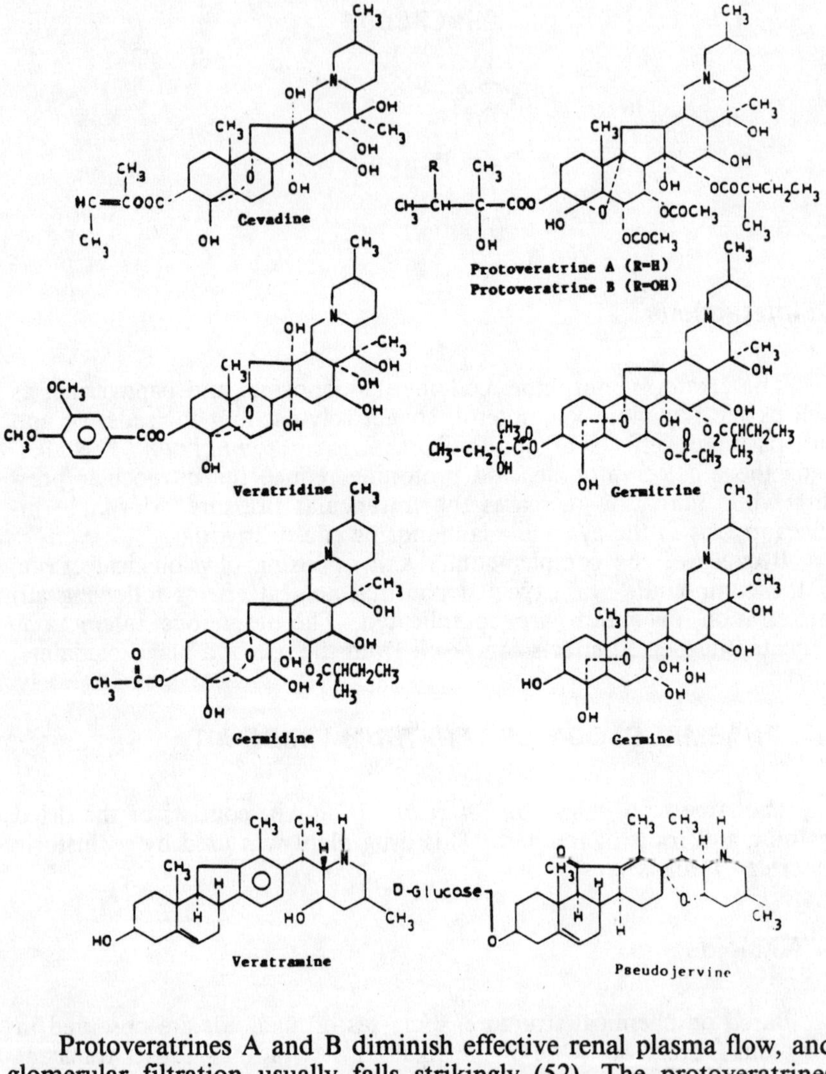

Protoveratrines A and B diminish effective renal plasma flow, and glomerular filtration usually falls strikingly (52). The protoveratrines produce hypotension (70) and cause arrhythmias (69). Injection of 0.1 µg of protoveratrine results in a decreased arterial blood pressure (55), and injection of protoveratrines at 3 µg/kg reduces output in laboratory animals, indicating that the protoveratrines stimulate release of vasopressin (7). These compounds also demonstrate some anesthetizing action and inhibit vomiting (41). Intravenous injection of veratridine

(60-70 µg) causes a steady increase in urine flow and a decrease in systemic blood pressure (75).

The cardiovascular effects of the crude drug are due largely to the ester alkaloid germitrine, a compound that produces high hypotensive activity in humans (24). Germitrine is less toxic and is less active than germidine (51). Germidine has a hypotensive effect (83) and causes transient stimulation of the intestine (16). Germine is effective in treatment of hypertension (86) and is a CNS stimulant (72).

Veratramine demonstrates a negative inotropic effect and nonspecifically depresses smooth muscle (23), causing a peculiar excitation of which convulsive struggling is the chief sign (72). Pseudojervine has a specific and selective action antagonistic to the positive chronotropic effect of epinephrine on the pacemaker tissue of the heart (44). When large amounts of veratrosine are infused, there is a concomitant increase in electroencephalogram wave amplitude. This treatment also reduces respiration and stimulates skeletal muscle and gastrointestinal activity. A hyperglycemic effect is also observed (12).

B. Interactions

Each of the alkaloids in the plant exhibits variable properties. The alkaloids cevadine, protoveratrine, veratridine, germitrine, germidine, and germine cause reduction in blood pressure. Cevadine and protoveratrine cause stimulation of heart and tachycardia. Veratramine has a negative chronotropic effect on the heart, and pseudojervine has an antagonistic effect on the positive chronotropism induced by epinephrine on the heart. Cevadine and protoveratrine increase respiration, whereas veratrosine reduces respiration.

Note

This article was conceived and the original manuscript was prepared by Professor Mohamed Izaddoost. Contact with Professor Izaddoost has been lost and the second author is responsible for this final version.

IX. REFERENCES

1. Alles, G.A. and H. Charles. 1952. A comparative study of the pharmacology of certain cryptopine alkaloids. J. Pharmacol. Exp. Ther. 104:253-263.

2. Alyukina, L.S. 1955. *Ephedra* as a tanning plant. Izvest. Akad. Nauk Kazakh. SSR, Ser. Biol. 9:55-64.

3. Arora, R.B., S.L. Agarwal, P.C. Dandiya, and K. P. Singh. 1956. Chemical structure of *Cinchona* alkaloids and cupreines responsible for its negative intropic action in isolated amphibian and mammalian hearts. Ind. J. Med. Res. 44:645-648.

4. Atsuji, C. 1955. Comparative study on the action of various derivatives of Cinchona alkaloids upon the electrically produced ventricular fibrillation of isolated frog's heart. Folia Pharmacol. Japan 51:218-228.

5. Bach, E., B. Robert, and L. Robert. 1951. Action of quinine and quinidine on cholinesterase. Boll. soc. Chim. biol. 33:1805-1812.

6. Benforado, J. M. 1957. *Veratrum* alkaloids. XXVI. Comparison of the cardiac action of various tertiary amine ester alkaloids. J. Pharmacol. Exp. Ther. 120:412-425.

7. Blackmore, W.P. 1955. The antidiuretic action of protoveratrine, and its mechanism in dogs. J. Pharmacol. Exp. Ther. 114:87-89.

8. Bluthgen, U. and P. Marquardt. 1950. Therapeutic use and pharmacology of emetine. Pharmazie 5:415-420.

9. Borkowski, B. 1960. Diuretic action of several flavone drugs. Planta Med. 8:95-104.

10. Borkowski, B. and K. Szpunar. 1960. Spasmolytic effects of some natural flavonoids. Pharm. Zentralhalle 99:280-284.

11. Boyd, E.M. and L. M. Knight. 1964. The expectorant action of cephaline, emetine, and 2-dehydroemetine. J. Pharm. Pharmacol. 12:118-124.

12. Buck, W.B., R.F. Keeler, and W. Binns. 1966. Some pharmacologic effects of *Veratrum* alkaloids in sheep and goats. Am. J. Vet. Res. 27:140-154.

13. Buultoi, N. P. 1966. The problem of chemotherapy in prediabetes. Hypoglycemic effects of aromatic and heterocyclic acids. Med. Pharmacol. Exptl. 14:576-584.

14. Claus, E.P. and V.E. Tyler, Jr. 1965. *Pharmacognosy*. 5th Ed. Lea and Febiger, Philadelphia. p. 45.

15. Cotten, M. deV. and R. P. Walton. 1951. The nature of the cardiac stimulation produced by veratrine alkaloids. Arch. Intern. Pharmacodynamie 87:473-492.

16. Courzis, J.T. and R.O. Bauer. 1951. Effect of *Veratrum* derivatives on the isolated intestine of the rabbit and on the intact intestine of the trained, unanesthetized dog. J. Pharmacol. Exp. Ther. 103:471-478.

17. Covello, M., O. Schettino, M.I. LaRotonda, and P. Forgione. 1970. Chromatographic identification and quantitative determination of anthraquinones of plant origin. Boll. Soc. Ital. Biol. Sper. 46:500-503.

18. DeCarneri, I. 1970. Drug sensitivity of Hartmannella and *Naegleria*, causative agents of meningoencephalitis. Riv. Parasitol. 31:1-8.

19. Dipalma, J.R. and J.J. Lambert. 1948. Importance of the methoxy group in antifibrillation compounds. Science 107:66-68.

20. Duquenois, B. 1957. Caffeic acid and its esters (chlorogenic acid, etc.) considered as antibacterial of native plant origin. Acad. Natl. Med. 141:71-74.

21. Endo, K., M. Tamada, C. Konno, H. Hikino, and C. Kabuto. 1979. Structures of ephedradines, hypotensive principles of *Ephedra* roots. Koen Yoshishu-Tennen Yuki Kagobutsu Toronkai 22:517-524.

22. Farrell, K.W. and L. Wilson. 1984. Tubulin-colchicine complexes diferentially poison opposite microtubule ends. Biochemistry 23:3741-3748.

23. Fleming, W.W. and D.F. Hawkins. 1965. *Veratrum* alkaloids XXXVIII. The effects of L-ethomoxane and of veratramine on isolated mammalian and invertebrate hearts and on the isolated guinea pig ileum. J. Pharmacol. Exp. Ther. 148:218-224.

24. Fries, E.D., J.R. Stanton, and F.C. Maister. 1950. Assay in man of the chemical fractions of *Veratrum* viride, and identification of the pure alkaloids germitrine and germidine as potent hypotensive principles derived from the drug. J. Pharm. Exp. Ther. 98:166-173.

25. Gennaro, A.R., D. Chase, M.R. Gibson, C.B. Grandberg, S.C. Harvey, R.E. King, A.N. Martin, T. Medwick, E.A. Swinyard, and G.L. Zinc, eds. 1985. *Remington's Pharmaceutical Sciences*, 17th Ed. Mack Pub., Easton, PA.

26. Gillespie, E., R.J. Levine, and S.E. Malawista. 1968. Histamine release from rat peritoneal mast cells: inhibition by colchicine and potentiation by deuterium oxide. J. Pharmacol. Exp. Ther. 164:158-165.

27. Guillaume, V. and H. Morin. 1969. Pharmacological effects of chlorogenic acid. Colleg. Inst. Chim. Cafes Verts, Torrefies Leurs Deriv. 4:248-253.

28. Gyermek, L. 1951. The cholinergic blocking substances, site of action. Acta. Physiol. Acad. Sci. Hung. 2:511-517.

29. Harada, M. and Nishimura, M. 1981. Contribution of alkaloid fraction topressor and hyperglycemic effect of crude *Ephedra* extract in dogs. J. Pharmacobio-Dyn. 4:691-699.

30. Harashi, Y. 1959. Histamine receptor of the guinea pig small intestine from the standpoint of the curve analysis of drug antagonism. Kobe Ike. Daigakukiyo 16:172-184.

31. Hartwell, J.L., M.J. Shear, J.M. Johnson, and S.R.L. Kornberg. 1946. Selection and synthesis of organic compounds (for action against tumors in mice). Cancer Res. 6:489 (proceedings).

32. Hava, M. and I. Janku. 1958. Bronchodilator action of apigenin. Arch. Intern. Pharmacodynamie 117:23-29.

33. Hicks, N.M. 1964. The effect of uremic blood constituents on certain cerebral enzymes. Clin. Chim. Acta 9:228-235.

34. Hikino, H., C. Konno, H. Takata, and M. Tamada. 1980. Studies on the constituents of Ephedra. VI. Anti-inflammatory principle of *Ephedra* herbs. Chem. Pharm. Bull. 28:2900-2904.

35. Horsfall, G. and S. Rich. 1951. Fungi toxicity of heterocyclic nitrogencompounds. Contrib. Boyce Thompson Inst. 16:313-347.

36. Hotovy, R. 1954. The pharmacology of belladonine. Arzneimittel-Forsch. 4:287-292.

37. Inoue, K. 1957. A quantitative study of histamine release by chemical substances, using minced tissue of guinea pig lung. Nippon Yakurigaku Zasshi 53:797-818.

38. Janku, I. 1957. Apigenin, a spasmolytic substance from *Matricaria chamomilla*. Compt. Rend. Soc. Biol. 151:241.

39. Jequier, R., D. Branceni, and N. Peterfalvi. 1955. Antimitotic activity and toxicity of certain derivatives of colchicine and of thiocolchicine. Arch. Inter. Pharmacodyn. 103:243-255.

40. Jobin, F. and F. Tremblay. 1969. Platelet reactions and immune processes. II. Inhibition of platelet aggregation by complement inhibitors. Thromb. Diath. Haemorrh. 22:466-481.

41. Kanno, T. 1956. The central and vomiting actions of *Veratrum* ester alkaloids. Yonazo Izaku Zasshi 7:407-429.

42. Karp, D. 1948. Effect of quinine and atabrin on gastric secretory function in dogs. Rev. Can. Biol. 7:508-531.

43. Koltai, M. and E. Minkey. 1969. Effect of various nucleic acids and protein synthesis inhibitors on anaphylactoid inflammation in rats. J. Pharmacol. 6:175-182.

44. Krayer, O. 1950. *Veratrum* alkaloids. XII. A quantitative comparison of the antiaccelerator cordis action of veratramine, veratrosine, jervine, and pseudojervine. J. Pharmacol. Exp. Ther. 98:427-436.

45. Kriegar, G. 1952. Comparative determinations of the tannin content of various drugs. Deut. Apoth. Ztg. Ver. Süddeut. Apoth.-Ztg. 92:849-851.

46. Lambin, S. and J. Bernard. 1953. Sterility test of injectable official alkaloid solutions. Ann. Pharm. Fran. 11:336-346.

47. Laubender, W. and H. Ballmaier. 1965. Differences in the effects of galenic preparation and pure alkaloids of belladonna leaves. Arzneimittel-Forsch. 15:905-910.

48. Lewis, R.A. 1946. Enteric infections and their sequelae. N.E.J. Med. 235:571-581.

49. Luduena, F.P. 1938. Pharmacology of cryptopine. Rev. Soc. Argentina Biol. 14:339-352.

50. Maison, G.L., E. Gotz, and J.W. Stutzman. 1951. Relative hypotensive activity of certain *Veratrum* alkaloids. J. Pharmacol. Exp. Ther. 103:74-78.

51. Marchetti, G. 1954. Action of two new alkaloids from *Veratrum viride* on the circulatory apparatus. Arch. Ital. Soc. Farmacol. 4:15-27.

52. Meilman, E. 1953. Clinical studies on *Veratrum* alkaloids. III. The effect of protoveratrine on renal function in man. J. Clin. Invest. 32:80-89.

53. Mercier, F. 1938. Action of cryptine on the isolated intestine. Compt. Rend. Soc. Biol.127:1018-1022.

54. Mercier, J. and E. Mercier. 1955. Action of some secondary alkaloids of opium on the electrocardiogram of the dog. Compt. Rend. Soc. Biol. 149:760-762.

55. Moran, N.C., M.E. Perkins, and A.P. Richardson. 1954. Veratridine blockade of the carotid sinus pressor receptors. J. Pharmacol. Exp. Ther. 111:459-468.

56. Nada, M.-J. 1957. Cardiac and vascular action of luteolin in animals. Arzneimittel-Forsch. 7:442-445.

57. Ng, K.K.F. 1966. A new pharmacological action of emetine. Brit. Med. J.1(5498):1278-1279.

58. Nicola, P. De and D. Fumarola. 1959. Action of cytostatic drugs on antibody production. Arzneimittel-Forsch. 9:27-30.

59. Oelkers, H.A. 1962. Studies on anthelmintics. Arzneimittel-Forsch. 123:810-812.

60. Radomski, J.L., E.C. Hagan, H.N. Fuyat, and A.A. Nelson. 1952. Pharmacology of ipecac. Pharmacol. Exp. Ther. 104:421-426.

61. Rosztoczy, I. 1969. Effect of emetine on the multiplication of *Pseudoralies* and *Semliki* forest viruses and on the interferon production by cultured cells. Acta Microbiol. 16:227-235.

62. Ryakhovskii, V.V. and T.A. Seidakhanova. 1971. Properties of leucoanthocyanidins from *Polygonum* species and *Ephedra* species. Tr. Inst. Fiziol., akad. Nauk Kaz. SSR 16:28-32. [Chem. Abstr. 76:94604].

63. Shibata, S. and M. Harada. 1960. Constituents of Japanese and Chinese crude drugs. Antispasmodic action of flavonoids and anthraquinones. Yakugaku Zasshi 80:620-624.

64. Shoji, R. and S. Makino. 1966. Preliminary notes on the teratogenic and embryocidal effects of colchicine on mouse embryos. Proc. Jap. Acad. 42:822-827.

65. Shoji, S. 1960. Constituents of Japanese and Chinese crude drugs—antispasmodic action of flavonoids and anthraquinones. Yakugaku Zasshi 80:620-624.

66. Sirtori, C., P. Truffini, and F. Talamazzi. 1952. Evaluation of certain antimitotic substances. Cong. Intern. Biochim., 2e Cong., Paris. p. 841.

67. Sneddon, J.M. 1971. Effect of mitosis inhibitors on blood platelet microtubules and aggregation. J. Physiol. 214:145-158.

68. Steinegger, E., D. Sonanini, and K. Tsingaridas. 1964. The Solanaceae flavones. IV. Constitution of glycosides C and F from belladonna leaves. Pharm. Acta Helv. 39:450-456.

69. Swain, H.H. and D.A. McCarthy. 1957. Veratrine, protoveratrine, and andromedotoxin arrhythmias in the isolated frog heart. J. Pharmacol. Exp. Ther. 121:379-388.

70. Swiss, E.D. and G.L. Maison. 1952. The site of cardiovascular action of *Veratrum* derivatives. J. Pharmacol. Exp. Ther. 105:87-95.

71. Tamada, M., K. Endo, and H. Hikino. 1978. Studies on the constituents of *Ephedra*. II. Maokonine, hypertensive principle of *Ephedra* roots. Planta Med. 34:291-293.

72. Tanaka, K. 1955. *Veratrum* alkaloids. XX. Actions of *Veratrum* alkaloids on the central nervous system of mice. J. Pharmacol. Exp. Ther. 113:89-99.

73. Taraskina, K.V., T.K. Chumbalov, L.N. Chekmeneva, and T. Chukenova. 1973. Polyphenols of some species of *Ephedra*. Fenol'nye Soedin. Ikh. Fiziol. Svoistva, Mater. Vses. Simp. Fenol'nym Soedin., 2nd 1971. [Chem. Abstr. 81:166323].

74. Theobald, W. 1955. The anti-inflammatory action of drugs on formalin edema in the rat. Arch Intern. Pharmacodyn. 103:17-20.

75. Thomas, S. 1967. Reflex increase in urine flow by veratridine. Quart. J. Exp. Physiol. 52:313-318.

76. Toth, C.E., M. Ferrari, A.R. Contessa, and R. Santi. 1966. Mechanism of spasmolytic action of some isoquinoline drugs. Arch. Intern. Pharmacol. Therap. 162:123-139.

77. Tyler, V.E., L.R. Brady, and J.E. Robbers. 1981. *Pharmacognosy*, 8th Ed. Lea and Febiger, Philadelphia.

78. Ullsperger, R. 1953. The mode of action of a new active body from hawthorn and of several pure anthocyanins. Pharmazie 8:923-926.

79. Vacher, J., P. Duchene-Marullaz, and P. Barbot. 1964. About some common products. Comparison of two methods of evaluation of analgesics. Med. Exptl. 11:51-58.

80. Vincent, D. and G. Segonzac. 1956. Antiacetylcholine and spasmolytic action of apoatropine. Arch. Intern. Pharmacodyn. 105:136-144.

81. Wallace, H.O. 1963. Inhibition of human plasma cholinesterase in vitro by alkaloids, glycosides, and other neutral substances. Lloydia 11:36-43.

82. Wallace, S.L. 1959. Colchicine analogues in the treatment of acute gout. Arthritis Rheumatism 2:389-395.

83. Weisenborn, F.L. 1954. Synthetic hypotensive esters from germine. J. Am. Chem. Soc. 76:1792-1795.

84. Wilhelmi, G. 1964. The analgesic effects of anti-inflammatory drugs from the point of view of different pharmacological test methods. Acta Med. Okayama 18:297-310.

85. Williams, A.W. 1963. Experimental production of altered jejunal mucosa. J. Pathol. Bacteriol. 85:467-472.

86. Windholz, M., S. Badawari, R.F. Blumetti, and E.S. Otterbein, Eds. 1983. *Merck Index*, 10th Ed. Merck and Co., Rahway, NJ.

87. Wolfgang, A.L. and H. Joachim. 1956. Papaveraceae alkaloids and eye pressure. Monatsbl. Augenheilk. 128:686-705.

88. Yukio, K. 1957. Quantitative study of histamine release by chemical substances, using minced tissue of guinea pig lung. Yakurigaku Zashi 53:836-849.

89. Zipf, H.F., E.C. Dittmann, and H. Marquardt. 1963. Local and endoanesthetic effects of tropeines. Arzneimittel-Forsch. 13:1097-1100.

Vegetative Propagation of Aromatic Plants of the Mediterranean Region

Michael Raviv
Department of Ornamental Horticulture, Agricultural Research Organization, Newe Ya'ar Experiment Station, Haifa, Israel

Eli Putievsky
Department of Medicinal, Aromatic and Spice Plants, Agricultural Research Organization, Newe Ya'ar Experiment Station, Haifa, Israel

CONTENTS

I. INTRODUCTION

Vegetative propagation has been used in plant production since early historical times. One of the first Western accounts of this standard horticultural technique is in reference to Noah and the biblical phrase "He planted a vineyard" (Genesis 9:20) following the "world-wide" flood. The source of grapes, figs, and olives of the vineyard is assumed to be cuttings Noah carried with him on the Ark. As early as 1633, Gerarde (33) wrote about tarragon in his reference, *The Herbal or General Historie of Plant*, that "the root is long and fibrous, creeping farre abroad under the earth ... by which sprouting forth is increaseth." This description clearly refers to the possibility of propagation by division, a technique still used for tarragon and for many other aromatic plant species.

Vegetative propagation of plants has served and continues to serve as an important means of plant production for aromatic plants such as scented geranium (*Pelargonium* spp.), lavender (*Lavandula* spp.), lemon balm (*Melissa officinalis* L.), mint (*Mentha* spp.), marjoram or oregano (*Origanum* spp.), rosemary (*Rosmarinus officinalis* L.), sage (*Salvia* spp.), and thyme (*Thymus* spp.). The objective of this review is to examine the utilization and importance of vegetative propagation as related to aromatic plant production in the Mediterranean region.

A. Basis of Vegetative Propagation

The genetic information encoded in the deoxyribonucleic acid (DNA) of all cells of an organism is considered to be uniform, allowing a cell or group of cells removed from a parent organism to form, through regeneration processes, a completely new organism that normally would be identical to the original parent (70). This asexual production of new plants, identical to a "mother plant," is termed vegetative propagation with the descendants of the "mother plant" known as clones. Although plants, even within the same species, differ greatly in their regeneration ability (93), cloning allows the rapid increase in plant material having desirable chemical and horticultural characteristics. Clones that become horticulturally important are termed cultivars and are named according to the International Code of Nomenclature Cultivated Plants (10).

Although methods for vegetative propagation of plants differ, the unifying principle in all methods is the regeneration of plants by mitosis. This process almost always begins with the formation of adventitious roots on the parent material followed by development of vegetative tissue (41). Current horticultural techniques for vegetative propagation include:

1. rooting of stem, leaf, or root cuttings;

2. grafting and budding;

3. layering, stool bedding, and other methods that regenerate tissue from parts attached to "mother plants";

4. planting of bulbs, corms, rhizomes, stolons, suckers, off-shoots, or other vegetative parts that serve for plant propagation in nature;
5. culturing of sterile selections of cells, tissues, or organs.

Of these techniques, rooting of cuttings, planting of vegetative parts, and *in vitro* culturing of sterile selections are the important vegetative propagation techniques used with aromatic plants.

The main advantage of asexual, as compared with sexual, propagation comes from the homogeneity that characterizes the offspring of vegetatively propagated plants. One of the preconditions to the development of modern agricultural and marketing systems has been the domestication of plant species with uniform development. Optimizing crop production during a growing season requires successful application of cultural tasks such as irrigation, fertilization, pest control, growth regulation application, and mechanical harvesting to fields where the majority of plants are at an identical, well-defined stage of growth. Uniformity of size, color, taste, smell, and other qualities of the desired plant product (fruit, leaf, root, essential oil, or other component), determined by the genome of the plant, is needed to provide processors and consumers with a defined product, particularly when the plant material is used for industrial purposes. Only a relatively few crop species have either the pure lines or the properties that will propagate through an F_1-hybrid to ensure uniformity. The offspring of a heterozygous genotype via sexual propagation generally maintain a high level of growth variability. This characteristic is especially noticeable with most aromatic plants that have not been subjected to long-term breeding programs, leaving high levels of heterogeneity that produce non-uniform populations.

In many instances, plant cultivars cannot be propagated by seeds, making vegetative propagation the only possible means of reproducing these plants. Selected examples of this situation include cultivars of *Mentha spicata* L. (for example, cv. 'Micham') and lavandin (*Lavandula angustifolia* Mill. x *Lavandula latifolia* Medic.) that were obtained by chromosome duplication through interspecies hybridization. Other aromatic plant species such as ginger (*Zingiber officinale* Roscoe) and lemongrass (*Cymbopogon citratus* [DC. ex Nees] Stapf and *Cymbopogon Nardus* [L.] Rendle) do not regularly produce seeds when transferred to locations different from their natural habitats. In some cases, such as with lavender (*Lavandula* spp.), rosemary (*Rosmarinus officinalis* L.), *Origanum* spp., and other slow-growing perennial herbs, the vegetative propagation is more rapid and economical than the sexual propagation. Vegetative propagation tends to shorten the juvenile period and hence induce precocity, a phenomenon that has been observed with *Lavandula* spp. and *Origanum* spp.

There are disadvantages to establishing horticultural uniformity with vegetative propagation. Under acute environmental stress situations like frost, flooding, or pest epidemics, entire crops can potentially be destroyed because all plants are equally susceptible. A heterogenous population established with different genotypes under the same environmental stress may well have resistant specimens that survive. In addition, vegetative propagation from the same parent plant material does not always ensure complete uniformity of development as the morphological form and metabolic response, including essential oil synthesis, are a result of the interaction between the genotype and the ecological growing conditions. Clone aging, considered an inevitable, detrimental problem of vegetatively propagated plants in the past, is now attributed to the accumulation of various intercellular pathogens (6) for which known *in vitro* procedures can be routinely used to clean the infected plant material. None of these problems need to interfere with the agricultural value of uniform plant material, but suggest that professionals and growers must be aware of such circumstances during the early stages of introduction and selection of new crops.

Mutations that occur during the mitotic process are a relatively rare event but can be expected periodically. These types of mutation, termed somatic mutations or sports, have, in most cases, a negligible effect and are generally easily eliminated by selection during propagation. Somatic mutations, however, may occasionally be valuable for the plant breeder, leading to the development of new cultivars, such as those of the various *Mentha* spp. In these situations, vegetative propagation may be the only way to conserve the desired mutation (45, 75, 76, 77, 110).

Steps to achieve production of true-to-type, pathogen-free plant material include:

1. using only individual plants that meet all characteristics typical of the cultivar as parent material for propagation;
2. using only healthy plants as sources of propagation material and having appropriate checks conducted at regular intervals to prevent the introduction of infected plant material into propagation and to trace any latent contamination appearing in offspring;
3. using only plants that have been cleared of pathogens and that have been maintained in growing conditions that prevent recontamination.

B. Aspects of Regeneration

A drastic shift from the usual predetermined sequence of cellular activities is necessary before a differentiated adult cell in a vegetative cutting will or can initiate the cellular division and organization into the new organs necessary for successful vegetative propagation. While the control of gene expression is exercised at several levels, including the rate of transcription, the rate of RNA processing and transport, the stability of RNA, and the rate of translation and post-translational modifications, changes in these activities can be triggered and/or modified by exogenous factors. A relevant example of a triggering episode is the separation of a cutting from a "mother plant" and the subsequent loss to the cutting of a regular supply of water, minerals, growth hormones, and, in some cases, photosynthate. To survive, the new cutting must alter cellular gene expression to regenerate and compensate for lost tissue. In an unknown but crucial manner, the signal for regeneration and the metabolic adjustments to alleviate immediate stress must be coordinated to enable tissue to initiate and continue regeneration until the process is complete.

The sequence of events leading to adventitious root formation, detailed by Haissig (37), begins with dedifferentiation, a process where a predifferentiated cell becomes meristematic with vigorous cell division. The newly formed cells are small, dense, isodiametric, and without vacuoles, but, following a few cell divisions, congregate into a dome-like root primordium resembling the shape of a root cap. As the dome approaches final size (in terms of number of cells), a connection develops between the root primordium and the plant vascular system. Subsequently (and sometimes simultaneously) primordium formed by dedifferentiated internal cells elongate outward towards the external surface of the tissue. The emergence of the root primordia at the tissue surface may be slowed or stopped by a hard, lignous, sclerenchyma layer (23). In some plants like oregano, the growing roots tear and penetrate the external layer of cells, while in other plants, like carnations, the growing root primordia turn downward and exit through the base of the cutting. Indeed, the cutting of the tissue surface during vegetative propagation may facilitate rooting by providing an opportunity for adventitious roots to grow outside the plant when a schlerenchyma cell layer acts as a mechanical barrier (93).

Stems of many plants, especially of the *Lamiaceae* (formerly *Labiatae*) family, contain preformed root primordia. In these cases, cuttings are usually easy to root as rooting is merely an elongation of the root primordia. This phenomenon is demonstrated through observations on the rooting ability of oregano stem cuttings with or without preformed root primordia as reported by Kuris *et al.* (56) (Table 1). Auxin application readily promoted rooting in cuttings with preformed root primordia but had no promotive effect on cuttings without preformed roots.

The anatomical site of root primordium formation is different in various types of plants. Herbaceous plants generally originate root primordia in parenchymatic tissues adjacent to vascular elements, from the pericycle, or, in some instances, from the epidermis and lateral buds. Woody plants produce adventitious roots in several areas includ-

TABLE 1. Development of Roots in Oregano Stem Cuttings as Related to Preformed Root Primordia

Treatment	Roots/Cutting*
Cuttings with preformed roots	
Control	3.5 ± 1.4
IBA, 1000 mg/l	11.4 ± 2.6
IAA, 1000 mg/l	9.3 ± 2.1
IAA, 2000 mg/l	11.1 ± 2.0
Cuttings without preformed roots	
Control	4.2 ± 1.5
IBA, 1000 mg/l	3.5 ± 1.3
IAA, 500 mg/l	5.1 ± 1.6
IAA, 2000 mg/l	1.7 ± 0.8

* Mean ± S.E. at 7 days after planting. Adapted from Kuris et al. (56).

ing the cambium, wound callus, and bud phloem. Monocotyledons form adventitious roots in perivascular positioned parenchyma cells.

II. THE REGENERATION PROCESS

A. Selection of Plant Material

The juvenile and adult phases of plant development differ distinctly in their ability to be rooted. The most common distinction between the 2 phases is that juvenile plants are easier to root than adult plants. Returning the difficult-to-root species to a juvenile stage of growth will generally greatly facilitate rooting of plant cuttings. This rejuvenation can be aided by gibberellin treatments (99) or by growing new shoots from etiolated parts of a plant (29). Shoots developing leaves while their bases are kept in the dark will behave as juvenile stems and will readily form adventitious roots.

Juvenile characteristics are usually exhibited by the lower parts of perennial plants like bay laurel (Table 2). Severe and repeated pruning of this plant can therefore serve as a means of inducing partial rejuvenation of mature plants. Higher concentrations of rooting promoters have been observed in juvenile lavender cuttings as compared with the respective adult cuttings (46). Further aspects of ontogenetical age and rooting ability have been reviewed by Hackett (36).

TABLE 2. Rooting of Bay Laurel Stem Cuttings as Affected by In-Tree Position

Tree Position	Rooted Cuttings (%)	Number of Roots Per Cutting
Upper	29 a*	1.4 b
Lower	51 b	2.4 b

* Means followed by the same letter within a column do not differ significantly at $P \leq 0.01$ using Duncan's Multiple Range Test.

Generally, vegetative cuttings from vigorous, well-fertilized plants have the greatest rooting potential. As the regeneration processes are energy consuming, the availability of carbohydrate reserves near the site of cell division is necessary (116). The initial starch level is particularly significant in cuttings that do not photosynthesize simultaneously with regeneration and thus can only utilize pre-existing reserves. A low starch content within a cutting usually results in poor regeneration (123). The carbohydrate requirement of a cutting can be fulfilled in some cases by soaking the plant material in a concentrated sucrose solution (up to 5%) (61) or, alternatively, girdling the stem prior to excision, allowing the accumulation of carbohydrates in the shoot (111). In cuttings that can maintain active photosynthesis, environmental conditions that promote the accumulation of photosynthate will enhance rooting (67).

In some cases, like with sage, removal of flower buds will considerably improve rooting of cuttings (92). This undoubtedly reflects the reduction in the intensive photosynthate consumption and a change in the hormonal balances seasonally associated with the flowering process that reduce the ability of a cutting to root. Some negative seasonal effects may be reduced by continuously maintaining pruned "mother plants" and by growing the "mother plants" within a daylength- and temperature-controlled greenhouse that regulates photoperiod and temperature.

While most of the evergreens and herbaceous species can best be rooted at the end of a growth cycle when the new flush of growth starts to lignify, deciduous plants may be rooted when dormant and as leafy cuttings under mist. *Lippia* spp., although botanically not a true deciduous plant, has been rooted in our laboratory as a "dormant" leafless cutting or as leafy cutting. Root cuttings of tarragon can be propagated during dormancy (34). Other more difficult-to-root plants should be rooted during the optimal growth period to take advantage of natural seasonal effects on rooting potential. Studies with *Salvia officinalis* L. indicate rooting is highest in the spring just after the flush of new shoots complete growth and before the beginning of flowering (92). *Laurus nobilis* L. stem cuttings root better in July through August, under Mediterrean conditions, than in any other season, although the optimal rooting period can be extended by bottom heating from May until September (91). Stem cuttings of tarragon can be rooted in the spring and late autumn or while dormant in the winter, but rooting percentage is low in the summer (96).

B. Types of Cuttings

Theoretically, every organ (leaf, stem, and root) of an aromatic plant could, under suitable conditions, be regenerated to form a completely new plant. However, rates of regeneration from different tissues vary, and for practical purposes, more rapid regeneration rates ensure better rooting of cuttings. The abundance of the different organs available for propagation and the ease of their detachment and use must also be considered. For example, root cuttings are normally the most difficult to obtain, and the necessity of maintaining the correct polarity of the root sections make them difficult to use. Therefore, root cuttings are used with only a few aromatic plants, such as *Papaver orientale* L. (41) and French tarragon (*Artemisia dracunculus* L. var. *sativa*) (58, 112).

While leaf cuttings are commonly used for some foliage plants, like *Begonia* and *Peperomia* spp., use with aromatic plants is negligible. This type of vegetative cutting requires a great deal of care, and frequently, shoots are not formed even after a long rooting period (102). Instead, the most commonly used type of cutting in aromatic plant propagation is the stem cutting. Either dormant (leafless) or active (leafy) cuttings can be used, but since all Mediterranean aromatic plants are either herbaceous or evergreens, leafy cuttings (herbaceous, softwood, or semihardwood) are most frequently utilized. The presence of leaves is beneficial for rooting of the leafy cuttings, and up to a critical limit, there appears to be a positive correlation between the number of leaves and the rooting capacity of a cutting (18, 85).

The effects of other tissue properties on rooting, such as degree of lignification, part of stem, or existence of an active terminal bud, need to be studied for each specific plant. Usually, these properties cannot be evaluated separately from other seasonal and environmental factors that prevail during both their formation and rooting. As an example, the observed rooting response of apical and subapical stem sections of tarragon cuttings are similar under favorable conditions, while cuttings from the subapical region, which are less prone to rapid water loss, have a pronounced advantage when rooted in a field limited to 3 irrigations per day (Table 3). Ligneous, subapical stem cuttings of bay laurel have a higher rooting percentage than herbaceous, apical cuttings (Table 4), probably as a result of reduced water deficit that, in the case of bay laurel, may be critical due to the very long rooting period (4 to 5 months) required (93).

TABLE 3. Rooting Conditions and Root Development in Tarragon Cuttings*

Type of Cutting	Field Planting		Mist Planting	
	Rooting %	Roots/Cutting	Rooting %	Roots/Cutting
Apical	65	5.8	95	32.3
Subapical	87	7.9	92	23.7

* The effect of rooting conditions measured one month after planting on subsequent yield have not been determined. Data of Raviv et al. (96).

TABLE 4. The Effect of Plant Material on Rooting of Stem Cuttings from Bay Laurel

Type of Cutting	Rooting (%)	No. of Roots/Cutting
Subapical, lignous	85 a*	4.3 a
Apical, lignous	75 ab	3.6 a
Apical, herbaceous	63 b	3.3 a

* Means followed by the same letter do not differ significantly at P ≤0.01 using Duncan's Multiple Range Test. Data of Raviv et al. (93).

C. Rooting Media

The type of material best used as the rooting medium for various species has been the subject of numerous studies and reviews (80, 88). The rooting media can be classified as soil and soilless substrates. Mainly for economic reasons, but also due to adherence to known traditions, soil was, for many years, the only rooting medium used with aromatic plants throughout the world.

Various types of soils differ greatly in their properties relevant to rooting of cuttings with the most important of these being air space, available water, and hydraulic conductivity. Since rooting, as an energy-consuming process, is dependent upon adequate oxygen supply for respiration, the rate of air penetration into the large pores of the soil has a profound effect on the metabolic activity of the section of the cutting producing the adventitious roots. Under the frequent irrigations that are mandatory to avoid dessication prior to the root emergence, the drainage capacity of the soil determines when anaerobic conditions develop.

Optimal values for air and water in growth media for propagation have been determined by De Boodt and Verdonck (19) as 20 to 30 percent air and 50 to 60 percent water on a volumetric basis. Unfortunately, the optimal levels of both air and water probably cannot exist simultaneously in any soil. In addition, special situations or plant material may require adjustment of the air-to-water ratio. Where frequent watering of cuttings is required, even a higher percentage of air space generally promotes root development. Both root initiation and elongation in *Pelargonium graveolens* L'Her. ex Ait. cuttings are significantly higher in well-aerated media such as peat, perlite, or a mixture of these media, but few roots develop in local soil that has less air space (4). In a similar manner, the rooting of bay laurel cuttings is known to be affected by the amount of air space in the medium (89).

Soilless substances are being used to overcome the inherent disadvantages of soils. Optimal contents of air, water, and nutrient levels can be achieved in the soilless substrates almost immediately following irrigation due to the high hydraulic conductivity, the high total porosity, and the desired distribution of small and large pores.

D. Use of Hormones

The involvement of plant hormones in regeneration processes was one of the first growth regulator activities to be discovered (114). The native auxin, indole-3-acetic acid (IAA), has been identified as a natural rooting promoter. Nevertheless, our understanding of the mode of action of hormones in regeneration processes is still fragmentary, probably due to the many hormonal requirements that need to be satisfied

(41). Stem cuttings of bay laurel excised during the winter, a season characterized by low rootability, can serve as a good example of multiple hormone requirements. Auxin, at concentrations as high as one percent in talc powder, failed to promote root initiation as compared with the nontreated control (93).

No promotive role in differentiation has been reported for any of the known plant hormones, and early assumptions about the involvement of auxin as the causative agent in the change of mature cells to meristematic cells have been dismissed (38, 47, 95). Other natural rooting promoters are now suggested as the dedifferentiation agents in cuttings (65, 94, 118). These natural rooting promoters belong to various chemical groups and include the bicyclic diterpene portulal (124), an aliphatic rooting compound from avocado consisting of 17 carbons (87), and a dihydrocholesterol rooting promoter extracted from *Picea* species (118). However, no convincing evidence concerning the generality of action for these compounds exists.

The primary mediators of various morphogenetic processes are suggested by Albersheim and Darvill (3) to be oligosaccharins, secreted by damaged cells. However, investigations with wounded tomato leaf tissues indicate these compounds are not translocated (9) and thus cannot be regarded as a long-distance wound hormone initiating dedifferentiation. These oligosaccharins may stimulate the dispatch of a second, more soluble messenger that initiates the dedifferentiation.

The second and third stages of primordium formation are positively affected by auxins. Either natural auxin flowing from the buds and young leaves to a base of a cutting or synthetic auxins [such as indole-butyric acid (IBA) and naphthalene acetic acid (NAA)] exogenously applied to the base of a cutting will stimulate root formation (39). While external application of IAA does not consistently lead to increased rooting, due to rapid oxidation of the auxin in plant tissues by the enzyme IAA-oxidase, the more difficult to metabolize synthetic auxins, which are widely used in aromatic plant propagation, increase rooting percentages (52, 53, 79) and early establishment of cuttings (55). IBA and NAA are the most useful compounds for this purpose (Table 5).

More recently, the action of auxin in rooting has been explained through the stimulatory effects the compound has on ethylene formation in tissue (1, 98, 100). Presumably, the wounding at the base of a cutting may also facilitate rooting via induction of wound ethylene production (98). Ethylene has also been previously associated with adventitious root formation observed with waterlogged plants (113, 119).

The relationship of auxin and ethylene in promoting root formation, however, remains unclear. No correlation between ethylene or auxin-induced ethylene formation and rooting has been observed (8, 33, 69). Nordstrom and Eliasson (73) report that auxin-induced ethylene formation exerts a negative effect on rooting of pea stem cuttings, and very high concentrations of auxin are required to counteract this

TABLE 5. The Use of Rooting Hormones in Aromatic Plant Propagation

Species	Rooting Hormone	Concentration	Reference No.
Elsholtzia stauntonii	IAA	1000	74
Lavandula officinalis	IBA	1000	49
	IBA	500	43
Lavandula vera	NAA	500	12
Mentha citrata	IAA	500	53
	IBA	1000	
Pelargonium graveolens	IAA	500	54
	Boric acid	500	17
Pelargonium roseum	IBA	1000	64
Satureja montana	IAA	1000	74
Thymus vulgaris	IAA	500	74

effect. Jackson (44), in a recent review dealing with the responses of plants to soil waterlogging, suggests that both exogenous ethylene and ethylene formed as a response to waterlogging only enhances the emergence of preformed root primordia occurring in plants such as tomato, willow, and many members of the *Lamiaceae* family.

Exogenous applications of cytokinins exert a negative effect on rooting over a wide range of concentrations and at all stages of root formation (107, 122). Gibberellins at high concentrations also hinder the rooting process, but GA_3 can enhance rooting when applied immediately following root initiation (105, 107). Abscisic acid is inhibitory to emergence and elongation of root primordia (122). The role of plant hormones in rooting was most recently viewed by Hartmann and Kester (41).

E. Maintenance of the Propagation Environment

The rooting potential of many plant species changes throughout the year, as the effects of daylength, temperature, irradiance, and humidity alter endogenous hormone content (108), hormone sensitivity (28), and photosynthate accumulation (13, 15). To ensure successful rooting, proper control over the environmental conditions is essential to maintain the plant in a status conducive for rooting. For each of the environmental factors, a determined optimum needs to be established for the plant species, the type of plant material, and the season.

Generally, mineral nutrition appears to be of minimal importance in regard to vegetative propagation. Only the borate ion is known to exert a consistent beneficial effect on rooting (17). Usually, supplying large amounts of nitrogen to stock plants results in the formation of herbaceous, "leggy" new shoots from which cuttings are frequently difficult to root (7). A high content of manganese in the plant tissue may also be deleterious to rooting, probably due to its function as a cofactor for IAA oxidase (97).

The uptake of nutrients by cuttings is negligible prior to root emergence, but the use of mist systems on many rooting benches, can cause considerable leaching of nutrients from the leaves of cuttings (59). In these situations, both foliar sprays with mineral solutions and regular liquid fertilization of cuttings have enhanced root development in aromatic plants (51, 90). The inclusion of slow-release fertilizers in the rooting medium has also been suggested to be advantageous for subsequent establishment of the rooted plant (90). The nutritional aspects of plant propagation have been previously reviewed by Haissig (39).

Although turgidity is indispensable for cell division and hence for root primordium formation, negative water potentials can be measured in the tissue shortly after the detachment of the cutting from the "mother plant," resulting in a decrease of rooting activity (60, 64). While water loss can be minimized by the aid of antitranspirant polymers, by lowering the temperature, or by altering the vapor pressure gradient, decreasing leaf water conductance by these means has not proven effective for promoting rooting under nursery conditions (31, 60, 103). For leafy and softwood cuttings under Mediterranean conditions, intermittent mist serves as an adequate means of maintaining a continuous water film on the leaves, avoiding water loss.

Vegetative cuttings of many Mediterranean plants such as *Melissa officinalis, Rosmarinus officinalis, Salvia officinalis, Salvia fruticosa,* and *Origanum syriaca* that can be propagated directly in the field during the winter will usually root faster and at a higher percentage under indoor propagating conditions where there is less water loss. The removal of the upper, herbaceous part of the stem helps minimize water loss and increases rooting in semihardwood cuttings of sage and laurel under mist (92, 93). Mist propagation of tarragon, as compared with direct field planting of cuttings, results in a higher percentage of cuttings with roots and more roots per cutting (Table 3) (96).

When mist systems are not economical and direct planting usually leads to poor root development, alternative systems such as irrigation to raise the ambient humidity and a shade net to reduce photon flux by 30 to 60 percent can aid in providing more adequate environmental conditions for rooting of aromatics (83). In conditions where the ambient humidity is low, a shaded polyethylene tent will maintain water-saturated air around the cuttings, reducing water loss considerably (60). The inherent disadvantage of these alternatives is a considerable reduction in the amount of photosynthetically active radiation and thus carbohydrate synthesis necessary for cellular energy.

Optimal air and leaf temperatures for rooting aromatic plants are usually very close to the optimal growing temperatures for each specific cultivar, but the rooting medium should be considerably warmer than the air temperature (81, 82). Rapid and efficient rooting of *Origanum vulgare* L., *Salvia officinalis* L., and *Laurus nobilis* L. occurs at a rooting medium temperature of 20°C to 30°C, especially during the winter when, if not heated, both the medium and air temperatures are less than 15°C in the Mediterranean region (83, 91).

III. TISSUE CULTURE IN PROPAGATION OF AROMATIC PLANTS

The development of sterilization techniques in the second half of the 19th century has provided for the emergence of tissue culture—the growing of plant cells, tissues, or organs in nutrient media under aseptic conditions, as a method of propagation of plants. In 1902, Haberlandt (35) was the first to show the possibility of maintaining plant tissues in sterile culture for long periods of time. By the early 1950s, plant tissue culture became a widely used laboratory technique and, following the elucidation of the role of auxins and cytokinins in the differentiation process of unorganized tissues by Skoog and Miller (106), *in vitro* methods became practical for mass propagation of plants.

Propagation of plants using tissue culture is routinely employed with several species to obtain very large numbers of identical plants in a relatively short period of time. Standard methods for the mass propagation of aromatic plants with tissue culture have been suggested for sweet basil (2), turmeric (71), lavender (84), rosemary (14), tarragon (30), fennel (22), and ginger (78). These species can be regenerated from leaf blades (30), shoot tips (22), rhizome sections (78), and various other tissues. The media used in propagation are generally first supplemented with cytokinin to initiate shoot formation and subsequently (through transfer of the new plantlets to a fresh medium) with auxin to initiate root formation.

Propagation via tissue culture also offers a technique for producing aromatic plants free of endopathogens. While the problem of endopathogens is not yet a limiting factor in the production of aromatics, a plethora of endopathogens native to these plants has been described (16, 20, 63), and as the culture intensifies, the importance of obtaining disease-free plants will increase. The more vigorous growth and higher yields exhibited by endopathoge..-free plants via the commercial cleaning procedures and sterile culture techniques used in many countries for propagation of carnations, chrysanthemums, potatoes, strawberries, and other horticultural plants (70). Virus- and mycoplasm-free plantlets in tissue culture have been observed in the laboratory for lavandin (62) and garlic (72).

By growing cells, tissues, or organs for propagation under controlled conditions, the interference of most environmental factors can be minimized. Pathogen-free cultivars and large genetic banks of plant material can be preserved for prolonged periods of time as cell cultures requiring only occasional subculturing under sterile conditions, or, when appropriate systems are developed, as tissue samples stored under cryogenic conditions (117, 121). In addition, plant improvement can be accelerated and facilitated using aseptic tissue culture methods (21, 115) as biochemical (5, 25), morphogenetic (27, 40), and physiological parameters (11, 26, 104, 120) are easily studied under these conditions. Selective pressure in tissue cultures should isolate traits such as cold-hardiness, salt tolerance, and herbicide resistance in a controllable, accurate, rapid, and economical fashion (68, 120). The potential of developing completely homozygous plant material for propagation exists by initiating cell cultures from pollen grains *in vitro* after diploidization (46, 86). The somatic fusion of protoplasts in culture may rapidly yield new and improved cultivars as the production of F_1-plants is avoided and the difficulty of crossing certain plants is eliminated.

While not central to this review, cell and callus cultures may serve as sources for the production of natural compounds having pharmaceutical and industrial value (42, 109). Although this technique is not yet employed commercially, aromatic compounds have been observed to be produced *in vitro* by cell culture of *Salvia miltiorrhiza* (66), callus and tissues of peppermint (49, 50) and coriander (101), and by tissue culture of *Ruta* species (57). The essential oils produced by tissue cultures of *Ruta* species have the same quality as the naturally produced essential oils. Alkaloids are produced *in vitro* by cell cultures of *Papaver* species (24). The production of natural plant chemicals by cell and organ culture offers exciting prospects and opportunities.

IV. CONCLUSIONS AND PERSPECTIVES

Until recently, herbal plant material was primarily collected in the wild. Now, with the increase in cultivation and use of herbal plants, a fundamental understanding of the processes involved in vegetative propagation of aromatic plants is important. Many problems can be anticipated as new herbs or spice plants are domesticated and introduced into culture. These problems include:

1. the nonuniform germination of seeds that extends over long periods of time due to natural inhibitory mechanisms in species collected from wild populations;

2. the difficulty in applying agrotechnical treatments to plants due to differences in age and genetic composition of newly domesticated populations;

3. the potential difference in aromatic characteristics of plants taken from their native habitats and grown under modern agricultural conditions (even if grown within the same geographic area).

The development of successful techniques for vegetative propagation allows for the consistent production of highly uniform plant material. Simultaneously, the processing industry can clearly define product requirements as related to the desired chemical composition. While the completion of a shift to standardized plant may require the consumer to adapt to a presumably slightly different aroma produced by uniform plant materials, the food, fragrance, wine, and pharmaceutical industries will receive well-defined chemotypes instead of crude mixtures that vary from lot to lot and country to country. Striking examples of the benefits that can result from this change are the use of either thymolic or carvacrolic types of clones of oregano rather than the existing mixtures, or the use of clones of *Salvia officinalis* L. that have a high content of α- and β- thujones. Vegetative propagation has an important role in opening up a new era for the herb and spice industry.

V. REFERENCES

1. Abeles, F.B. 1973. *Ethylene in Plant Biology.* Academic Press, Inc., New York. pp. 58-63.

2. Ahuja, A. and S. Grewal. 1982. Clonal propagation of *Ocimum* species by tissue culture. Indian J. Exp. Biol. 20:455-458.

3. Albersheim, P. and A.G. Darvill. 1985. Oligosaccharins. Sci. Am. 253(3):44-50.

4. Altman, A. and D. Freudenberg. 1983. Quality of *Pelargonium graveolens* cuttings as affected by the rooting medium. Sci. Hortic. (Amsterdam) 19:379-385.

5. Aviv, D., E. Krochmal, A. Dantes, and E. Galun. 1981. Biotransformation of monoterpenes by mentha cell lines: conversion of menthone to neomenthal. Planta Med. 42:236-243.

6. Baily, S. 1963. Effect of exocortis and xyloporosis viruses on growth of nucellar grapefruit on different rootstocks. J. Rio Grande Val. Hortic. Soc. 17:180-211.

7. Basu, R.N. and S.K. Ghosh. 1974. Effect of nitrogen nutrition of stock plants of *Justicia gendarussa* L. on the rooting of cuttings. J. Hort. Sci. 49:245-252.

8. Batten, D.J. and M.G. Mullins. 1978. Ethylene and adventitious root formation in hypocotyl segments of etiolated mung bean seedlings. Planta 138: 193-197.

9. Baydoun, E.A.H. and S.C. Fry. 1985. The immobility of pectic substances in injured tomato leaves and its bearing on the identity of wound hormone. Planta 165:269-276.

10. Brickell, C.D., E.G. Voss, A.F. Kelly, F. Schneider, and R.H. Richens, eds., 1980. *International Code of Nomenclature of Cultivated Plants.* (Regnum Vegetable Vol. 104.) Bohn, Scheltema, and Holkema, Utrecht. 72 p.

11. Bricout, J. and C. Paupardin. 1985. The composition of essential oil of *Mentha piperita* L. cultured *in vitro*: influence of several factors on its synthesis. C.R. Acad. Sci. Ser. D. 281:383 (in French).

12. Cen, E.Z. and V.C. Van. 1965. Trials on the propagation and cultivation of *Lavendula vera.* Sborn. Statej. Introd. Akkum. Rast. Peking. 71-85 (in Chinese with English summary).

13. Champagnol, F. 1981. Relation entre la formation de pousse et de racines par une bouture de vigne et la quantite d'amidon. C. R. Seances Acad. Agric. Fr. 67:1398-1405.

14. Chaturvedi, H.C., P. Misra, and M. Sharma. 1984. *In vitro* multiplication of *Rosmarinum officinalis* L. Z. pflanzenphysiol. 113:301-304.

15. Cormack, D.B. and G.C. Bate. 1976. Seasonal changes in carbohydrate levels and rooting efficiency of macadamia. Acta Hort. 57:21-28.

16. Cousin, M.T., J.P. Moreau, and M. Bassino. 1972. Yellow wilt of lavandin: a mycoplasma disease. Actas do III Congresso da Vniao Fitopatologica Mediterranea. Oieras, Portugal. pp. 19-28.

17. Dass, S.M., A.K. Mani, and V. Sampath. 1982. Boron for improved root characters in geranium cuttings. Madras Agr. J. 69:398-399.

18. Dass, S.M., A.K. Mani, and V. Sampath. 1983. Rooting response of geranium cuttings as influenced by number of leaves. Madras Agr. J. 70:347-348.

19. De Boodt, M. and O. Verdonck. 1971. The physical properties of the substrates used in horticulture. Acta Hort. 26:37-44.

20. Debrot, E.A., J.M. Acosta, and R.C. Uzcategui. 1974. Natural infection of *Salvia splendens* with cucumber mosaic virus. Phytopathol Z. 80:193-198.

21. Dore, C., ed. 1980. Application of *in vitro* culture of improvement of culinary plants. Publ. Versailles, France, INRA (in French with English abstract).

22. Du Manoir, J., P. Desmarest, and R. Savssay. 1985. *In vitro* propagation of fennel (*Foeniculum vulgare* Miller). Sci. Hort. 27:15-19.

23. Edwards, R.A. and M.B. Thomas. 1980. Observation on physical barriers to root formation in cutting. Plant Propagator 26:6-8.

24. Eilert, V., W.G.W. Kurz, and F. Constabel. 1985. Stimulation of sanguinarine accumulation in *Papaver somniferum* cell cultures by fungal elicitors. J. Plant Physiol. 119:65-76.

25. Ellis, B.E. 1984. Probing secondary metabolism in plant cell cultures. Can. J. Bot. 62:2912-2917.

26. Ernst, D. and D. Oesterhelt. 1985. Changes of cytokinin nucleotides in an anise cell culture (*Pimpinella anisum* L.) during growth and embryogenesis. Plant Cell Rep. 4:140-143.

27. Ernst, D., D. Oesterhelt, and W. Schafer. 1984. Endogenous cytokinins during embryogenesis in an anise cell culture (*Pimpinella anisum* L.) Planta 161:240-245.

28. Fernqvist, I. 1966. Studies on factors in adventitious root formation. Lant. Ann. 32:109-244.

29. Gardner, F.E. 1937. Etiolation as a method of rooting apple variety stem cuttings. Proc. Am. Soc. Hortic. Sci. 34:323-329.

30. Garland, P. and L.P. Stoltz. 1980. *In vitro* propagation of tarragon. HortScience 15:739.

31. Gay, A.P. and K. Loach. 1977. Leaf conductance changes on leafy cuttings of *Cornus* and *Rhododendron* during propagation. J. Hortic. Sci. 52:509-516.

32. Geneve, R.C. and C.W. Heuser. 1983. The relationship between ethephon and auxin on adventitious root initiation in cuttings of *Vigna radiata* (L.) R. Wilcz. J. Am. Soc. Hortic. Sci. 108:330-333.

33. Gerarde, J. 1633. *The Herbal or General Historie of Plants*. Lib. 2 Chap. Whitakers, London. p. 249.

34. Grieve, M. 1977. *A Modern Herbal*. Penguin Books, Harmondsworth, Middlesex. 839 p.

35. Haberlandt, G. 1902. Culturversuche mit isolierten Pflanzenzellen, Sitzungsbero. Math. Naturwiss. Kl. Keis. Akad. Wiss. Wien, 111:69-92.

36. Hackett, W.P. 1984. Juvenility, phase change and rejuvenation in woody plants. Hort. Rev. 7:109-155.

37. Haissig, B.E. 1974. Origins of adventitious roots. N.Z.J. For. Sci. 4:299-310.

38. Haissig, B.E. 1974. Influence of auxins and auxin synergists on adventitious root primordium initiation and development. N.Z.J. For. Sci. 4:311-323.

39. Haissig, B.E. 1974. Metabolism during adventitious root primordium initiation and development. N.Z.J. For. Sci. 4:324-337.

40. Hara, S., II. Falk, and H. Kleinig. 1985. Starch and triacylglycerol metabolism related to somatic embryogenesis in *Papaver orientale* tissue cultures. Planta 164:303-307.

41. Hartmann, H.T. and D.E. Kester. 1983. *Plant Propagation, Principles and Practice*. 4th ed. Prentice-Hall, Inc., Englewood Cliffs, NJ.

42. Heinstein, P.F. 1985. Future approaches of secondary natural products in plant cell suspension cultures. J. Nat. Prod. 48(1):1-10.

43. Iliev, L., E. Varanov, M. Tsolova, and S. Zlatev. 1984. Improved rooting of lavender cuttings with growth regulators. Rastenievud. Navki. 21:34-38.

44. Jackson, M.B. 1985. Ethylene and responses of plants to soil waterlogging and submergence. Annu. Rev. Plant Physiol. 36:145-174.

45. Jankulov, J.K., T.D. Stoeva, I.N. Ivanov and A.N. Zuzulova. 1979. Production of peppermint oils with new aroma components. C. R. Acad. Bulg. Sci. 32:981-983.

46. Kaio, M., T. Suga, and S. Teoumous. 1980. Effect of 2.4-D and NAA on callus formation and haploid production in anther culture of *Pelargonium roseum.* Mem. Coll. of Agric. Ehime Univ. 24:199-207.

47. Kefford, N.P. 1973. Effect of a hormone antagonist on the rooting of shoot cuttings. Pl. Physiol. 51:214-216.

48. Kireeva, S.A. and A.Z. Bylda. 1973. The physiology of root formation in lavender softwood cuttings. Efirnomaslichnykh kul'tur. 5:35-40 (in Russian).

49. Kireeva, S.A., V.N. Mel'nikov and S.A. Reznikova. 1978. Accumulation of essential oil in callus tissue of peppermint. Fizologiya Rastenil. 25:564-570 (in Russian).

50. Korasawa, D. and S. Shimizu. 1980. Triterpene acid in callus tissues form *Mentha arvensis* var. piperasens Mal. Agric. Biol. Chem. 44:1203-1205.

51. Koseva, D. and R. Decheva. 1972. The effect of endogenous factors on rooting of two lavender varieties. Fiziologia Rastenil. 19:748-751 (in Russian).

52. Kumar, N. and R. Arumugan. 1980. Effect of growth regulators on rooting of rosemary (*Rosmarinum officinalis* L.) Indian Perfum. 24:210-213.

53. Kumar, N., R. Arumagan, S. Sambandamoorthy, and O.S. Kandasamy. 1980. Note on rooting of planting material of Bergamot mint (*Menta citrata* Ehrh.) Indian Perfum. 24:31-35.

54. Kumar, N., R. Arumugan, S. Sambandamoorthy, and O.S. Kandasamy. 1980. Effect of growth regulators on rooting of geranium (*Pelargonium graveolens* L. Herit). Indian Perfum. 24:36-39.

55. Kuris, A., A. Altman, and E. Putievsky. 1980. Rooting and initial establishment of stem cutting of oregano, peppermint and balm. Sci. Hortic. 13: 53-59.

56. Kuris, A., A. Altman, and E. Putievsky. 1981. Vegetative propagation of spice plants: root formation in oregano stem cuttings. Sci. Hortic. 14:151-156.

57. Kuzovkina, I.N., G.A. Kuznetsova, and A.M. Smirnov. 1975. Essential oils in isolated plant tissue culture. Izv. Akad. Nauk. SSSR Biol. 3:377-381 (in Russian).

58. Lammerink, J. 1985. French tarragon propagation. N.Z. Comml. Grow. 40(4):18.

59. Lee, C.I. and H.B. Tukey, Jr. 1971. Effect of intermittent mist on development of fall color in foliage of *Euonymus alatus.* Sieb Compactus. J. Am. Soc. Hortic. Sci. 97:97-101.

60. Loach, K. 1977. Leaf water potential and the rooting of cuttings under mist and polythene. Physiol. Plant. 40:191-197.

61. Loach, K. and D.N. Whalley. 1978. Water and carbohydrate relationships during the rooting of cuttings. Acta Hortic. 79:161-168.

62. Maia, E., B. Bettachini, D. Beck, P. Venard, and N. Maia. 1973. A contribution to improving the state of health of Abrial lavandin. Phytopathol. 2:115-124.

63. Maloy, O.C. and C.B. Skotland. 1969. Diseases of mint. Ext. Circ. Wash. St. Univ. 357:1-4.

64. Michellon, R. 1978. Rose geranium in reunion: intensifying growing and the possibilities of genetic improvement. Agron. Trop. (Maracay, Venez.) 33:80-89 (in French with English abstract).

65. Mitsuhashi, M., H. Shibaoka, and M. Shimokoriyama. 1969. Portulal: a rooting promoting substance in *Portulaca* leaves. Plant Cell Physiol. 10:715-723.

66. Miyasaka, H., M. Nasu, T. Yamanoto, and K. Yoneda. 1985. Production of ferruginol by cell suspension culture of *Salvia miltiorrhiza*. Phytochemistry 24:1931-1933.

67. Molnar, J.M. and W.A. Cumming. 1968. Effect of carbon dioxide on propagation of softwood, conifer and herbaceous cuttings. Can. J. Plant Sci. 48: 595-599.

68. Mossner, H. and F.C. Czygan. 1978. Tissue cultures and their importance in the breeding and cultivation of medicinal plants. Acta Hortic. 73:45-57.

69. Mudge, K.W. and B.T. Swanson. 1978. Effect of ethephon, IBA and treatment solution pH on rooting and on ethylene levels within mung bean cuttings. Pl. Physiol. 61:271-273.

70. Murashige, T. 1974. Plant propagation through tissue cultures. Ann. Rev. Plant Physiol. 25:135-166.

71. Nadgauda, R.S., A.F. Mascarenhas, R.R. Hender, and V. Jagannathan. 1978. Rapid multiplication of turmeric (*Curcuma longa* Linn) plants by tissue culture. Indian J. Exp. Biol. 16:120-122.

72. Nome, S.F., A. Abril, and R. Racca. 1981. Obtaining virus free garlic plants by apical meristem culture. Phyton. (Buenos Aires) 41:139-151.

73. Nordstrom, A.-C. and L. Eliasson. 1984. Regulation of root formation by auxin-ethylene interaction in pea stem cuttings. Physiol. Plant. 61:298-302.

74. Novikov, P.G. and I.G. Kapelev. 1983. Propagation of some essential oil-bearing plants of the *Labiateae* family by softwood cuttings. Byull. Gos. Nikitsk. Bot. Sada. 50:60-63 (in Russian with English abstract).

75. Ono, A. 1970. Studies on radiation breeding in the genus *Mentha*. VI. Dose response curve for root growth and interspecific in radiosensitivity. Sci. Rep. Fac. Agric. Okayama Univ. 35:1-6.

76. Ono, S. and N. Ikeda. 1970. Studies on radiation in the genus *Mentha*. VII. Sensitivity to rust in radiation induced varieties of Japanese mint. Sci. Rep. Fac. Agric. Okayama Univ. 35:7-10.

77. Ono, S. and N. Ikeda. 1970. Studies on radiation in the genus *Mentha*. VIII. The relationship between the water content of mint seeds and their sensitivity to different doses of γ-rays. Sci. Rep. Fac. Agric. Okayama Univ. 36:13-18.

78. Pillai, S.K. and K.B. Kumar. 1982. Note on the clonal multiplication of ginger *in vitro*. Indian J. Agr. Sci. 52:397-399.

79. Pillay, V.S., A.B.M. Ali, and K.C. Chandy. 1982. Effect of 3-indole butyric acid on root initiation and development in stem cuttings of pepper (*Piper nigrum* L.). Indian Cocoa, Areconut & Spices Journal 6:7-9.

80. Poole, R.T., C.A. Conover, and J.N. Joiner. 1981. Soils and potting mixtures. *In* J.N. Joiner, ed., *Foliage Plant Production*. Prentice-Hall, Inc., Englewood Cliffs, NJ. pp. 179-202.

81. Putievsky, E. 1983. Temperature and day-length influences on the growth and germination of sweet basil and oregano. J. Hortic. Sci. 58:113-117.

82. Putievsky, E. 1983. Effect of day-length and temperature on growth and yield components of three seed species. J. Hortic. Sci. 58:271-275.

83. Putievsky, E., M. Raviv, D. Sanderovich, and R. Ron. 1983. Vegetative propagation of three aromatic plants. Hassadeh 63:1148-1150 (in Hebrew with English abstract).

84. Quazi, M.H. 1980. *In vitro* multiplication of *Lavandula* spp. Ann. Bot. 45:361-362.

85. Rao, D.R., M.R. Narayana, and R.S.G. Rao. 1972. Optimum foliage as an important factor in the rooting of *Pelargonium graveolens* cuttings. Lal Baugh. 17:14-18.

86. Rashid, A. and H.E. Street. 1973. The development of haploid embryoids from anther cultures of *Atropa belladonna* L. Planta 113:263-270.

87. Raviv, M., D. Becker, and Y. Sahali. 1986. Chemical identification of root promoters in avocado tissue. Plant Growth Reg. (In press).

88. Raviv, M., Y. Chen, and Y. Inbar. 1986. Peat and peat substitutes as growth media for container grown plants. *In* Chen, Y. and Y. Avnimelech, eds., *Organic Matter in Modern Agriculture*. Martinus-Nijhof/Dr. W. Junk Publ., The Hague. pp. 255-287.

89. Raviv, M. and E. Putievsky. 1984. Rooting of bay laurel cuttings: rooting media and fungicidal treatments. Hassadeh 64:2247-2249 (in Hebrew with English abstract).

90. Raviv, M., E. Putievsky, and D. Amsalem. 1985. The effect of early fertilizer application on rooting and further development of cuttings and seedlings of aromatic plants. Hassadeh 65:2408-2410 (in Hebrew).

91. Raviv, M., E. Putievsky, U. Ravid, D. Sanderovich, N. Snir, and R. Ron. 1983. Bay laurel as an ornamental plant. Acta. Hortic. 132:35-42.

92. Raviv, M., E. Putievsky, and D. Sanderovich. 1984. Rooting stem cuttings of sage (*Salvia officinalis* L.) Plant Propagator 30:8-9.

93. Raviv, M., E. Putievsky, D. Sanderovich, and R. Ron. 1983. Rooting of bay laurel cuttings. Hassadeh 63:684-686 (in Hebrew).

94. Raviv, M. and O. Reuveni. 1984. Endogenous content of a leaf substance(s) associated with rooting ability of avocado cuttings. J. Am. Soc. Hortic. Sci. 109:284-287.

95. Raviv, M., O. Reuveni, and E.E. Goldschmidt. 1986. Evidence for the presence of a native non-auxinic rooting promoter in avocado. Plant Growth Regul. 4:95-102.

96. Raviv, M., R. Ron, E. Putievsky, E. Zuabi, Y. Michaelovitch, and D. Saadia. 1986. Rooting of tarragon cuttings. Hassadeh 66:2012-2013 (in Hebrew).

97. Reuveni, O. and M. Raviv. 1981. The importance of leaves retention and their contribution to rooting of avocado cuttings. J. Am. Soc. Hortic. Sci. 106:127-130.

98. Robbins, J.A., S.J. Kays, and M.A. Dirr. 1983. Enhanced rooting of wounded mung bean cuttings by wounding and ethephon. J. Am. Soc. Hortic. Sci. 108:325-329.

99. Rogler, C.E. and W.P. Hackett. 1975. Phase change in *Hedera helix*: induction of the mature to juvenile phase change by gibberellin A₃. Physiol. Plant 34:141-147.

100. Roy, B.N., R.N. Basu, and T. Bose. 1972. Interactions of auxins with growth-retarding, inhibiting and ethylene producing chemicals in rooting of cuttings. Plant Cell Physiol. 13:1123-1127.

101. Sardesai, D.L. and H.P. Tipnis. 1969. Production of flavouring principles by tissue culture of *Coriandrum sativum*. Curr. Sci. 38:545.

102. Schroder, F.J. 1978. Vegetative propagation and variability of *Marticaria chamomilla* L. Acta Hortic. 73:73-80.

103. Scott, M.A. 1974. Antitranspirants. Report of the Efford Experimental Horticulture Station for 1973. pp. 154-157.

104. Sharp. W.R., M.R. Sondahl, L.S. Caldas, and S.B. Maraffa. 1980. The physiology of *in vitro* asexual embryogenesis. Hort. Rev. 2:268-310.

105. Sircar, P.K. and S.K. Chatterjee. 1974. Physiological and biochemical changes associated with adventitious root formation in *vigna* hypocotyl cuttings. II. Gibberellin effects. Plant Propagator 20:15-22.

106. Skoog, F. and C.O. Miller. 1957. Chemical regulation of growth and organ formation in plant tissues cultured *in vitro*. Symp. Soc. Exp. Biol. 1:118-131.

107. Smith, D.R. and T.A. Thorpe. 1975. Root initiation in cuttings of *Pinus radiata* seedlings. II. Growth regulator interactions. J. Exp. Bot. 26:193-202.

108. Smith, N.G. and P.F. Wareing. 1972. The rooting of actively growing and dormant leafy cuttings in relation to endogenous hormone levels and photoperiod. New Phytol. 71:483-500.

109. Staba, E.J. 1980. *Plant Tissue Culture as a Source of Biochemicals*. CRC Press, Inc., Boca Raton, Florida.

110. Stanev, D. 1970. Induced mutation in *Mentha piperita* L. with the aid of colchicine. Genet. Selek. 3:131-137 (in Bulgarian with English abstract).

111. Stoltz, L.P. and C.E. Hess. 1966. The effect of girdling upon root initiation: carbohydrates and amino acids. Proc. Am. Soc. Hortic. Sci. 89:734-743.

112. Sutton, S., C. Humphries, and J. Hopkinson. 1985. Tarragon. Garden (U.K.) 110:237-240.

113. Tang, Z.C. and T.T. Kozlowski. 1984. Ethylene production and morphological adaptation of woody plants to flooding. Can. J. Bot. 62:1659-1664.

114. Thimann, K.V. and F.W. Went. 1934. On the chemical nature of the root forming hormone. Proc. Ned. Akad. Wet. 37:456-459.

115. Thomas, E., P.J. King, and I. Potrykus. 1979. Improvement of crop plants via single cells *in vitro* - an assessment. Z. Pflanzenzucht. 82:1-30.

116. Thorpe, T. and T. Murashige. 1970. Some histochemical changes underlying shoot initiation in tobacco callus cultures. Can. J. Bot. 48:277-285.

117. Tisseart, B., J.M. Ulrich, and B.J. Finkle. 1981. Cryogenic preservation and regeneration of date palm tissue. HortScience 16:47-48.

118. Tognoni, F. and R. Lorenzi. 1983. Identification of root-promoting substances from *Picea glauca* CV. Albertina. HortScience 18:893-894.

119. Tsukahara, H. and T.T. Kazlowski. 1985. Importance of adventitious roots to growth of flooded *Platanus occidentalis* seedlings. Plant Soil 88:123-132.

120. Watanabe, K., Y. Yamada, S. Ueno, and H. Mitsuda. 1985. Change of freezing resistance and retention of metabolic and differentiation potentials

in cultured green *Lavandula vera* cells which survived repeated freeze-thaw procedures. Agr. Biol. Chem. 49:1727-1731.

121. Wheelands, K. and L.A. Witlers. 1984. The IBPGR international database on *in vitro* conservation. Plant Genet. Resour. Newsl. 60:33-38.

122. Whitman, F., E.A. Schneider, and K.V. Thimann. 1980. Hormonal factors controlling the initiation and development of lateral roots. II. Effects of exogenous growth factors on lateral root formation in pea roots. Physiol. Plant 49:304-314.

123. Winkler, A.J. 1927. Some factors influencing the rooting of vine cuttings. Hilgardia 2:329-349.

124. Yamazaki, S., S. Tamura, F. Marumo, and Y. Saito. 1969. Structure of portulal. Tetrahedron Lett. 5:359-362.

Botanical Nomenclature of Commercial Sources of Essential Oils, Concretes, and Absolutes

Arthur O. Tucker
**Department of Agriculture and Natural Resources,
Delaware State College, Dover, DE 19901**

Brian M. Lawrence
**R.J. Reynolds Tobacco Company, Bowman Gray
Technical Center, Winston-Salem, NC 27102**

CONTENTS

I. INTRODUCTION

Recently the International Organization for Standardization (ISO) circulated the draft of a document which would set an international standard for the nomenclature of essential oils (80). This list of names, to be approved by the ISO Council, would form the backbone of industrial, technological, and commercial regulations on an international scale. While standardization of the nomenclature of essential oil plants is laudatory, the incomplete knowledge of many plants obviates any attempts to regulate absolute names.

The fragrance/flavor literature is replete with incorrect names. Perfumers consistently cite lavandin as *Lavandula hybrida*, but the correct name is *L. x intermedia* (177). The genus *Aeolanthus* is sometimes listed as a source of an oil, but the preferred spelling is *Aeollanthus* (48). Furthermore, chemists cite ninde as *A. graveolens* (7), a name which apparently has never been correctly published. The correct name of cloves, *Syzygium aromaticum*, is often stated incorrectly as *Eugenia carophyllata* (43). Often perfumers and flavorists base their nomenclatural knowledge upon Guenther's *The Essential Oils* (63), which was written between 1948 and 1952, or upon Gildemeister and Hoffmann's *Die ätherischen Öle* (60), which was written between 1956 and 1968. Many botanical revisions have been published in the last 20 to 40 years, and perfumers and flavorists are continually experimenting with new sources of essential oils, thereby adding new species to their vocabulary.

Many tropical genera still need revisionary work; a good example is the *Amomum-Aframomum-Elettaria* complex, especially in view of the illegitimate genera indicated by *Index Nominum Genericorum (Plantarum)* (48). While occasional revisions have been appearing on some Southeast Asian genera, correct citations of plants from Africa and tropical South America are hampered by a dearth of literature.

In addition, the botanical source of many essential oils still needs clarification. What are the botanical sources of sarsaparilla? What cultivars of roses are grown for attar? What are the botanical sources of oils labelled simply as rose geranium, linaloe, frankincense, myrrh, eucalyptus, copaiba, cabore, cosmos, or leribe? As long as the botanical sources remain incompletely known, adulteration and falsification are easy.

II. DELIMITATION OF INCLUDED TAXA

Many plants used for fragrance and flavor yield a product which fits the classic definition of an essential oil, while others yield resinoids, concretes, pomades, absolutes, and/or tinctures; adequate definitions of these preparations exist in the literature (7, 63) and need not be discussed here. While the title of this article limits this discussion to plants which yield commercial essential oils, concretes, and absolutes, a number of taxa which more commonly yield other products (for example, extract of vanilla) are also included because of their importance in fragrance and flavor work. Omitted from this discussion are fruit juices and preparations principally composed of alkaloids, iridoids, tannins, sweeteners, fixed oils, and/or saponins.

This list emphasizes materials which are currently available on the international commercial market. For this reason, we have omitted some items, such as matico oil (predominantly from *Piper angustifolium*), which only have historical significance. In contrast, many emerging materials are currently available in from hundreds to thousands of pounds but are not discussed in any current text (for example, louro nhamuy from *Nectandra elaiophopra* and Moroccan chamomile from *Ormenis* species).

III. ORGANIZATION OF LIST

This list is a continuation of the botanical nomenclature of culinary herbs and potherbs (178). The following list of additional taxa was compiled through a survey of many books on essential oils, perfumes, and flavor constituents (7, 21, 35, 37, 57, 60, 63, 64, 76, 82, 123, 132, 194, 202). Guides to the correct nomenclature (6, 30, 34, 42, 68, 78, 83, 86, 100, 103, 109, 117, 125, 136, 163, 164, 187, 188) included many regional floras. The list conforms to the rules listed in the *International Code of Botanical Nomenclature* (190) and *International Code of Nomenclature for Cultivated Plants* (18). Generic citations follow *Index Nominum Genericorum (Plantarum)* (48). Literature citations directly following the Latin names conform to *Taxonomic Literature-2* (160) and *B-P-H* (99); other literature references refer to citations in the reference section. Common names are listed as English (Eng.) (American, Amer., or British, Brit.), French (Fr.) (Canadian, Can.), German (Ger.), Italian (It.), Spanish (Sp.) (Mexican, Mex.), Japanese (Jap.), Russian (Rus.), Chinese (Chin.), Portuguese (Port.), Indian, Malay, and others (81).

The citations of authors may be shortened but must follow Article 46 of the *ICBN* (190). Recommendation 46D states that *Eucalyptus sideroxylon* A. Cunn. in T. Mitch. may be shortened to *Eucalyptus sideroxylon* A. Cunn. Recommendation 46E states that *Eucalyptus staigerana* F.v. Muell ex F.M. Bailey may be shortened to *Eucalyptus staigerana* F.M. Bailey. Recommendation 46C.2 states that more than 2 authors may be shortened to *et al.* (for example, *Armoracia* P. Gaertn., B. Mey., and Scherb. may be shortened to *Armoracia* P. Gaertn. *et al.*).

IV. LIST OF PLANTS USED AS COMMERCIAL SOURCES OF ESSENTIAL OILS, CONCRETES, AND ABSOLUTES

A. A Summary

This list is organized phylogenetically by family, but the genera and species within each family are arranged alphabetically. The following genera are included.

Parmeliaceae: *Parmelia*
Usneaceae: *Evernia, Ramalina, Usnea*
Pinaceae: *Abies, Cedrus, Picea, Pinus, Pseudotsuga, Tsuga*
Taxodiaceae: *Cryptomeria*
Cupressaceae: *Chamaecyparis, Cupressus, Juniperus, Neocallitropsis, Thuja, Thujopsis, Widdringtonia*
Podocarpaceae: *Dacrydium*
Araucariaceae: *Agathis*
Pandanaceae: *Pandanus*
Poaceae (Gramineae): *Anthoxanthum, Cymbopogon, Vetiveria*
Cyperaceae: *Cyperus*
Araceae: *Acorus*
Liliaceae: *Allium, Hyacinthus,*
Smilacaceae: *Smilax*
Amaryllidaceae: *Narcissus*
Agavaceae: *Polianthes*
Iridaceae: *Iris*
Zingiberaceae: *Alpinia, Curcuma, Elettaria, Hedychium, Zingiber*
Orchidaceae: *Vanilla*
Piperaceae: *Piper*
Betulaceae: *Betula*
Salicaceae: *Populus*
Moraceae: *Ficus, Humulus*
Santalaceae: *Santalum*
Aristolochiaceae: *Asarum*
Chenopodiaceae: *Chenopodium*
Caryophyllaceae: *Dianthus*
Magnoliaceae: *Michelia*
Illiciaceae: *Illicium*
Annonaceae: *Cananga*
Myristicaceae: *Myristica*
Monimiaceae: *Peumus*
Lauraceae: *Aniba, Cinnamomum, Cryptocarya, Laurus, Lindera, Litsea, Nectandra, Ocotea, Phoebe*
Brassicaceae (Cruciferae): *Armoracia, Brassica, Cheiranthus*
Resedaceae: *Reseda*
Grossulariaceae: *Ribes*

Hamamelidaceae: *Liquidambar*
Rosaceae: *Prunus, Rosa*
Mimosaceae: *Acacia*
Fabaceae (Leguminosae, *pro parte*): *Copaifera, Daniellia, Dipteryx, Glycyrrhiza, Melilotus, Myrocarpus, Myroxylon, Robinia, Spartium, Trifolium, Trigonella*
Geraniaceae: *Geranium, Pelargonium*
Zygophyllaceae: *Bulnesia*
Rutaceae: *Agathosma, Amyris, Boronia, Citrus, Dictamnus, Galipea, Luvunga, Ruta, Skimmia, Zanthoxylum*
Burseraceae: *Boswellia, Bursera, Canarium, Commiphora*
Meliaceae: *Aglaia, Cabralea, Cedrela*
Euphorbiaceae: *Croton*
Anacardiaceae: *Pistacia, Schinus*
Aquifoliaceae: *Ilex*
Malvaceae: *Abelmoschus*
Byttneriaceae: *Theobroma*
Theaceae: *Camellia*
Dipterocarpaceae: *Dipterocarpus, Dryobalanops*
Cistaceae: *Cistus*
Violaceae: *Viola*
Thymelaeaceae: *Aquilaria*
Myrtaceae: *Eucalyptus, Melaleuca, Myrtus, Pimenta, Syzygium*
Apiaceae (Umbelliferae): *Anethum, Angelica, Anthriscus, Apium, Carum, Coriandrum, Cuminum, Daucus, Dorema, Ferula, Foeniculum, Levisticum, Pastinaca, Petroselinum, Pimpinella, Trachyspermum*
Ericaceae: *Gaultheria*
Styracaceae: *Styrax*
Oleaceae: *Jasminum, Osmanthus, Syringa*
Boraginaceae: *Heliotropium*
Verbenaceae: *Aloysia, Lippia*
Lamiaceae (Labiatae): *Aeollanthus, Hedeoma, Hyssopus, Lavandula, Melissa, Mentha, Monarda, Nepeta, Ocimum, Origanum, Perilla, Pogostemon, Rosmarinus, Salvia, Satureja, Thymus*
Solanaceae: *Nicotiana*
Rubiaceae: *Anthocephalus, Coffea, Gardenia, Leptactina,*
Caprifoliaceae: *Lonicera, Sambucus*
Valerianaceae: *Nardostachys, Valeriana*
Asteraceae (Compositae): *Achillea, Arnica, Artemisia, Atractylodes, Baccharis, Balsamita, Blumea, Brachylaena, Carphephorus, Chamaemelum, Chamomilla, Conyza, Eriocephalus, Helichrysum, Ormenis, Pteronia, Saussurea, Solidago, Tagetes, Tanacetum*

B. The Plants

Parmeliaceae

Parmelia Achar., Methodus 153. t. 4, f. 3-6, 1803.
    Literature: 9
    Species:
    Parmelia cirrhata Fr., Syst. orb. veg. 283. 1825 (*P. nepalensis*
        Taylor): Indian moss (Eng.), jhoola (Indian), charilla (Indian).

Usneaceae

Evernia Achar. in Luyk., Tent. hist. lich. 90. 1809.
    Literature: 53, 126
    Species:
    Evernia furfuracea (L.) W. Mann, Lich. Bohemia 105. 1825: tree
        moss (Eng.), mousse d'arbre (Fr.), Baummoos (Ger.).
    Evernia prunastri (L.) Achar., Lichenogr. universalis 442. t. 10, f.
        1. 1810: oakmoss (Eng.), mousse de chêne (Fr.), Eichenmoos
        (Ger.), muschio di quercia (It.), musco de encina (Sp.).

Ramalina Achar. in Luyk., Tent. hist. lich. 95. 1809.
    Literature: 9
    Species:
    Ramalina fastigiata (Pers.) Achar., Lichenogr. universalis 603.
        1810: Chinese moss (Eng.).
    Ramalina subcomplanata Nyl., Bull. Soc. Linn. Normandie II,
        4:134. 1870: Indian moss (Eng.).
        Ramalina subcomplanata and *Usnea lucea* are harvested to-
        gether as haraphool (Indian).

Usnea (Dill.) Adans., Fam. pl. 2:7. 1763.
    Literature: 9, 53, 126
    Species:
    Usnea barbata (L.) Wigg., Prim. fl. Hols. 91. 1780.
        Usnea barbata is harvested with *Evernia furfuracea* as tree
        moss.
    Usnea lucea Motyka, Usnea 534. 1938: Indian moss (Eng.).
        Usnea lucea and *Ramalina subcomplanata* are harvested to-
        gether as haraphool (Indian).

Pinaceae

Abies Mill., Gard. dict. abr. ed. 4. 1754.
  Literature: 17, 24, 44, 45, 94, 95, 106, 108, 152
  Abies alba Mill., Gard. dict. ed. 8. 1768 [*Abies pectinata* (Lam.)
    Lam. ex DC]: silver fir (Eng.), white fir (Eng.), silver "spruce"
    (Eng.), white "spruce" (Eng.), sapin blanc (Fr.), sapin argenté
    (Fr.), Edeltanne (Ger.), Weisstanne (Ger.), Silbertanne (Ger.),
    abete argentato (It.), abete bianco (It.).
    The cones of *A. alba* yield templin oil. The needle/twig oil is
    commonly sold as fir needle oil.
  Abies balsamea (L.) Mill., Gard. dict. ed. 8. 1768: balsam fir
    (Eng.), sapin balsamier (Fr.), Balsamtanne (Ger.).
    The oleoresin of *A. balsamea* is sold as Canada balsam or
    balm of Gilead. The needle oil is sold as fir needle oil or
    balsam fir needle oil.
  Abies sachalinensis (F.W. Schmidt) Mast., Gard. Chron.
    1879(2):588. 1879: Sachalin fir (Eng.), sapin de l'Ile de
    Sakhaline (Fr.), Sachalintanne (Ger.), aka-todo-matsu (Jap.).
    The oil of the needles of *A. sachalinensis* is sold as Japanese
    pine needle oil, Japanese fir needle oil, or shin-yo-yu. Besides
    the typical variety, the following is also an important variety:
    var. *mayriana* Miyabe & Kudo, Trans. Sapporo Nat. Hist.
      Soc. 7:131. 1919 [*Abies mayriana* (Miyabe & Kudo)
      Miyabe & Kudo]: Mayr Sakhalin fir (Eng.), sapin de Mayr
      (Fr.), Mayr Tanne (Ger.), ao-todo-matsu (Jap.).
  Abies sibirica Ledeb., Fl. Altaic. 4:202. 1833: Siberian fir (Eng.),
    sapin de Sibérie (Fr.), sibirische Edeltanne (Ger.), pichta
    (Rus.).
    Two varieties exist, but var. *sibirica* is most often encoun-
    tered. The needle/twig oil of *A. sibirica* is sold as Siberian fir
    oil or Siberian pine needle oil.

Cedrus Trew, Cedr. lib. hist. 1757(1):6. 1757.
  Literature: 24, 44, 45, 94, 152
  Species:
  Cedrus atlantica G. Manetti, Cat. pl. hort. Modic. Suppl. 8. 1844:
    Atlantic cedar (Eng.), Atlas cedar (Eng.), cèdre de l'Atlas (Fr.),
    Atlas-Ceder (Ger.).
  Cedrus deodara (Roxb.) Loud., Hort. brit. 388. 1830: deodar cedar
    (Eng.), Himalayan cedar (Eng.), cèdre de l'Himalaya (Fr.),
    Himalaja Cedar (Ger.).
  Cedrus libani A. Rich. in Bory, Dict. class. hist. nat. 3:299. 1823:
    cedar of Lebanon (Eng.), cèdre du Liban (Fr.), Libanon-Ceder
    (Ger.).

Picea A. Dietr., Fl. Berlin 1(2):794. 1824
Literature: 24, 44, 45, 94, 106, 152
Species:
Picea abies (L.) H. Karst., Deut. Fl. 325. f. 155. 1881 [*P. excelsa*
(Lam.) Link]: Norway spruce (Eng., Amer.), common spruce
(Eng., Brit.), épicéa (Fr.), Fichte (Ger.), Rottanne (Ger.).
The needle oil of *P. abies* is sold as fir needle oil.
Picea abies also yields Burgundy pitch and Jura turpentine. *Picea
abies*, *Picea glauca*, and *Picea mariana* oils are often sold
simply as spruce oils.
Picea glauca (Moench) Voss, Mitt. Deutsch. Dendrol. Ges. 16:93.
1907 [1908] [*P. alba* Link, *P. canadensis* (Mill.) Britton, Sterns
& Poggenb.]: white spruce (Eng.), Canadian spruce (Eng.,
Amer.), epinette blanche (Fr.), Weissfichte (Ger.).
Picea jezoensis (Siebold & Zucc.) Carrière, Traité gén. conif. 255.
1855: yeddo spruce (Eng., Amer.), yezo spruce (Eng., Brit.),
kuro-ezo (Jap.), ezo-matsu (Jap.).
The needles/twigs of *P. jezoensis* are often mixed with those of
Abies sachalinensis to produce Japanese pine needle oil. *Picea
mariana* (Mill.) Britton, Sterns, & Poggenb., Prelim. cat. 71.
1888 (*P. nigra* Link): black spruce (Eng.), Canadian black
"pine" (Eng.), epinette noire (Fr.).

Pinus L., Sp. pl. 1000. 1753.
Literature: 24, 38, 44, 45, 94, 106, 107, 119, 149, 152, 161, 192
Species:
Pinus ayacahuite Ehrenb., Linnaea 12:492. 1838: Mexican white
pine (Eng.), pin blanc du Mexique (Fr.), pino blanco (Sp.),
pino de azucar (Sp., Mex.), acalocote (Sp., Mex.), pinabete
(Sp., Mex.). *P. ayacahuite* is used as a source of turpentine in
Mexico.
Pinus contorta Douglas ex Loud., Arbor. frutic. brit. 4:2292, f.
2210, 2211. 1838.
This species is known in 3 varieties, but the following is the
most important for commercial purposes:
var. *latifolia* Engelm. in Wats. in King, Rep. U.S. geol. expl.
40th par. 5:331. 1871: lodgepole pine (Eng.).
Pinus contorta var. *latifolia* is the source of "Tasmanian"
turpentine.
Pinus elliottii Engelm., Trans. Acad. Sci. St. Louis 4:186, t. 1-3.
1880 (*P. caribaea* auct., non Morelet): slash pine (Eng.).
P. elliottii is one leading source of American gum turpentine.
P. elliottii var. *elliottii* ranges from South Carolina to Louisiana, while *P. elliottii* var. *densa* Little & Dorman occurs in
southern Florida. *Pinus elliottii* was formerly included as
conspecific with *P caribaea*, Caribbean pine, and sometimes
with *P. palustris*.

Pinus halepensis Mill., Gard. dict. ed. 8. 1768: Aleppo pine (Eng.),
Jerusalem pine (Eng.).

Pinus insularis Endl., Syn. conif. 157. 1847 (*P. khasya* Royle, *P.
kesiya* Royle ex Gordon, *P. khasyana* Griff., *P. langbianensis*
A. Chev.): khasi pine (Eng.), benguet pine (Eng.).

Pinus insularis is one source of Indian turpentine.

Pinus koraiensis Sieb. & Zucc., Fl. jap. 2:28, t. 116, f. 5-6. 1844:
Korean pine (Eng.).

Pinus massoniana Lamb., Descr. Pinus 1:17, t. 12. 1803: Masson
pine (Eng.), southern red pine (Eng.).

Pinus merkusii Jungh. & de Vriese in de Vriese, Pl. nov. ind. bat.
5, t. 2. 1845 (*P. latteri* F. Mason): Merkus pine (Eng.).

Pinus mugo Turra, Fl. ital. prodr. 67. 1764 (*P. montana* Mill.):
mountain pine (Eng., Brit.), Swiss mountain pine (Eng.,
Amer.), pine de montagne (Fr.), Latschenkiefer (Ger.).

This species may be divided into 4 varieties, but the following
2 are the most important:

var. *mugo* [var. *mughus* (Scop.) Zenari, *P. mughus* Scop.]:
mugho pine (Eng., Brit.), mugho Swiss mountain pine
(Eng., Amer.), Krummholzkiefer (Ger.), pino mugo (It.,
Sp.).

var. *pumilio* (Haenke) Zenari, Boll. Soc. Bot. Ital. 1921:65.
1921 (*P. pumilio* Haenke): dwarf pine (Eng.), Zwergkiefer
(Ger.).

Pinus nigra J.F.X. Arnold, Reise Marizell 8. 1785: Austrian pine
(Eng.), black pine (Eng.), pin noir (Fr.).

Pinus nigra is very variable, but subsp. *nigra* is the typical
subspecies and usually encountered. Many cultivars exist.

Pinus palustris Mill., Gard., dict. ed. 8. 1768: longleaf pine (Eng.),
longleaf yellow pine (Eng.), southern yellow pine (Eng.), pitch
pine (Eng.), pitchpin du Sud (Fr.).

This is the leading source of American gum turpentine.

Pinus ponderosa Douglas ex C. Laws, Agric. Man. 354. 1836:
ponderosa pine (Eng.), western yellow pine (Eng.), pin à bois
lourd (Fr., Can.), pitchpin à bois lourd (Fr.), pinabete (Sp.,
Mex.), pino real (Sp., Mex.).

Three varieties exist, but var. *ponderosa* is most often encountered.

Pinus radiata D. Don, Trans. Linn. Soc. London 17:442. 1836:
Monterey pine (Eng.).

This is the source of "New Zealand" turpentine.

Pinus roxburghii Sarg., Silva 11:9. 1897: chir pine (Eng.).

This is another source of Indian turpentine.

Pinus strobus L., Sp. pl. 1001. 1753: white pine (Eng.), Canadian
white pine (Eng.), pin blanc (Fr.), pin de Lord Weymouth
(Fr.), Weymouthskiefer (Ger.).

Many cultivars of this species exist.

Pinus sylvestris L., Sp. pl. 1000. 1753: Scotch pine (Eng.), pin sylvestre (Fr.), Gemeine Kiefer (Ger.), weiss Förhe (Ger.), pino silvestre (It.), pino sylvestris (Sp.).
Many varieties, forms, and cultivars of this species are cultivated.

Pinus tabulaeformis Carrière, Traité gén. conif. ed. 2. 510. 1867: Chinese pine (Eng.).

Pinus yunnanensis Franch., J. Bot. (Morot) 13:253. 1899: Yunnan pine (Eng.), Chinese pine (Eng.).
Arguments have been advanced, pro and con, to include this as conspecific with *P. insularis*.

Pseudotsuga Carrière, Traité gén. conif. ed. 2. 256. 1867.
Literature: 24, 44, 45, 93, 106, 152
Species:

Pseudotsuga menziesii (Mirb.) Franco, Conif. Duar. Nom. 4. 1959; Bol. Soc. Brot. ser. 2. 24:74 1950 (*P. taxifolia* Lamb.): Douglas-fir (Eng.), sapin de Douglas (Fr.).
This species exists in 2 varieties, both yielding "Oregon fir balsam" or "Oregon balsam":
var. *menziesii*: coast Douglas-fir (Eng.), Douglas vert (Fr.).
var. *glauca* (Beissn.) Franco, Bol. Soc. Brot. ser. 2. 24:77. 1950: Rocky Mountain Douglas-fir (Eng.), Douglas bleu (Fr.), Douglas du Colorado (Fr.).

Tsuga Carrière, Traité gén. conif. 185. 1855.
Literature: 24, 44, 45, 94, 106, 152
Species:

Tsuga canadensis (L.) Carrière, Traité gén. conif. 189. 1855: hemlock (Eng.), eastern hemlock (Eng.), pruche de l'Est (Fr.), Hemlocktanne (Ger.).
Numerous cultivars of this species exist. The needle/twig oil is sometimes sold as fir needle oil, spruce oil, or hemlock oil.

Taxodiaceae

Cryptomeria D. Don, Ann. Nat. Hist. 1(3):233. 1838.
Literature: 24, 44, 45, 94, 152
Species:

Cryptomeria japonica D. Don, Trans. Linn. Soc. London 18:166. 1841: cryptomeria (Eng., Amer.), Japanese cedar (Eng., Brit.), sugi (Eng., Brit.; Jap.).
Many cultivars of this species exist.

Cupressaceae

Chamaecyparis Spach, Hist. nat. vég. 11:329. 1841.
Literature: 24, 44, 45, 94, 101, 106, 152
Species:
Chamaecyparis funebris (Endl.) Franco, Agros (Lisbon) 24:93. 1941
(*Cupressus funebris* Endl.): mourning cypress (Eng.), Chinese
weeping cypress (Eng.).
Oil of *C. funebris* is sometimes sold as Chinese cedarwood oil.
Chamaecyparis lawsoniana (Andr. Murray) Parl. in DC, Prodr.
16(2):464. 1868: Port-Orford-cedar (Eng.), Oregon-cedar
(Eng.), Lawson false cypress (Eng.), cyprès de Lawson (Fr.).
Numerous cultivars of this species exist.
Chamaecyparis nootkatensis (D. Don) Spach, Hist. nat. vég.
11:333. 1841: Alaska-cedar (Eng.), Alaska yellow-cedar (Eng.),
yellow-cedar (Eng.).
Chamaecyparis obtusa (Siebold & Zucc.) Endl., Syn. conif. 63.
1847.
Two varieties exist:
var. *obtusa*: hinoki false cypress (Eng.), Hinokibaum (Fr.),
hinoki (Jap.).
var. *formosana* (Hayata) Rehd. in L. H. Bailey, Stand. cycl.
hort. 2:731. 1914 (*C. taiwanensis* Masamune & Suzuki):
Formosan hinoki (Eng.), arisan hinoki (Chin.).

Cupressus L., Sp. pl. 1002. 1753.
Literature: 24, 44, 45, 94, 106, 112, 150, 151, 152
Species:
Cupressus sempervirens L., Sp. pl. 1002. 1753: Mediterranean
cypress (Eng.), cypres commun (Fr.), Cypresse (Ger.).
Many cultivars exist, but the most commonly cultivated is
'Stricta,' the Italian cypress (Eng.).
Cupressus torulosa D. Don in Lamb., Descr. Pinus 2:18; D. Don,
Prodr. fl. nepal. 55. 1825: Himalayan cypress (Eng.), cyprès du
Bhoutan (Fr.).

Juniperus L., Sp. pl. 1038. 1753.
Literature: 24, 44, 45, 49, 94, 106, 112, 152, 161, 208
Species:
Juniperus ashei Buchholz, Bot. Gaz. (Crawfordsville) 9:329. 1930
(*J. mexicana* auct.): mountain cedar (Eng.), rock cedar (Eng.),
Mexican cedar (Eng.), Mexican juniper (Eng.).
The name *J. mexicana* has been erroneously applied to many
species of *Juniperus* of the southwestern U.S. and Mexico, but
J. ashei appears to be the principal species under this name.
Juniperus communis L., Sp. pl. 1040. 1753: common juniper
(Eng.), genévrier (Fr.), genièvre commun (Fr.), Wacholder
(Ger.), ginepro (It.), enebro (Sp.).

Many cultivars of this species are raised. *Juniperus communis* L. var. *depressa* Pursh, Canadian juniper (Eng.), produces an oil from the fleshy cones ("juniper berries") inferior to that from var. *communis* (var. *erecta* auct. chem.).

Juniperus oxycedrus L., Sp. pl. 1038. 1753: prickly juniper (Eng.), cade juniper (Eng.), genévrier cade (Fr.), genévrier epineux (Fr.), Kade (Ger.).

The empyreumatic wood oil of *J. oxycedrus* is known as oil of cade or juniper tar.

Juniperus phoenicea L., Sp. pl. 1040. 1753: Phoenician juniper (Eng.).

This species is the source of Phoenician savin oil.

Juniperus procera Hochst. ex. Endl., Syn. conif. 26. 1847: East African cedar (Eng.), Kenyan cedar (Eng.), cèdre de l'Afrique Orientale (Fr.).

Juniperus sabina L., Sp. pl. 1039. 1753: savin juniper (Eng., Amer.), savin (Eng., Brit.), sabine (Fr.), Sadebaum (Ger.).
Many cultivars of this species exist.

Juniperus squamata F. Ham. ex Lamb., Descr. Pinus 2:17. 1824 [*J. recurva* F. Ham. ex D. Don var. *squamata* (F. Ham. ex Lamb.) Parl.]: single-seed juniper (Eng., Amer.), scaly-leaved Nepal juniper (Eng., Brit.).
Several cultivars exist in cultivation.

Juniperus virginiana L., Sp. pl. 1039. 1753: eastern red cedar (Eng., Amer.), red cedar (Eng., Brit.), genévrier de Virginie (Fr.), cèdre rouge de l'Est des États-Unis (Fr.).
Many cultivars of this species exist.

Neocallitropsis (R.H. Compton) Florin, Palaeontographica, Abt. B, Paläophytol. 85B:590. 1944.
Literature: 24, 44, 94, 152
Species:

Neocallitropsis pancheri (Carriére) de Laubenfels, Fl. N. Caléd. & Dépend. 4:161. 1972. [*N. araucarioides* (R.H. Compton) Florin, *Callitropsis araucarioides* R.H. Compton]: Pancher neocallitropsis (Eng.).
Oil from the wood of this species is marketed as "oil of araucaria."

Thuja L., Sp. pl. 1002. 1753.
Literature: 24, 44, 45, 94, 106, 152
Species:

Thuja occidentalis L., Sp. pl. 1002. 1753: northern white-cedar (Eng.), white cedar (Eng.), eastern arborvitae (Eng.), thuja (Eng.), swamp cedar (Eng.), cèdre blanc (Fr., Can.), thuya du Canada (Fr.), Thuja (Ger.), Lebensbaum (Ger.), thuja (It., Sp.).

Many cultivars of this species exist. Oil of *T. occidentalis* is often loosely called cedar leaf oil. Cedarwood oil is derived from *Juniperus virginiana*, while white cedarwood oil is derived from *T. occidentalis*.

Thuja plicata Donn ex D. Don in Lamb., Descr. Pinus 2:[19].
    1824: western red cedar (Eng.), western arborvitae (Eng.), thuya géant (Fr.), thuya de Lobb (Fr.), Washington-Ceder (Ger.).

Thujopsis Siebold & Zucc. ex Endl., Gen. pl. Suppl. 2:24. 1842.
    Literature: 24, 44, 45, 94, 152
    Species:
Thujopsis dolobrata (L. fil.) Siebold & Zucc., Fl. jap. 2:32. 1844:
    hiba (Eng.).
    This species has 2 varieties:
    var. *dolobrata*: azunaro (Jap.)
    var. *hondae* Makino, Bot. Mag. (Tokyo) 15:104. 1901: hinoki-asunaro (Jap.).

Widdringtonia Endl., Cat. horti Vindob. 1:209. 1842.
    Literature: 24, 44, 94, 111, 152
    Species:
Widdringtonia cupressoides (L.) Endl., Cat. horti Vindob. 1:209.
    1842 (*W. dracomontana* Stapf, *W. whytei* Rendle): mountain widdringtonia (Eng.), mlange cedar (Eng.).

Podocarpaceae

Dacrydium Lamb., Descr. Pinus 1:93. 1807.
    Literature: 24, 44, 94, 152
    Species:
Dacrydium franklinii J.D. Hook. in Hook., London J. Bot. 4:152.
    t. 6. 1845: huon pine (Eng.), huon dacrydium (Eng.).

Araucariaceae

Agathis Salisb., Trans. Linn. Soc. London 8:311. 1807.
    Literature: 24, 44, 94, 152
    Species:
Agathis australis (Lamb.) Steud., Nomencl. bot. ed. 2. 1:34. 1840:
    kauri (Eng., Fr.), kauri pine (Eng.), New Zealand kauri (Eng.), Kaurikopal (Ger.).

Pandanaceae

Pandanus S. Parkinson, J. voy. South Seas 46. 1773.
Literature: 165
Species:
Pandanus fascicularis Lam., Encycl. 1:372. 1785 (*P. odoratissimus*
L. fil.): padang (Eng.).
The male flowers of *P. fascicularis* are macerated with sesame
oil to yield "attar of kewda" or "atar of keora." Other flower
oils or sandalwood oil may also be used for extraction or
co-distillation.

Poaceae (Gramineae)

Anthoxanthum L., Sp. pl. 28. 1753.
Literature: 186
Species:
Anthoxanthum odoratum L. Sp. pl. 28. 1753: sweet vernalgrass
(Eng.), flouve odorante (Fr.), Geruchgras (Ger.), paleo odoroso
(It.), grama de olor (Sp.).

Cymbopogon Spreng., Pl. min. cogn. pug. 2:14. 1815.
Literature: 33, 159, 162
Species:
Cymbopogon citratus (DC) Stapf, Bull. Misc. Inform. 1906:322.
357. 1906. (*Andropogon citratus* DC): West Indian lemongrass
(Eng.), lemongrass de l'Amerique Centrale (Fr.), Lemongras
(Ger.).
Cymbopogon flexuosus (Nees ex Steud.) Wats. in Atkinson, Gaz.
N.W. Prov. India 392. 1882 (*Andropogon flexuosus* Nees ex
Steud.): East Indian lemongrass (Eng.), lemongrass (Fr.),
Lemongras (Ger.).
Cymbopogon martinii (Roxb.) Wats. in Atkinson, Gaz. N.W. Prov.
India 392. 1882 (*Andropogon martinii* Roxb.): rosha (Indian),
rusha (Indian).
This species occurs in 2 eco-chemotypes which are not separa-
ble morphologically:
var. *martinii*: palmarosa (Eng., Fr., It., Sp.), motia (Eng.),
Palmarosa (Ger.), motiya (Indian).
var. *sofia* Gupta, Proc. Indian Acad. Sci. 71B:97. 1970:
gingergrass (Eng., Fr., It., Sp.), sofia (Eng.), Gingergras
(Ger.), sofiya (Indian).
Cymbopogon nardus (L.) Rendle, Cat. welw. afr. pl. 2:155. 1899
(*Andropogon nardus* L.).
This species can be distinguished as 2 varieties:
var. *nardus*: Ceylon citronella (Eng.), citronelle type Ceylan
(Fr.), Ceylon-Citronell (Ger.), lenabatu (Sinhal.).

var. *confertiflorus* (Steud.) N.L. Bor, J. Bombay Nat. Hist. Soc.
51:905. 1953.
Cymbopogon pendulus (Steud.) Wats. in Atkinson, Gaz. N.W. Prof.
India 392. 1882 (*Andropogon pendulus* Steud.): Jammu
lemongrass (Eng.).
Cymbopogon winterianus Jowitt, Ann. Roy. Bot. Gard.
(Peradeniya) 4:188. 1908: Java citronella (Eng.), citronelle type
Java (Fr.), Java-Citronell (Ger.), mahpengiri (Javanese).
Vetiveria Bory in Lem., Bull. Sci. Soc. Philom. Paris 1822:43. 1822.
Literature: 162
Species:
Vetiveria zizanoides (L.) Nash in Small, Fl. s.e. U.S. 67. 1903:
vetiver (Eng., It., Sp.), vétiver (Fr.), Vetiver (Ger.), khas-khas
(Indian), akar wangi (Javanese).

Cyperaceae

Cyperus L., Sp. pl. 44. 1753.
Literature: 92
Species:
Cyperus mitis Steud., Syn. pl. glumac. 2:316. 1855 (*C. scariosus
sensu* Koyama): nagar mustika (Sanskrit), nagar motha
(Hindi), cyperiol (Indian).
Cyperus rotundus L., Sp. pl. 45. 1753: nut-grass (Eng.), coco-grass
(Eng.), souchet rond (Fr.).

Araceae

Acorus L., Sp. pl. 324. 1753.
Literature: 139
Species:
Acorus calamus L., Sp. pl. 324. 1753: sweet flag (Eng.), calamus
(Eng., Fr.), acore (Fr.), Kalmus (Ger.), calamo (It., Sp.).
This species can be divided into 3 varieties [var. *calamus*
from Eurasia, var. *americanus* (Raf.) Wulff from North Amer-
ica and Siberia, and var. *angustatus* Besser from Southeast
Asia], but their correct nomenclature needs study.

Liliaceae

Allium L., Sp. pl. 295. 1753.
Literature: see 178
Species: see 178; add:

Allium cepa L., Sp. pl. 300. 1753: onion (Eng.), o(i)gnon (Fr.),
Zweibel (Ger.), cipolla (It.), cebolla (Sp.).
Numerous cultivars of the onion exist, but the following bo-
tanical varieties may be recognized:

var. *cepa*: this includes the onions with single bulbs; no bulbs
are produced in the inflorescence and it is usually propagated by seed. This is the source of commercial onion oil.

var. *viviparum* (Metzg.) Alef., Landw. fl. 301. 1866: this includes the Egyptian onion, top onion, tree onion, and
Catawissa onion; this variety is propagated by large
bulbils borne in the inflorescence.

var. *aggregatum* G. Don, Mem. Wern. Nat. Hist. Soc. 6:18.
1827: this includes the potato onion, multiplier onion,
ever-ready onion, and shallot; this lacks bulbils in the
inflorescence, is often sterile, and is propagated by lateral
bulbs.

Hyacinthus L., Sp. pl. 316. 1753.
Literature: 41, 72
Species:
Hyacinthus orientalis L., Sp. pl. 316. 1753: hyacinth (Eng.),
jacinthe (Fr.), Hyazinthe (Ger.), giacinto (It.), jacinto (Sp.).

Smilacaceae

Smilax L., Sp. pl. 1028. 1753.
Literature: 161
Species:
Smilax medica Schlechtend. & Cham., Linnaea 6:47. 1831 (*S.
aristolochiaefolia* auct., non Mill.): Mexican sarsaparilla (Eng.),
zarzaparilla (Sp., Mex.).
The species of *Smilax* which furnish the sarsaparilla of commerce are imperfectly known. *Smilax medica* is also known as
Vera Cruz or gray sarsaparilla. *Smilax regelii* Killip & Morton
may be the source of Honduras or brown sarsaparilla. *Smilax
febrifuga* Kunth may be the source of Ecuadoran sarsaparilla.
The species which furnish the other sarsaparillas (for example,
red Jamaica, Costa Rica, Lima, Guayaquil, and Virginian) are
not properly identified in the literature.

Amaryllidaceae

Narcissus L., Sp. pl. 289. 1753.
Literature: 197, 205
Species:
Narcissus jonquilla L., Sp. pl. 290. 1753: jonquil (Eng.), jonquille
(Fr.), Jonquille (Ger.).

Narcissus poeticus L., Sp. pl. 289. 1753: poet's narcissus (Eng.), pheasant's eye (Eng.), narcisse (Fr.), Narzisse (Ger.), narciso (It., Sp.).
Two subspecies exist:
subsp. *poeticus.*
subsp. *radiiflorus* (Salisb.) Baker, Handb. Amaryll. 12. 1888.

Agavaceae

Polianthes L., Sp. pl. 316. 1753.
Literature: 175.
Species:
Polianthes tuberosa L., Sp. pl. 316. 1753: tuberose (Eng.), tubéreuse (Fr.), Tuberose (Ger.), Nachthyazinthe (Ger.), tuberosa (It., Sp.).

Iridaceae

Iris L., Sp. pl. 38. 1753.
Literature: 47, 113, 198
Species:
Iris x *germanica* L., Sp. pl. 38. 1753: German iris (Eng.), flag (Eng.), orris (Eng.), iris (Fr., Sp.), Iris (Ger.), ireos (It.).
While orris is often cited as originating from *I.* x *germanica* var. *florentina* Dykes (*I. florentina* auct.), the morphological characters to distinguish it from the "typical" nothovariety do not appear to be constant. It is best named as a cultivar, 'Florentina'.
Iris pallida Lam., Encycl. 3:294. 1789: orris (Eng.), iris (Fr., Sp.), Iris (Ger.), ireos (It.).

Zingiberaceae

Alpinia Roxb., Asiat. Res. 11:350. 1810.
Literature: 23, 75, 155
Species:
Alpinia officinarum Hance, J. Linn. Soc., Bot. 13:6. 1873 [*Languas officinarum* (Hance) Farw.]: lesser galangal (Eng.), Chinese ginger (Eng.), petit galanga (Fr.), Kleiner Galangant (Ger.), galanga (It.), galangal (Sp.).

Curcuma L., Sp. pl. 2. 1753.
Literature: 22, 23, 75, 154
Species:

Curcuma longa L., Sp. pl. 2. 1753: turmeric (Eng.), curcuma (Eng., It., Sp.), curcuma longue (Fr.), Gelbwurzel (Ger.), Curcuma (Ger.), ukon (Jap.), zholty imbir' (Rus.), yü-chiu (Chin.), açafrâo-da-India (Port.).

Elettaria Maton, Trans. Linn. Soc. London 10:250. 1811.
Literature: 23, 75, 92, 158
Species:
Elettaria cardamomum (L.) Maton, Trans. Linn. Soc. London 10:254. t. 5. 1811.
Two varieties are listed:
var. *cardamomum* (var. *minus* Watt, var. *minuscula* Burkill); Mysore cardamom (Eng.), cardamom (Eng.), cardamome de Malabar (Fr.), cardamome de Sri Lanka (Fr.), Malabar-Cardamomen (Ger.), Ceylon-Malabar-Cardamomen (Ger.), cardamomo (It., Sp.).
var. *major* Thwaites, Enum. pl. zeyl. 318. 1861: wild cardamom (Eng.), Ceylon-Cardamomen (Ger.).

Hedychium J.G. Konig in Retz., Observ. bot. 3:61 ("73"). 1783.
Literature: 23, 75, 157
Species:
Hedychium flavescens [Carey ex] Roscoe, Monandr. pl. Scitam. t. 50. 1824. (*H. flavum* auct., non Roxb.): longoze (Eng., Fr.).
Hedychium spicatum Sm. in Rees, Cycl. 17:n. 3. 1811: sanna (Jap.), ekangi (Indian), Kapur kachri (Indian).

Zingiber Boehmer in Ludw., Def. gen. pl. ed. 3. 89. 1760.
Literature: 23, 75, 98, 156
Species:
Zingiber officinale Roscoe, Trans. Linn. Soc. London 8:348. 1807: ginger (Eng.), gingembre (Fr.), Ingwer (Ger.), zenzero (It.), jengibre (Sp.), shōga (Jap.), imbir' (Rus.), hiang (Chin.), gengibre (Port.).

Orchidaceae

Vanilla Mill., Gard. dict. abr. ed. 4. 1754.
Literature: 15, 28, 66, 130
Species:
Vanilla planifolia Andr., Bot. repos. t. 538. 1808 [*Vanilla fragrans* (Salisb.) Ames]: vanilla (Eng.), Bourbon vanilla (Eng.), Mexican vanilla (Eng.), Vanille (Ger.), vaniglia (It.), vainilla (Sp.), banira (Jap.), vanil' (Rus.), hsiang-ts'ao (Chin.), baunilha (Port.).
Vanilla pompona Schiede, Linnaea 4:573. 1829: West Indian vanilla (Eng.), Guadeloupe vanilla (Eng.), vanillon (Eng.), pompona vanilla (Eng.), vannilon des Antilles (Fr.).

Vanilla tahitensis J.W. Moore, Bernice P. Bishop Mus. Bull.
102:25. 1933: Tahitian vanilla (Eng.), vanille de Tahiti (Fr.).

Piperaceae

Piper L., Sp. pl. 28. 1753.
Literature: see 178; add 174
Species:
Piper cubeba L. fil., Suppl. pl. 90. 1782: cubeb (Eng)., cubebe (Fr.),
Cubebe (Ger.), cubebe (It.), cubeba (Sp.).
Piper nigrum L., Sp. pl. 28. 1753: pepper (Eng.), black pepper
(Eng.), white pepper (Eng.), poivre noir (Fr.), poivre blanc
(Fr.), Pfeffer (Ger.), pepe (It.), pimienta (Sp., Port.), koshō
(Jap.), pyerets (Rus.), hu-chiao (Chin).

Betulaceae

Betula L., Sp. pl. 982. 1753.
Literature: 55, 106
Species:
Betula lenta L., Sp. pl. 983. 1753: sweet birch (Eng.), black birch
(Eng.), cherry birch (Eng.), betula dulce (Sp.).
Betula papyrifera Marsh., Arbust. amer. 19. 1785: paper birch
(Eng.).
    Betula papyrifera is one source of birch bud oil. At least 6
    varieties can be distinguished, but var. *papyrifera* is the
    one usually encountered.
Betula pubescens Ehrh., Beitr. Naturk. 6:98. 1791 (*B. alba* L., *B.
odorata* Bechst.).
    Betula pubescens is one source for birch bud oil and birch tar.
    Many cultivars exist.
Betula verrucosa Ehrh., Beitr. Naturk. 6:98. 1791 (*B. alba* L., *B.
pendula* L.).
    Betula verrucosa is one source for birch bud oil and birch tar.
    Many cultivars exist.

Salicaceae

Populus L., Sp. pl. 1034. 1753.
Literature: 1, 16, 106, 116, 140, 141
Species:
Populus balsamifera L., Sp. pl. 1034. 1753 (*P. tacamahacca* Mill.):
    hackmatack (Eng.), tacamahac (Eng.), poplar (Eng.), peuplier
    (Fr.), Pappel (Ger.), pioppo (It.), alamo (Sp.).
    Two subspecies exist, but subsp. *balsamifera* is most often
    encountered.

Populus x *gileadensis* Rouleau, Rhodora 50:235. 1948 (*P. candicans sensu* Michx., non Aiton): balm-of-Gilead (Eng.). This is a hybrid of *P. balsamifera* x *P. deltoides* Bartram ex Marsh. ssp. *deltoides*.

Moraceae

Ficus L., Sp. pl. 1059. 1753.
Literature: 167, 182
Species:
Ficus carica L., Sp. pl. 1059. 1753: fig (Eng.), figue (Fr.), Feige (Ger.), fico (It.), higo (Sp.).

Humulus L., Sp. pl. 1028. 1753.
Literature and Species: see 178; add 124

Santalaceae

Santalum L., Sp. pl. 349. 1753.
Species:
Santalum album L., Sp. pl. 349. 1753: East Indian sandalwood (Eng.), white sandalwood (Eng.), white saunders (Eng.), yellow sandalwood (Eng.), yellow saunders (Eng.), santal des Indes (Fr.), Ostindisches Sandelhoz (Ger.), sandalo Indias Orientales (Sp.).

Aristolochiaceae

Asarum L., Sp. pl. 442. 1753.
Species:
Asarum canadense L., Sp. pl. 442. 1753: wild ginger (Eng.), Canadian snakeroot (Eng.), serpentaire du Canada (Fr.), Canadische Schlangenwurzel (Ger.), asaro (It., Sp.), serpentaria (Sp.).

Chenopodiaceae

Chenopodium L., Sp. pl. 218. 1753.
Literature and Species: see 178; add:
ansérine vermifuge (Fr.) and Amerikanisches-Wurmsamen (Ger.) to *Chenopodium ambrosioides* L.

Caryophyllaceae

Dianthus L., Sp. pl. 409. 1753.
Literature and Species: see 178

Magnoliaceae

Michelia L., Sp. pl. 536. 1753.
Species:
Michelia champaca L., Sp. pl. 536. 1753: champaca (Eng.),
Champaca (Ger.).
Michelia figo Spreng., Syst. veg. 2:643. 1825.

Illiciaceae

Illicium L., Syst. nat. ed. 10. 2:1042, 1050, 1370. 1759.
Species:
Illicium verum J.D. Hook., Bot. Mag. t. 7005. 1888: star anise
(Eng.), badiane de Chine (Fr.), anise etoilé (Fr.), Sternanis
(Ger.), anice stellato (It.), anis estrallado (Sp.).

Annonaceae

Cananga (DC) J.D. Hook. & T. Thomson, Fl. ind. 129. 1855.
Species:
Cananga odorata (Lam.) J.D. Hook. & T. Thompson, Fl. ind. 130.
1855 (*Canangium odoratum* Baill.).
Two forms may be distinguished, [f. *odorata*, or ylang ylang
(Eng., Fr., Sp., Malay), Ylang Ylang (Ger.); and f.
macrophylla Koolhaas, or cananga (Eng., Fr., It., Sp.),
Cananga (Ger.)] but their correct nomenclature needs
study.

Myristicaceae

Myristica Gronov., Fl. orient. 141. 1755.
Literature: 97, 153
Species:
Myristica fragrans Houtt., Nat. Hist. 2(3):333. 1774 (*M. officinalis*
L. fil., *M. moschata* Thunb., *M. aromatica* O. Schwartz, *M.
amboinensis* Gand.): nutmeg & mace (Eng.), noix muscade &
macis (Fr.), Muskatnuss & Macis (Ger.), noce moscata &
macis (It.), nuez moscada & macis (Sp.).

Monimiaceae

Peumus Molina, Sag. stor. nat. Chili 185, 350. 1782.
Species:
Peumus boldus Molina, Sag. stor. nat. Chili 185, 350. 1782: boldo
(Eng., Fr., It., Sp), Boldo (Ger.).

Lauraceae

Aniba Aubl., Hist. pl. Guiane 327. 1775.
　　Literature: 88, 89, 90, 91
　　Species:
　　Aniba duckei Kosterm., Recueil. Trav. Bot. Néerl. 35:924. 1938:
　　　　Brazilian rosewood (Eng.), bois de rose type Brésil (Fr.).
　　Aniba parviflora (Meisn.) Mez, Jahrb. Königl. Bot. Gart. Berlin
　　　　5:56. 1889: Brazilian rosewood (Eng.), bois de rose type Brésil
　　　　(Fr.), Brasilianisches Rosenholz (Ger.).
　　Aniba rosaeodora Ducke, Rev. Int. Bot. Appl. Agric. Trop. 8:845.
　　　　1928.
　　　　Besides the typical variety, the principal variety harvested is:
　　　　var. *amazonica* Ducke, Arch. Jard. Bot. Rio de Janeiro 5:110.
　　　　　　f. 6. 1930: Brazilian rosewood (Eng.), bois de rose type
　　　　　　Brésil (Fr.), Brasilianisches Rosenholz (Ger.), legno di rose
　　　　　　(It.), bois de rosa (Sp.).

Cinnamomum Schaeff., Bot. exped. 74. 1760.
　　Literature: 88, 89, 90, 91
　　Species:
　　Cinnamomum burmannii (Nees & T. Nees) Blume, Bijdr. fl. Ned.
　　　　Ind.11:569. 1826 (*C. pedunculata* J. Presl): Indonesian cassia
　　　　(Eng.), Padang cassia (Eng.), Padang cinnamon (Eng.), Batavia
　　　　cassia (Eng.), Java cassia (Eng.), Korintje cassia (Eng.),
　　　　cannelle type Indonésia (Fr.).
　　Cinnamomum camphora (L.) J. Presl, Prir. Rostl. 2:36, 47-56. t. 8.
　　　　1825 (*Laurus camphora* L.): camphor tree (Eng.), camphre
　　　　(Fr.), Campher (Ger.), canfora (It.), alcanfor (Sp.), kuso-no-ki
　　　　(Jap.).
　　　　At least 12 varieties have been published but their synonymy
　　　　still remains to be fully assessed. The 13 chemical subvarieties
　　　　of Hirota (73) were not validly published according to the
　　　　ICBN (190) and are difficult to appraise in terms of the
　　　　previously published taxa of *C. camphora*.
　　Cinnamomum cassia J. Presl, Prir. Rost. 2:36, 44-45. t. 6. 1825.
　　　　(*C. aromaticum* Nees): cassia (Eng.), canelle de Cochinchine
　　　　(Fr.), Cassia (Ger.), Zimtcassie (Ger.), canela de la China
　　　　(Sp.), kashia-keihi (Jap.), keui (Chin.).
　　Cinnamomum cecidodaphne Meisn. in DC, Prodr. 15(1):25. 1864:
　　　　Nepalese tejpat (Eng.).
　　Cinnamomum culiliban J. Presl, Prir. Rostl. 2:45. 1825 [*C.
　　　　culiliwan* (Roxb.) J. Presl.]: lawang (Indonesian).
　　Cinnamomum micranthum (Hayata) Hayata, Icon. pl. formos.
　　　　3:160, 246. 1913: Chinese sassafras (Eng.), sassafras de Chine
　　　　(Fr.), ohba-kusu (Jap.), pha-chium (Chin.).

Cinnamomum tamala (F. Ham.) T. Nees & Eberm., Handb.
med.-pharm. Bot. 2:426, 428. 1831: Indian cassia (Eng.),
tejpat (Indian).

Cinnamomum zeylanicum Blume, Bijdr. 568. 1825-1826 (*Laurus*
cinnamomum L., *C. verum* J. Presl): cinnamon (Eng.), Sri
Lanka (or Ceylon) cinnamon (Eng.), Seychelles cinnamon
(Eng.), Madagascar cinnamon (Eng.), cannelle (Fr.), cannelle
type Sri Lanka (Fr.), cannelle type Seychelles (Fr.), cannelle
type Madagascar (Fr.), Zimt (Ger.), cannella (It.), canela (Sp.,
Port.), seiron-nikkei (Jap.), koritsa (Rus.), jou-kuei (Chin).

Cryptocarya R.Br., Prodr. 402. 1810.
Literature: 88, 89, 90, 91
Species:
Cryptocarya massoy (Oken) Kosterm., New crit. Mal. pl. 3:21. f. 9,
10. 1955 (*Massoia aromatica* Becc.): massoi (Eng.), Massoi
(Ger.).

Laurus L., Sp. pl. 369. 1753.
Literature and Species: see 178

Lindera Thunb., Nova gen. pl. 64. 1783.
Literature: 88, 89, 90, 91
Species:
Lindera umbellata Thunb., Nova Acta Regiae Soc. Sci. Upsal.
4:40. 1783.
This species may be broken into 7 varieties, but the 3 most
important are:
var. *umbellata*: kuro-moji (Jap.).
var. *lancea* Momiyama, J. Jap. Bot. 28(10):317. 1953: hime-
kuro-moji (Jap.)
var. *membranacea* Makino, Bot. Mag. (Tokyo) 14:185. 1900:
ōba-kuro-moji (Jap.).

Litsea Lam., Encycl. 3:574. 1792.
Literature: 88, 89, 90, 91
Species:
Litsea cubeba (Lour.) Pers., Syn. pl. 2:4. 1806 (*L. citrata* Blume):
May-Chang (Ger.), sambal (Javanese).

Nectandra Rolander ex Rottb., Acta Lit. Univ. Hafn. 1:279. 1778.
Literature: 88, 89, 90, 91
Species:
Nectandra elaiophora Barb. Rodr., Vellosia ed. 2. 1:64. t. 18. 1891:
louro nhamuy (Port., Brazil).

Ocotea Aubl., Hist. pl. Guiane 780. 1775.
Literature: 88, 89, 90, 91
Species:

Ocotea caudata (Nees) Mez, Jahrb. Königl. Bot. Gard. Berlin
   5:378. 1889 (*Licaria guianensis* Aubl.): Cayenne rosewood
   (Eng.), bois de rose de Cayenne (Fr.), Cayenne Rosenholz
   (Ger.), Cayenne-Linaloe (Ger.).
Ocotea cymbarum Humb., Bonpl. & Kunth, Nov. gen. sp. 2:166.
   1817 (*Mespilodaphne sassafras* Meisn.): Amazonian sassafras
   (Eng.).
Ocotea pretiosa (Nees) Benth. & J.D. Hook., Gen. pl. 3:158. 1880:
   Brazilian sassafras (Eng.), sassafras du Brésil (Fr.).

Phoebe Nees, Syst. laur. 98. 1836.
   Literature: 88, 89, 90, 91
   Species:
Phoebe nanmu Gamble in Sarg., Pl. wilson. 2:72. 1914.

Brassicaceae (Cruciferae)

Armoracia P. Gaertn., B. Mey. & Scherb. Oekon. Fl. Wetterau 2:426.
   1800.
   Literature and Species: see 178
Brassica L., Sp. pl. 666. 1753.
   Literature and Species: see 178; add 176
Cheiranthus L., Sp. pl. 661. 1753.
   Literature: 5
   Species:
Cheiranthus cheiri L., Sp. pl. 661. 1753: wallflower (Eng.),
   revenelle (Fr.), Goldlack (Ger.), violacciocca (It.).

Resedaceae

Reseda L., Sp. pl. 448. 1753.
   Literature: 206
   Species:
Reseda odorata L., Syst. nat. ed. 10. 2:1046. 1759: reseda (Eng.),
   common mignonette (Eng.), mignonette (Fr.), Reseda (Ger.).

Grossulariaceae

Ribes L., Sp. pl. 200. 1753.
   Literature: 84, 195
   Species:
Ribes nigrum L., Sp. pl. 201. 1753: black currant (Eng.), cassis
   (Fr.), groseillier noir (Fr.), Schwarze Johannisbeere (Ger.),
   ribes nero (It.), grosella negra (Sp.).
   A number of forms and cultivars exist. Black currant oil is
   also known as "niribine" oil.

Hamamelidaceae

Liquidambar L., Sp. pl. 999. 1753.
    Literature: 106
    Species:
Liquidambar orientalis Mill., Gard. dict. ed. 8. 1768: oriental
        sweetgum (Eng.), Levant styrax (Eng.), Asiatic styrax (Eng.),
        styrax (Fr.), Storax (Ger.).
Liquidambar styraciflua L., Sp. pl. 999. 1753: sweetgum (Eng.),
        American styrax (Eng.).

Rosaceae

Prunus L., Sp. pl. 473. 1753.
    Literature: 106, 196
    Species:
Prunus dulcis (Mill.) D.A. Webb, Feddes Repert. 74:24. 1967
        [*Amygdalus communis* L.; *A. dulcis* Mill.; *P. communis* (L.)
        Arcang., non Huds.; *Prunus amygdalus* Batsch.].
    Two varieties may be distinguished:
    var. *dulcis*: sweet almond (Eng.).
    var. *amara* (DC) H.E. Moore, Baileya 19:169. 1975: bitter
        almond (Eng.), amandes amères (Fr.), Bittermandel (Ger.),
        mandorla amara (It.), almendras amargas (Sp.).

Rosa L., Sp. pl. 491. 1753.
    Literature and Species: see 178

Mimosaceae

Acacia Mill., Gard. dict. abr. ed. 4. 1754.
    Literature: 2, 106
    Species:
Acacia caven (Molina) Molina, Sag. stor. nat. Chili ed. 2. 163, 299.
        1810. (*A. cavenia* Hook. & Arnott): Roman cassie (Eng.),
        cassie Romaine (Fr.).
Acacia dealbata Link, Enum. hort. berol. alt. 2:445. 1822: mimosa
        (Eng., Fr., It., Sp.), Mimose (Ger.).
Acacia farnesiana (L.) Willd., Sp. pl. ed. 4. 4:1083. 1806:
        sweetacacia (Eng.), cassie (Eng.), cassie ancienne (Fr.), Cassie
        (Ger.), gaggia (It.), acacia (Sp.), huisache (Sp., Mex.).

Fabaceae (Leguminosae, *pro parte*)

Copaifera L., Sp. pl. ed. 2. 557. 1762.
Species:
  Copaifera coricea Mart., Reise Bras. 1:285. 1823: copaiba (Eng.,
    Sp.), copahu (Fr.), Copaiva (Ger.).
  Copaifera guyanensis Desf., Mem. Mus. Paraná 7:376. 1821:
    copaiba (Eng., Sp.), copahu (Fr.), Copaiva (Ger.).
  Copaifera lansdorffinii Desf., Mem. Mus. Paraná 7:377. 1821:
    copaiba (Eng., Sp.), copahu (Fr.), Copaiva (Ger.).
  Copaifera martii Hayne, Getreue Darstell. Gew. 10:t 15. 1827:
    copaiba (Eng., Sp.), copahu (Fr.), Copaiva (Ger.).
  Copaifera multijuga Hayne, Getreue Darstell. Gew. 10:sub t. 15.
    1827: copaiba (Eng., Sp.), copahu (Fr.), Copaiva (Ger.).
  Copaifera officinalis (Jacq.) L., Sp. pl. ed. 2. 557. 1762: copaiba
    (Eng., Sp.), copahu (Fr.), Copaiva (Ger.).
    Copaifera officinalis yields a resin called Maracaibo balsam or
    balsam copaiba.
  Copaifera reticulata Ducke, Arch. Jard. Bot. Rio de Janeiro
    1:22.1915: copaiba (Eng., Sp.), copahu (Fr.), Copaiva (Ger.).

Daniellia Benn., Pharm. J. Trans. 14:252. 1854.
Literature: 78
Species:
  Daniellia thurifera Benn., Pharm. J. Trans. 14:252. 1854.
    The resin of *D. thurifera* is variously sold as ogea gum,
    frankincense, illorin gum, or balsam copaiba or balsam Sierra
    Leone (Eng.).

Dipteryx Schreb., Gen. 485. 1791.
Literature: 133
Species:
  Dipteryx odorata (Aubl.) Willd., Sp. pl. 3:910. 1802 (*Coumarouna
    odorata* Aubl.): Dutch tonka bean (Eng.), fève de tonka (Fr.),
    Tonkabohne (Ger.), fava tonka (It.), haba tonca (Sp.).

Glycyrrhiza L., Sp. pl. 741. 1753.
Literature: 207
Species:
  Glycyrrhiza glabra L., Sp. pl. 742. 1753: licorice (Eng., Amer.),
    liquorice (Eng., Brit.), réglisse (Fr.), Lakritze (Ger.), Süssholz
    (Ger.), liquirizia (It.), regaliz (Sp.).

Melilotus Mill., Gard. dict. abr. ed. 4. 1754.
Literature: 65
Species:
  Melilotus officinalis (L.) Pall., Reise russ. Reich. 3:537. 1776:
    yellow melilot (Eng.), mélilot officinal (Fr.), Gelber Steinklee
    (Ger.), meliloto giallo (It.), meliloto amarillo (Sp.).

Myrocarpus Alemâo, Pl. novas Brasil [no. 5]. 1847.
Species:
Myrocarpus fastigiatus Allemâo, Pl. novas Brasil [no. 5]. 1847:
cabreuva (Eng.).
Myrocarpus frondosus Allemâo, Pl. novas Brasil [no. 8]. 1848:
cabreuva (Eng.).

Myroxylon L. fil., Suppl. pl. 34, 233. 1782.
Literature: 142
Species:
Myroxylon balsamum (L.) Harms, Notizbl. Königl. Bot. Gart.
Berlin 5:94. 1908 (*Toluiferum balsamum* L., *M. toluiferum*
Humb., Bonpl. & Kunth).
This species may be divided into at least 3 varieties:
var. *balsamum* (var. *genuinum* Baill.): opobalsam (Eng.), tolu
(Eng., Fr., Sp.), Tolu (Ger.), tolu (It.).
var. *pereirae* (Royle) Harms, Notizbl. Königl. Bot. Gart. Berlin
5:95. 1908 [*Myrospermum pereirae* Royle, *Myroxylon
pereirae* (Royle) Klotsch, *Toluifera pereirae* (Royle) Baill.]:
balsam Peru (Eng.), baume de Pérou (Fr.), Perubalsam
(Ger.), balsamo del Peru (It.), balsamo Peru (Sp.),
vermelho (Port., Brazil).
var. *punctatum* (Klotsch) Harms, Notizbl. Konigl. Bot. Gard,
Berlin 5:97. 1908 (*Myroxylon punctatum* Klotsch in
Hayne).

Robinia L., Sp. pl. 722. 1753.
Literature: 12, 106
Species:
Robinia pseudo-acacia L., Sp. pl. 722. 1753: black locust (Eng.),
false acacia (Eng.), yellow locust (Eng.).

Spartium L., Sp. pl. 708. 1753
Literature: 70
Species:
Spartium junceum L., Sp. pl. 708. 1753: Spanish broom (Eng.),
weaver's broom (Eng.), genêt d'Espagne (Fr.), Spanischer
Ginster (Ger.), ginstra (It., Sp.).

Trifolium L., Sp. pl. 764. 1753.
Literature: 31
Species:
Trifolium pratense L., Sp. pl. 768. 1753: red clover (Eng.).
This species includes 5 varieties, but var. *pratense* is most
commonly encountered.

Trigonella L., Sp. pl. 776. 1753.
Literature and Species: see 178

Geraniaceae

Geranium L., Sp. pl. 676. 1753.
   Literature: 56, 199
   Species:
   Geranium macrorrhizum L., Sp. pl. 680. 1753: Bulgarian geranium
      (Eng.), zdravetz (Bulgarian).

Pelargonium L'Hér. ex Aiton, Hort. kew. 2:417. 1789.
   Literature: 120, 121, 189
   Species:
   Pelargonium graveolens L'Hér. ex Aiton, Hort. kew. 2:423. 1789:
      rose geranium (Eng.), geranium (Eng.), géranium (Fr.),
      Geranium (Ger.), geranio (It., Sp.).
      While numerous species [*P.* x *asperum* Ehrh. ex Willd., *P.
      capitatum* (L.) L'Hér. ex Aiton, *P. odoratissimum* (L.) L Hér.
      ex Aiton, and *P. radens* H.E. Moore] have been cited in the
      chemical literature as sources of rose geranium oil, *P.
      graveolens* seems to be the only species commercially cul-
      tivated.

Zygophyllaceae

Bulnesia Gay Fl. Chil. 1:474. 1846.
   Species:
   Bulnesia sarmientii Lorentz ex Griseb., Abh. Königl. Ges.
      Wiss.Göttingen 24:75. 1879: guaiac wood (Eng.), bois de gaiac
      (Fr.), Guajakholz (Ger.), guaico (It.), guajaco (Sp.).

Rutaceae

Agathosma Willd., Enum. pl. hort. Berol. 259. 1809.
   Literature: 58, 129
   Species:
   Agathosma betulina (Bergius) Pillans, J.S. African Bot. 16:75. 1950
      [*Barosma betulina* (Bergius) Bartil & Wendl.]: mountain buchu
      (Eng.), short buchu (Eng.), bucco (Fr., It.), Bucco (Ger.), buchu
      (Sp.).
   Agathosma crenulata (L.) Pillans, J.S. African Bot. 16:73. 1950.
      [*Barosma crenulata* (L.) Hook.]: oval buchu (Eng.), crenate
      buchu (Eng.), bucco (Fr., It.), Bucco (Ger.), buchu (Sp.).

Amyris P. Br., Civ. nat. hist. Jamaica 208. 1756.
   Literature: 161
   Species:

Amyris balsamifera L., Syst. nat. ed. 10. 1000. 1759: amyris (Eng.,
Fr.), West Indian sandalwood (Eng.), West Indian rosewood
(Eng.), bois de santal de l'Amérique Centrale (Fr.), sandalo
delle India Occidental (It.).

Boronia Sm., Trans. nat. hist. 288. 1798.
Species:
Boronia megastigma Nees ex Bartt. in Lehm., Pl. Preiss. 2:227.
1848: boronia (Eng., Fr., It., Sp.), Boronia (Ger.).

Citrus L., Sp. pl. 782. 1753.
Literature: 13, 74, 110, 131, 144, 145, 146, 147, 166, 168, 169,
170, 171, 173
Species:
Citrus aurantifolia (Christm. & Panz.) Swingle, J. Wash. Acad. Sci.
3:465. 1913 (*C. latifolia* Tan.): lime (Eng., Fr.), Limette (Ger.),
lima (It., Sp.).
The small-fruited acid limes probably involve ramets of one
clone known as Mexican in California and either Key or West
Indian in Florida; the cultivar designation 'West Indian' seems
to be preferred. The large-fruited acid limes, or Persian limes,
usually refer to either the 'Tahiti' or 'Bearss' clones.
Citrus aurantium L., Sp. pl. 782. 1753.
The fruit of *C. aurantium* is known as bitter orange (Eng.),
sour orange (Eng.), Seville orange (Eng.), bigarade (Fr.), orange
amère (Fr.), Bittere Pomeranze (Ger.), arancio amaro (It.), or
naranga amarga (Sp.), or daidai (Jap.).
The flowers of *C. aurantium* yield neroli (Eng., Fr., It., Sp.),
Neroli (Ger.), or orange flower concrete and absolute (Eng.).
Cultivars which are raised for their flowers include 'Bouquet'
('Bouquet des Fleurs'), 'Bouquetier à Grandes Fleurs'
('Bouquetier à Peau Epaisse'), and 'Bouquetier de Nice a
Fleurs Doubles' ('Bouquetier de Nice a Fruits Plats,'
'Bouquetier de Nice').
The leaves of *C. aurantium* yield petitgrain (Eng., Fr., It., Sp.),
Petitgrain (Ger.), or petitgrain bigardier (Fr.).
A "water oil" extracted from a mixture of orange flower water
and petitgrain bigarade water is known as "eau de brouts."
Citrus bergamia Risso & Poit., Hist. nat. orangers 111. 1818 [*C.
aurantium* L. subsp. *bergamia* (Risso & Poit.) Wight &
Walker-Arn.]: bergamot (Eng.), bergamote (Fr.), Bergamot
(Ger.), bergamotto (It.), bergamota (Sp.).
'Castagnaro' and 'Femmenillo' are 2 preferred cultivars of
bergamot.
Citrus hystrix DC, Cat. pl. horti monsp. 97. 1813: leech-lime
(Eng.), Mauritius papeda (Eng.), combava (Eng.).
Citrus jambhiri Lush., Indian Forester 36(6/7):342. 1910: rough
lemon (Eng.), jamberi (Indian).

Citrus jambhiri represents stabilized hybrid taxa of *C. medica* x. *C. reticulata* with introgression from *C. limon*, *C. sinensis*, and *C. aurantium*. Two cultivars, 'Estes' and 'Milam,' are noted.

Citrus limon (L.) N. L. Burm., Fl. indica 173. 1768: lemon (Eng.), citron (Fr.), Zitrone (Ger.), limone (It.), limón (Sp.).

Many cultivars are noted: 'Berna' is preferred in Spain; 'Eureka' and 'Lisbon' are preferred in California; 'Femminello Ovale' and 'Femminello Sfusato' are preferred in Italy.

Citrus medica L., Sp. pl. 782. 1753: citron (Eng.), cedrat (Eng., Fr.), cedrat petitgrain (Eng., Fr.), Zitrone (Ger.), Cedrat (Ger.).

A number of cultivars are noted; 'Diamante' is the leading cultivar in Italy and probably elsewhere.

Citrus x *paradisi* Macfady., Bot. Misc. 1:304. 1830 [*C. maxima* (L.) Osbeck var. *racemosa* (Roem.) Stone]: grapefruit (Eng.), pamplemousse (Fr.), Pampelmuse (Ger.), pompelmo (It.), toronja (Sp.).

Citrus x *paradisi* is a relatively recent hybrid of *C. maxima* x *C. sinensis*. Many cultivars are noted; 'Duncan' is a standard in Florida.

Citrus reticulata Blanco, Fl. Filip. 610. 1837 (*C. deliciosa* Ten.; *C. nobilis* Andr., non Lour.; *C. unshiu* Marcovitch): mandarin (Eng.), tangerine (Eng.), mandarine (Fr.), Mandarine (Ger.), mandarino (It.), mandarina (Sp.).

Many cultivars are noted. This species, defined here according to Swingle (168), includes 4 groups: satsuma mandarin or unshû mikan (Jap.) (*C. unshiu*); king mandarin (*C. nobilis*); Mediterranean mandarin (*C. deliciosa*); and common mandarin (*C. reticulata*). 'Cravo' ('Laranja Cravo'), a selection of the common mandarin, is sometimes cited in the chemical literature as a separate taxon.

Citrus sinensis (L.) Osbeck, Dagb. Ostind. resa 41. 1757: sweet orange (Eng.), orange douce (Fr.), orange du Portugal (Fr.), Süsses Orange (Ger.), arancio dolce (It.), naranja dulce (Sp.).

Many cultivars are noted, but 'Valencia' is the most important.

Citrus jambhiri x *C. aurantifolia*: lem'n lime (Eng.).

Citrus limon x *C. sinensis*: lemonange (Eng.).

This hybrid includes the 'Meyer' "lemon."

Citrus reticulata x *C.* x *paradisi*: tangelo (Eng.).

Many cultivars are noted; 'Minneola' and 'Orlando' are 2 of the most important cultivars in the U.S.

Dictamnus L., Sp. pl. 383. 1753.

Literature: 172

Species:

Dictamnus albus L., Sp. pl. 383. 1753: dittany (Eng.), fraxinella (Eng., Sp.), burning bush (Eng.), gas plant (Eng.), dictame (Fr.), fraxinelle (Fr.), Weisser Diptam (Ger.), Ascherwurz (Ger.), dittamo (It.), dictamo blanco (Sp.).

Galipea Aubl., Hist. pl. Guiane 662. 1775.
Species:
Galipea trifoliata Aubl., Hist. pl. Guiane 662. 1775 [*G. officinalis* Hancock, *G. cusparia* St. Hil., *Cusparia trifoliata* (Aubl.) Engl.]: angostura (Eng., Fr., It.), Angostura (Ger.), cuspa (Sp.).

Luvunga F. Ham. ex R. Wight & Arnott, Prodr. 90. 1834.
Species:
Luvunga scandens (Roxb.) R. Wight, Ill. Indian pl. 1:108. 1840 sugandh kokila (Indian).

Ruta L., Sp. pl. 383. 1753.
Literature: 178
Species: see 178; add:
Ruta angustifolia Pers., Syn. pl. 1:464. 1805: Sardinian rue (Eng.), North African rue (Eng.).
Ruta chalepensis L., Mant. pl. 69. 1767 (*R. bracteosa* DC): winter rue (Eng.), North African rue (Eng.), Sicilian rue (Eng.).
Ruta montana (L.) L., Amoen. acad. 3:52. 1756: summer rue (Eng.), Spanish rue (Eng.), North African rue (Eng.).

Skimmia Thunb, Nova gen. 3:57. 1783.
Species:
Skimmia laureola (DC) Sieb. & Zucc. ex Walp., Repert. bot. syst. 5:405. 1846.

Zanthoxylum L., Sp. pl. 270. 1753.
Literature: 54, 166, 193
Species:
Zanthoxylum alatum Steudel, Nom. ed. 2. 2:796. 1841: tomarseed (Eng.).
This species may be one source for Szechuan pepper.
Zanthoxylum piperitum DC, Prodr. 1:725. 1824: prickly ash (Eng.), san-shō (Jap.).
Zanthoxylum rhetsa (Roxb.) DC, Prodr. 1:728. 1824 [*Zanthoxylum bodrunga* (Roxb.) DC]: mulilam (Indian).
Zanthoxylum schinifolium Sieb. & Zucc., Abh. Math.-Phys. Cl. Königl. Bayer. Akad. Wiss. 4(2):1846 (*Zanthoxylum mantchuricum* Benn.): pepperbush (Eng.), inuzanshō (Jap.).
Zanthoxylum simulans Hance, Ann. Sci. Nat. Bot. ser. 5. 5:208. 1866 (*Zanthoxylum bungei* Planch.): Chinese pepper (Eng.), Szechuan pepper (Eng.), hua-chiao (Chin.).

Burseraceae

Boswellia Roxb. ex Colebr., Asiat. Res. 9:379. 1807.
Literature: 69, 179
Species:
Boswellia bhau-dajiana Birdwood, Trans. Linn. Soc. London
27:144. t. 31. 1870: frankincense (Eng.).
Boswellia carteri Birdwood, Trans. Linn. Soc. London 27:143. t.
29. 1870: frankincense (Eng.), olibanum (Eng.), encens oliban
(Fr.), Weibrauch (Ger.), Olibanum (Ger.), olibano (It., Sp.).
Boswellia frereana Birdwood, Trans. Linn. Soc. London 27:146. t.
32. 1870: African elemi (Eng.), elemi frankincense (Eng.).
Boswellia papyrifera (Del.) Hochst., Flora 26:81. 1843: Sudanese
frankincense (Eng.).
Boswellia sacra Fluckiger, Lehrb. Pharmakog. Pflanzenreichs 31.
1867 (*B. thurifera sensu* Carter): Saudi frankincense (Eng.).
Boswellia serrata Roxb. ex Colebr., Asiat. Res. 9:379. 1870: Indian
frankincense (Eng.), Indian olibanum (Eng.).

Bursera Jacq. ex L., Sp. pl. ed. 2. 471. 1762.
Literature: 115
Species:
Bursera aloexylon (Schiede) Engl. in DC, Monogr. phan. 4:52.
1883. linaloe (Eng., Sp.), linaloé (Fr.), Linaloe (Ger.).
Bursera fagaroïdes (Humb., Bonpl. & Kunth) Engl. in Engl., Bot.
Jahrb. Syst. 1:44. 1881: linaloe (Eng., Sp.), linaloé (Fr.),
Linaloe (Ger.).
Bursera glabrifolia (Humb., Bonpl. & Kunth) Engl. in Engl. &
Prantl, Nat. Pflanzenfam. III. 4:251. 1896 (*B. delpechiana*
Poisson): linaloe (Eng., Sp.), linaloé (Fr.), Linaloe (Ger.).
Bursera penicillata (Sesse & Moc. ex DC) Engl. in Engl., Bot.
Jahrb. Syst. 1:44. 1881: linaloe (Eng., Sp.), linaloé (Fr.),
Linaloe (Ger.).
Bursera simaruba (L.) Sarg., Gard. & Forest 3:260. 1890 [*B.
gummifera* L., *Elaphrium simaruba* (L.) Rose]: West Indian
birch (Eng.), West Indian elemi (Eng.), gumbo limbo (Eng.),
incense tree (Eng.), almácigo (Sp.).
The gum of *B. simaruba* is known as elequeme or tacamahaca
in Costa Rica.

Canarium L., Amoen. acad. 4:121. 1759.
Species:
Canarium luzonicum Miq., Fl. Ned. Ind. 1^2:651. 1859: elemi (Eng.,
It., Sp.), elémi (Fr.), Elemi (Ger.).

Commiphora Jacq., Pl. hort. schoenbr. 2:66. 1797.
Literature: 179, 203
Species:

Commiphora erythraea (Ehrenb.) Engl. in DC, Monogr. phan. 4:20.
1883: opopanax (Eng., Fr., It.), bisabol myrr (Eng.), Opopanax
(Ger.), opopónaco (Sp.).

Commiphora madagascariensis Jacq., Pl. hort. schoenbr. 2:66.
1797 (*Balsamodendron habessinica* O. Berg., *C. abyssinica*
Engl.): Abyssinian myrrh (Eng.).

Commiphora molmol Engl. ex Tschirch, Handb. pharmakogn.
3:117. 1925: Somalian myrrh (Eng.).

Commiphora myrrha (Nees) Engl. in DC, Monogr. phan. 4:10.
1883: common myrrh (Eng.), hirabol myrrh (Eng.), myrrhe
(Fr.), Myrrhe (Ger.), mirra (It., Sp.).

Meliaceae

Aglaia Lour., Fl. cochinch. 173. 1790.
Species:
Aglaia odorata Lour., Fl. cochinch. 173. 1790.

Cabralea Adr. Juss., Mem. Mus. Nat. Hist. 19:229. 1830.
Species:
Cabralea cangerana Saldanha, Ann. Sci. Nat. Bot. 19:210. 1874:
cangerana (Eng.).

Cedrela P. Br., Civ. nat. hist. Jamaica 158. 1756.
Species:
Cedrela odorata L., Syst. nat. ed. 10. 940. 1759: West Indian cedar
(Eng.), Spanish cedar (Eng.), cigar-box cedar (Eng.), Barbados
cedar (Eng.), Cedrela (Ger.).

Euphorbiaceae

Croton L., Sp. pl. 1004. 1753.
Literature: 34
Species:
Croton eluteria (L.) Swartz, Nov. gen. & sp. pl. 100. 1788:
cascarilla (Eng., It., Sp.), cascarille (Fr.), Kaskarillbaum (Ger.).

Anacardiaceae

Pistacia L., Sp. pl. 1025. 1753.
Literature: 184
Species:
Pistacia lentiscus L., Sp. pl. 1026. 1753: mastic (Eng.).

Schinus L., Sp. pl. 388. 1753.
Literature: 161
Species:

Schinus molle L., Sp. pl. 388. 1753: Peruvian pepper tree (Eng.), Peruvian mastic (Eng.), California pepper tree (Eng.), molée des jardins (Fr.), Weichpfeffer (Ger.), schino (It.), pimenta falsa (Sp.), arvoiera (Sp.).

Aquifoliaceae

Ilex L., Sp. pl. 125. 1753.
Literature: 59
Species:
Ilex paraguayensis St. Hil., Mém. Mus. Hist. Nat. 9:351. 1822: Paraguay tea (Eng.), yerba maté (Sp.).

Malvaceae

Abelmoschus Medik., Malvenfam. 45. 1787.
Literature: 14
Species:
Abelmoschus moschatus Medik., Malvenfam. 45. 1787. (*Hibiscus abelmoschus* L.): ambrette (Eng., Fr.), Moschuskörner (Ger.), ambretta (It.), abelmosco (Sp.).

Byttneriaceae

Theobroma L., Sp. pl. 782. 1753.
Literature: 32, 40
Species:
Theobroma cacao L., Sp. pl. 782. 1753: chocolate (Eng., Sp.), chocolat (Fr.), Schokolade (Ger.), cioccolata (It.).
Two subspecies [ssp. *cacao*, with 4 *formae*, and ssp. *sphaeocarpum* (A. Chev.) Cuatrecasas] exist, but ssp. *cacao* is most important. The cultivar groups represented by 'Criollo Morris' and 'Forastero Morris' are most frequently cultivated, but the latter supplies a lower quality of cocoa.

Theaceae

Camellia L., Sp. pl. 698. 1753.
Literature: 148
Species:
Camellia sinensis (L.) Kuntze, Um de Erde 500. 1881. tea (Eng.), thé (Fr.), Tee (Ger.), tè (It.), té (Sp.).
Two varieties exist:
var. *sinensis*: China tea (Eng.).
var. *assamica* (Mast.) Kitam., Acta Phytotax. Geobot. 14:59. 1950: Assam tea (Eng.).

Dipterocarpaceae

Dipterocarpus Gaertn., Fruct. sem. pl. 3:50. 1805.
Species:
Dipterocarpus alatus Roxb., Hort. bengal. 42. 1814: gurjun (Eng.,
Fr.), May-Nhang (Ger.).
Dipterocarpus jourdainii Pierre ex Laness., Pl. util. col. franç. 298.
1886: gurjun (Eng., Fr.), Gurjun (Ger.).
Dipterocarpus tuberculatus Roxb., Hort. bengal. 93. 1814: gurjun
(Eng., Fr.), Gurjun (Ger.), in (Burmese).
Dipterocarpus turbinatus C. F. Gaertn., Suppl. carp. 51. t. 188.
1805: gurjun (Eng., Fr.), East Indian copaiba balsam (Eng.),
kanyin (Burmese).

Dryobalanops Gaertn., Fruct. sem. pl. 3:49. 1805.
Species:
Dryobalanops aromatica Gaertn., Fruct. sem. pl. 3:49. 1805:
Borneo camphor (Eng.).

Cistaceae

Cistus L., Sp. pl. 523. 1753.
Literature: 19
Species:
Cistus ladanifer L., Sp. pl. 523. 1753. labdanum (Eng., Fr.),
Labdanum (Ger.), labdano (It., Sp.).
Cistus incanus L., Sp. pl. 524. 1753. (*C. villosus* auct. vix L., incl.
C. polymorphus Willk.).
This species may be divided into 3 subspecies:
subsp. *incanus* (*C. tauricus* K. Presl, *C. polymorphus* Willk.
subsp. -villosus- Willk. var. -vulgaris- Willk.).
subsp. *corsicus* (L.) Heywood, Feddes Repert. 79:60. 1968. [*C.
villosus* Willk. subsp. *corsicus* (Loisel.) Rouy & Foucaud].
subsp. *creticus* (L.) Heywood, Feddes Repert. 79:60. 1968. (*C.
creticus* L.): Cretan labdanum (Eng.).

Violaceae

Viola L., Sp. pl. 933. 1753.
Literature and Species: see 178

Thymelaeaceae

Aquilaria Lam., Encycl. 1:49. 1783.
Species:
Aquilaria agallocha Roxb., Hort. bengal. 33. 1814: agarwood
(Eng.), aloës wood (Eng.), Agar (Eng.).

Aquilaria malaccensis Lam., Encycl. 1:49. 1783: Indonesian agarwood (Eng.).

Myrtaceae

Eucalyptus L'Hér., Sert. angl. 18. 1789.
Literature: 19, 85, 128, 135
Species:
Eucalyptus citriodora Hook. in T. Mitch., J. exped. trop. Austral. 235. 1848: lemon-scented gum (Eng.), citron-scented gum (Eng.), spotted gum (Eng.).
Eucalyptus cneorifolia DC, Prodr. 3:220. 1828: Kangaroo Island narrow-leaved mallee (Eng.).
Eucalyptus dives Schauer in Walp., Repert. bot. syst. 2:926. 1843: broad-leaved peppermint (Eng.), blue peppermint (Eng.), peppermint (Eng.).
   A strain rich in 1,8-cineole ("var. c") is cultivated.
Eucalyptus dumosa A. Cunn. ex Schauer in Walp., Repert. bot. syst. 2:925. 1843: mallee (Eng.), congoo mallee (Eng.).
Eucalyptus elata Dehnh., Cat. horti camald. 26. 1829: (*E. andreana* Naudin, *E. lindleyana* DC, *E. longifolia* Lindl., *E. numerosa* Maiden): river peppermint (Eng.), river white gum (Eng.).
Eucalyptus globulus Labill., Voy. rech. Pérouse 1:153. t. 13. 1800: blue gum (Eng.), Tasmanian blue gum (Eng.), southern blue gum (Eng.), eucalyptus (Eng., Fr.), Eucalyptus (Ger.), eucalipto (It., Sp.).
Eucalyptus goniocalyx F.v. Muell., Fragm., 2:48. 1860 (*E. elaeophora* F.v. Muell.): long-leaved box (Eng.), bundy (Eng.), apple jack (Eng.), olive-barked box (Eng.).
Eucalyptus leucoxylon F.v. Muell., Trans. Vict. Inst. 2:33. 1855: yellow gum (Eng.), white ironbark (Eng.), white gum (Eng.).
   Three subspecies exist, but subsp. *leucoxylon* is most common.
Eucalyptus macarthurii H. Deane & Maiden, Proc. Linn. Soc. New South Wales 24:448. 1900: Camden woollybut (Eng.), Paddy's river box (Eng.).
Eucalyptus oleosa F.v. Muell., Fragm. 2:56. 1860: red mallee (Eng.), glossy-leaved red mallee (Eng.).
Eucalyptus polybractea R.T. Baker, Proc. Linn. Soc. New South Wales 25:692. 1901: blue-leaved mallee (Eng.).
Eucalyptus radiata Sieber ex DC, Prodr. 3:218. 1828 (*E. australiana* R.T. Baker & H.G. Sm., *E. phellandra* R.T. Baker & H.G. Sm.): narrow-leaved peppermint (Eng.), gray peppermint (Eng.).
   Two subspecies exist, but subsp. *radiata* has a broader geographical range.

Eucalyptus sideroxylon A. Cunn. in T. Mitch., J. exped. trop.
Austral. 339: 1848: red ironbark (Eng.), ironbark (Eng.),
mugga (Eng.).
Two subspecies exist, but subsp. *sideroxylon* is most often
encountered.

Eucalyptus smithii R.T. Baker, Proc. Linn Soc. New South Wales
12:561. 1888: gully gum (Eng.), gully peppermint (Eng.),
blackbutt peppermint (Eng.).

Eucalyptus staigerana F.v. Muell, ex F.M. Bailey, Syn. Queensl. fl.
176. 1883.

Eucalyptus viminalis Labill., Nov. Holl. pl. 2:12, t. 151. 1806.
Two subspecies exist, but subsp. *viminalis* is more common.

Eucalyptus viridis R.T. Baker, Proc. Linn. Soc. New South Wales
25:316. 1911: green mallee (Eng.).

Melaleuca L., Syst. nat. ed. 12. 2:509. 1767.
Literature: 127
Species:

Melaleuca alterniflora (Maiden & Betche) Cheel, J. & Proc. Roy.
Soc. New South Wales 58:195. 1924 (*M. linariifolia* Sm. var.
alterniflora Maiden & Betche): tea tree (Eng.).

Melaleuca cajaputi Roxb., Hort. bengal. 59. 1814: cajuput (Eng.),
cajeput (Eng., Fr., It., Sp.), Cajeput (Ger.).

Melaleuca leucadendra (L.). L., Syst. nat. ed. 12. 2:509. 1767.
(*Myrtus leucodendra* L.): cajuput (Eng.), cajeput (Eng., Fr., It.,
Sp.), river tea tree (Eng.), weeping tea tree (Eng.), Cajeput
(Ger.).

Melaleuca linariifolia Sm., Trans. Linn. Soc. London 3:278. 1797:
tea tree (Eng.).

Melaleuca minor Sm. in Rees, Cycl. 23:n. 2. 1812: cajuput (Eng.),
cajeput (Eng., Fr., It., Sp.), Cajeput (Ger.).

Melaleuca viridiflora Sol. ex Gaertn., Fruct. sem. pl. 1:175. t. 35.
1788: niaouli (Eng.), cajuput (Eng.), cajeput (Eng., Fr., It.,
Sp.), Cajeput (Ger.).

Myrtus L., Sp. pl. 471. 1753.
Literature: 25
Species:

Myrtus communis L., Sp. pl. 471. 1753: myrtle (Eng.), myrte
commun (Fr.), Myrte (Ger.), mirto (It., Sp.).
At least 2 subspecies exist, but subsp. *communis* is most often
encountered.

Pimenta Lindl., Coll. bot. ad t. 19. 1821.
Literature: 96, 118
Species:

Pimenta dioica (L.) Merr., Contr. Gray Herb. 165:37. 1947. (*P. officinalis* Lindl.): allspice (Eng.), pimento (Eng., It., Sp.), Jamaica pepper (Eng.), piment (Fr.), piment type Jamaïque (Fr.), Piment (Ger.).

Pimenta racemosa (Mill.) J.W. Moore, Bernice P. Bishop Mus. Bull.102:33. 1933. (*P. acris* Wight): bay (Eng., Fr., It.), West Indian bay (Eng.), Bay (Ger.), bay malagueta (Sp.).

Syzygium Gaertn., Fruct. sem. pl. 1:166. 1788.
Literature: 8, 79, 96, 143
Species:

Syzygium aromaticum (L.) Merr. & L.M. Perry, Mem. Amer. Acad. Arts 18:196. 1939 [*Eugenia aromatica* (L.) Baill., *E. caryophyllata* Thunb.]: clove (Eng.), clou de girofle (Fr.), Nelken (Ger.), Gewürznelken (Ger.), garofano (It.), jerofle clavo (Sp.), choji (Jap.), gvozdika (Rus.), ting-hsiang (Chin.), cravo (Port.).

Apiaceae (Umbelliferae)

Anethum L., Sp. pl. 263. 1753.
Literature and Species: see 178

Angelica L., Sp. pl. 250. 1753.
Literature and Species: see 178; add 201

Anthriscus Pers., Syn. pl. 1:320. 1805.
Literature and Species: see 178

Apium L., Sp. pl. 264. 1753.
Literature: 183
Species:

Apium graveolens L., Sp. pl. 264. 1753: celery (Eng.), céleri (Fr.), Sellerie (Ger.), sedano (It.), apio (Sp.).
At least 4 varieties are noted, but var. *graveolens* is grown for its seed oil.

Carum L., Sp. pl. 263. 1753.
Literature and Species: see 178

Coriandrum L., Sp. pl. 256. 1753.
Literature and Species: see 178

Cuminum L., Sp. pl. 254. 1753.
Literature and Species: see 178

Daucus L., Sp. pl. 242. 1753.
Literature: 71
Species:

Daucus carota L., Sp. pl. 242. 1753: carrot (Eng.), carotte (Fr.),
Möhre (Ger.), carota (It.), zanahoria (Sp.).
This species may be divided into at least 12 subspecies, but
the following is most commonly cultivated:
subsp. *sativus* (Hoffm.) Arcang., Comp. fl. ital. 299. 1882.

Dorema D. Don, Philos. Mag. Ann. Chem. 9:47. 1831.
Species:
Dorema ammoniacum D. Don, Philos. Mag. Ann. Chem. 9:47.
1831: ammoniac (Eng.), Bombay sumbul (Eng.), boi (Eng.),
Ammoniacum (Ger.).

Ferula L., pl. 246. 1753.
Literature: see 178; add 87
Species: see 178; add:
Ferula diversivittata Regel & Schmalhausen, Izv. Imp. Obšč.
Ljubit. Estestv. Moskovsk. Univ. 34(2):33. 1882 (*F. suavolens*
Aitch. & Hemsl.): sumbul (Eng., Fr., Sp.), muskroot (Eng.),
Sumbul (Ger.), Moschus (Ger.).
Ferula galbaniflua Boiss. & Buhse, Nov. Mem. Moskovsk. Obšč.
Isp. Prir. 12:99. 1860: galbanum (Eng., Fr.), Galbanum (Ger.),
galbano (It., Sp.).
Ferula jaeschkeana Vatke, Ind. sem. hort. Berol. append. 2. 1876.
Four varieties of this polymorphic species are reported.
Ferula moschata (Reinsch) Kosol-Pol., Bjull. Obšč. Estestvposp.
Voroneszsk. Gosud. Univ. 1:94. 1925 (*F. sumbul* J.D. Hook.):
sumbul (Eng., Fr., Sp.), muskroot (Eng.), Sumbul (Ger.),
Moschus (Ger.).

Foeniculum Mill., Gard. dict. abr. ed. 4. 1754.
Literature and Species: see 178

Levisticum J. Hill, Brit. herb. 423. 1756.
Literature and Species: see 178

Pastinaca L., Sp. pl. 262. 1753.
Literature: 185
Species:
Pastinaca sativa L., Sp. pl. 262. 1753: parsnip (Eng.), panais (Fr.),
Pastinak (Ger.), pastinaca (It.), chiriváa (Sp.).
This species can be divided into 4 subspecies, but subsp.
sativa is most commonly encountered.

Petroselinum J. Hill, Brit. herb. 424. 1756.
Literature and Species: see 178

Pimpinella L., Sp. pl. 263. 1753.
Literature and Species: see 178

Trachyspermum Link, Enum. hort. berol. alt. 1:267. 1821.
Literature and Species: see 178

Ericaceae

Gaultheria L., Sp. pl. 395. 1753.
Species:
Gaultheria procumbens L., Sp. pl. 395. 1753: wintergreen (Eng.),
tea berry (Eng.), gaulthérie (Fr.), Wintergrün (Ger.), gaulteria
(It., Sp.).

Styracaceae

Styrax L., Sp. pl. 444. 1753.
Species:
Styrax benzoin Dryander, Philos. Trans. 77(2):308. t. 12. 1787:
Sumatra benzoin (Eng.), benjoin de Sumatra (Fr.), Benzoë
(Ger.), benzoino (It.), benjui (Sp.).
styrax macrothyrsus Perkins, Bot. Jahrb. Syst. 31:485. 1901:
Vietnam styrax (Eng.).
Styrax paralleloneurus Perkins, Bot. Jahrb. Syst. 31:484. 1901:
haminjon toba (Indonesian).
Styrax tonkinense (Pierre) Craib ex Hartwich, Apotheker-Zeitung
28:698. 1913: Siam styrax (Eng.), benjoin officinal (Fr.).

Oleaceae

Jasminum L., Sp. pl. 7. 1753.
Literature: 62
Species:
Jasminum auriculatum Vahl, Symb. 3:1. 1794: Indian jasmine
(Eng.).
Jasminum grandiflorum L., Sp. pl. ed. 2. 9. 1762 [*J. officinale* L.
var. *grandiflorum* (L.) Stokes, *J. officinale* L. f. *grandiflorum*
(L.) Kobuski]: Catalonian jasmine (Eng.), royal jasmine (Eng.),
Spanish jasmine (Eng.), jasmin à grandes fleurs (Fr.), Jasmin
(Ger.), gelsomino (It.), jazmin (Sp.).
Jasminum sambac (L.) Aiton, Hort. kew. 1:8. 1789: Arabian
jasmine (Eng.), sambac (Eng.).
Two cultivars with double flowers are recorded: 'Maid of
Orleans' with semi-double flowers and 'Grand Duke'
('Grand Duke of Tuscany') with fully double flowers.

Osmanthus Lour., Fl. cochinch. 17. 1790.
Literature: 100
Species:
Osmanthus fragrans Lour., Fl. cochinch. 29. 1790: sweet olive
(Eng.), fragrant olive (Eng.), tea olive (Eng.).

Syringa L., Sp. pl. 8. 1753.
   Literature: 114, 134, 138
   Species:
   Syringa vulgaris L., Sp. pl. 9. 1753: common lilac (Eng.), lilas (Fr.),
      Spanischer Flieder (Ger.), lilla (It.), lila (Sp.).
   Numerous cultivars exist.

Boraginaceae

Heliotropium L., Sp. pl. 130. 1753.
   Literature: 109
   Species:
   Heliotropium arborescens L., Syst. nat. ed. 10. 913. 1759 (*H.
      peruvianum* L.): heliotrope (Eng.).

Verbenaceae

Aloysia Juss., Ann. Mus. Natl. Hist. Nat. 7:75. 1806.
   Literature and Species: see 178

Lippia L., Sp. pl. 633. 1753.
   Literature and Species: see 178

Lamiaceae (Labiatae)

Aeollanthus Mart. ex K. P.J. Sprengel, Syst. Veg. 2:678, 750, 1825.
   Literature: 122
   Species:
   Aeollanthus gamwelliae G. Taylor, J. Bot. 70:106. 1932 (*A.
      graveolens* auct. chem.): ninde (Eng.).

Hedeoma Pers., Syn. pl. 2:131. 1806.
   Literature and Species: see 178

Hyssopus L., Sp. pl. 569. 1753.
   Literature and Species: see 178

Lavandula L., Sp. pl. 572. 1753.
   Literature and Species: see 178

Melissa L., Sp. pl. 592. 1753.
   Literature and Species: see 178

Mentha L., Sp. pl. 576. 1753.
   Literature and Species: see 178

Monarda L.. Sp. pl. 22. 1753
   Literature: See 178
   Species: see 178; add:

Monarda fistulosa L., Sp. pl. 22. 1753: wild bergamot (Eng.), horsemint (Eng.), beebalm (Eng.).
Four varieties exist, but the most important for essential oils is:
var. *menthifolia* (J. Graham) Fernald, Rhodora 3:15. 1901.

Nepeta L., Sp. pl. 570. 1753.
Literature and Species: see 178

Ocimum L., Sp. pl. 597. 1753.
Literature and Species: see 178; add 122

Origanum L., Sp. pl. 588. 1753.
Literature and Species: see 178

Perilla L., Gen. pl. ed. 6. 578. 1764.
Literature and Species: see 178

Pogostemon Desf., Mem. Mus. Hist. Nat. 2:154. 1815.
Literature: 10, 36, 117
Species:
Pogostemon cablin (Blanco) Benth. in DC, Prodr. 12:156. 1848 (*P. patchouly* Pellet.): patchouly (Eng., Fr.), patchouli (Eng., It.), Patchouli (Ger.), patchuli (Sp.).
Pogostemon heyneanus Benth. in Wall., Pl. asiat. rar. 1:31. 1830. (*P. patchouli* J.D. Hook.): false patchouly (Eng.).

Rosmarinus L., Sp. pl. 23. 1753.
Literature: 5, 180
Species:
Rosmarinus officinalis L., Sp. pl. 23. 1753: rosemary (Eng.), romarin (Fr.), Rosmarin (Ger.), rosmarino (It.), ramerino (It.), romero (Sp.), mannenrû (Jap.), rozmarin (Rus.), mi-tieh-hsiang (Chin.), alecrim (Port.).
This species is known by the following cultivated infraspecific taxa:
var. *officinalis*
Derived from this variety are the cultivars 'Arp,' 'Aureus' ('Gilded'), 'Collingwood Ingram' ('Majorca'), 'Constance de Baggio,' 'Dark Logee Blue,' 'Dutch Mill,' 'Gorizia,' 'Herb Cottage' ('Foresteri'), 'Holly Hyde,' 'Huntington Blue,' 'Joyce de Baggio,' 'Light Logee Blue,' 'Lottie de Baggio,' 'Romance Vivace,' 'Severn Sea,' 'Very Oily,' 'Well Sweep,' and 'Well Sweep Golden.' *Rosmarinus officinalis* var. *officinalis* is the source of the commercial rosemary oil, but no cultivar names have been attached to the myriad clones.
f. *albiflorus* Béguinot in Fiori & Paol., Fl. Italia 3:14. 1903 ('Albus'): white-flowered rosemary (Eng.).
f. *erectus* Pasq. ex Béguinot in Fiori & Paol., Fl. Italia 3:14. 1903: upright rosemary (Eng.).

Derived from this *forma* is 'Miss Jessopp's Upright' ('Corsicus,' 'Fastigiatus,' 'Pyramidalis,' 'Trusty'). 'Blue Spire' also seems to be derived from this *forma.*

var. *angustifolius* Sweet, Hort. brit. 311. 1826 [*R. angustifolius* Mill.; *R. tenuifolius* Jord. & Fourr.; *R. officinalis* L. var. *angustissimus* Foucaud & Mand, var. *angustifolius* (Mill.) Gus.]: pine-needled rosemary (Eng.), pine-scented rosemary (Eng.).

Similar to this variety is the cultivar 'Benenden Blue' ('Corsican Blue').

var. *lavandulaceus* (De Noé in Balansa) Munby, Cat. Pl. Algeria 24. 1859 (*R. officinalis* L. *f. humilis* Ten., f. *procumbens* Pasq., var. *rupestris* Pasq. ex Béguinot, var. *prostratus* Pasq.): prostrate rosemary (Eng.).

Derived from this variety are the cultivars 'Alida Hyde,' 'Blue Boy,' 'Lockwood de Forest,' and 'Taylor's Blue.' A number of names have proliferated from prostrate selections which are probably not distinct from the typical variety, but the oldest name is 'Prostratus': 'Dwarf Prostrate,' 'Golden Prostrate,' 'Huntington Carpet,' 'Kenneth Prostrate,' and 'Santa Barbara.'

var. *pubescens* Pamp., Boll. Soc. Bot. Ital. 1914:16. 1914; Pl. tripol. 16. 1914.

f. *roseus* Pamp., Boll. Soc. Bot. Ital. 1914:16; Pl. tripol. 16. 1914: pink-flowered rosemary (Eng.).

Derived from this *forma* are the cultivars 'Majorca Pink' and 'Pinkie.'

var. *rigidus* (Jord. & Fourr.) Cariot & St. Lag., Étude fl. 2:657. 1889 (*R. rigidus* Jord. & Fourr.)

Derived from this variety is the cultivar 'Tuscan Blue.'

Salvia L., Sp. pl. 23. 1753.
Literature: see 178; add 104
Species: see 178; add:
Salvia stenophylla [Burch. ex] Benth., Labiat. gen. spec. 306. 1833.

Satureja L., Sp. pl. 567. 1753.
Literature and Species: see 178

Thymus L., Sp. pl. 590. 1753.
Literature and Species: see 178

Solanaceae

Nicotiana L., Sp. pl. 180. 1753.
Literature: 61
Species:
Nicotiana tabacum L., Sp. pl. 180. 1753: tobacco (Eng.), tabac (Fr.), Tabak (Ger.), tabacco (It.), tabaco (Sp.).

Rubiaceae

Anthocephalus A. Rich., Mém. Rubiac. 157. 1830.
Species:
Anthocephalus indicus A. Rich., Mém. Soc. Hist. Nat. Paris 5:237.
1834 (*A. cadamba* Miq.): cadamba (Eng.), kadamba (Eng.).

Coffea L., Sp. pl. 172. 1753.
Literature: 26, 27, 29, 52
Species:
Coffea arabica L., Sp. pl. 172. 1753: coffee (Eng.), common coffee
(Eng.), Arabian coffee (Eng.), café (Fr., Sp.), Kaffee (Ger.),
caffè (It.).
Many cultivars exist, but the most important are 'Bourbon
Amarelo,' 'Bourbon Vermelho,' 'Laurina,' 'Mundo Novo,'
and 'Sumatra.'
Coffea canephora Pierre ex Froehner, Notizbl. Königl. Bot. Gard.
Berlin 1:237. 1895 (*C. robusta* L. Linden): robusta coffee
(Eng.).
Many cultivars exist including 'Kouillou' ('Quillou'),
'Laurentii,' 'Robusta,' and 'Uganda.'

Gardenia J. Ellis, Philos. Trans. 51:935. t. 23. 1761.
Species:
Gardenia jasminoides J. Ellis, Philos. Trans. 51:935. t. 23. 1761
(*G. florida* L., *G. grandiflora* Lour., *G.radicans* Thunb.):
common gardenia (Eng.), cape jasmine (Eng.), gardénia (Fr.),
Gardenien (Ger.).

Leptactina J.D. Hook., Icon. pl. 11:t. 1092. 1871.
Literature: 78
Species:
Leptactina senegambica J.D. Hook., Icon. pl. 11:74. 1871.
karo-karoundé (Fr.).

Caprifoliaceae

Lonicera L., Sp. pl. 173. 1753.
Literature: 20, 204
Species:
Lonicera etrusca Santi, Viagg. Montamiata 1:113, t. 1. 1795.
The cultivar 'Superba' (*L. gigantea* Carriére) is occasionally
harvested with *L. periclymenum*.
Lonicera periclymenum L., Sp. pl. 173. 1753: common honeysuckle
(Eng.), chevrefeuille (Fr.), Geissblatt (Ger.), caprifoglio (It.),
madreselva (Sp.).
This species is sometimes confused with *L. caprifolium* L.

Sambucus L., Sp. pl. 269. 1753.
Literature: 50
Species:
Sambucus nigra L., Sp. pl. 269. 1753: elderberry (Eng.), elderflower
(Eng.), sureau (Fr.), Holunder (Ger.).

Valerianaceae

Nardostachys DC, Prodr. 4:624. 1830.
Literature: 200
Species:
Nardostachys chinensis Batalin, Trudy Imp. S.-Peterbursk. Bot.
Sada 13:376. 1894: Chinese spikenard (Eng.).
Nardostachys jatamansi (D. Don) DC, Prodr. 4:624. 1830: nard
(Eng.), spikenard (Eng.), jatamansi (Hindi).

Valeriana L., Sp. pl. 31. 1753.
Literature: see 178
Species: see 178; add:
Valeriana fauriei Briq., Annuaire Conserv. Jard. Bot. Genève
17:327. 1914 (*V. officinalis* auct. Jap., non L.; *V. officinalis* L.
var *angustifolia* Miq.; *V. officinalis* L. var. *latifolia* (Miq.):
Japanese valerian (Eng.), kesso (Eng.), kanoko-sō (Jap.).
Valeriana wallichii DC, Prodr. 4:460. 1830: Indian valerian (Eng.).

Asteraceae (Compositae)

Achillea L., Sp. pl. 896. 1753.
Literature: 137
Species:
Achillea millefolium L., Sp. pl. 899. 1753: common yarrow (Eng.),
milfoil (Eng.), achillée millefeuille (Fr.), Gemeine Schafgarbe
(Ger.), millefoglio (It.), milenrama (Sp.).
This is a very polymorphic species which may be divided into
at least 2 subspecies, with subsp. *millefolium* most commonly encountered.
Achillea erba-rotta All., Mélanges Philos. Math. Soc. Roy. Turin
5:69. 1774.
This is a very polymorphic species, but the most important is
the following:
subsp. *moschata* (Wulfen) I.B.K. Richardson, J. Linn. Soc.,
Bot. 71:271. 1976 (*A. moschata* Wulfen): iva (Eng.), musk
yarrow (Eng.), achillea musquée (Fr.), Feldgarbe (Ger.),
achillea muschiata (It.), achillea musgada (Sp.).

Arnica L., Sp. pl. 884. 1753.
Literature: 46, 51
Species:

Arnica montana L., Sp. pl. 884. 1753: arnica (Eng., It., Sp.),
arnique montagnard (Fr.), Arnika (Ger.).
This species can be divided into 2 subspecies, but subsp.
montana is most common.

Artemisia L., Sp. pl. 845. 1753.
Literature: see 178
Species: see 178; add:
Artemisia afra Jacq., Pl. hort. schoenbr. 4:34. t. 467. 1804: African
wormwood (Eng.), lanyana (Eng.), wildeals (Eng.).
Artemisia annua L., Sp. pl. 847. 1753: annual wormwood (Eng.),
sweet Annie (Eng.), qing hao (Chin.).
Artemisia herba-alba Asso, Syn. Stirp. Arag. 117. 1779 (*A.
sieversiana* auct. chem.): armoise (Eng., Fr.).
Artemisia maritima L., Sp. pl. 846. 1753: Levant wormseed (Eng.).
Artemisia pallens Wall. ex DC, Prodr. 6:120. 1838: davana (Eng.,
Fr., It., Sp.), Davana (Ger.).
Artemisia vestita Wallich, Num. list 3301. 1831.

Atractylodes DC, Prodr. 7:48. 1838.
Literature: 77
Species:
Atractylodes lancea (Thunb.) DC, Prodr. 7:48. 1838.
This species has 2 important varieties:
  var. *lancea* (*Atractylodes ovata* Thunb., *Atractylis ovata*
  Thunb., *Atractylis lancea* DC): atractylis (Eng.), cangzhu
  (Chin.), changzhu (Chin.).
  var. *chinensis* (Bunge) Kitam., Trans. Sapporo Nat. Hist. Soc.
  16:63. 1940 [*Atractylodes chinensis* (Bunge) Koidz.,
  Atractylis chinensis (Bunge) DC]: atractylis (Eng.), cangzhu
  (Chin.), changzhu (Chin.).

Baccharis L., Sp. pl. 860. 1753.
Species:
Baccharis dracunculifolia DC, Prodr. 5:421. 1836: vassoura (Port.,
Brazil).
Baccharis genistelloides Pers., Syn. pl. 2:425. 1807: carqueja (Port.,
Brazil).

Balsamita Mill., Gard. dict. abr. ed. 4. 1754.
Literature and Species: see 178

Blumea DC, Arch. Bot. (Paris) 2:514. 1833.
Literature and Species: see 178

Brachylaena R.Br., Trans. Linn. Soc. London 12:115. 1817.
Species:
Brachylaena hutchinsii Hutch., Bull. Misc. Inform. 1910:126. 1910:
muhuhu (Eng.).

Carphephorus Cass., Bull. Sci. Soc. Philom. Paris 1816:198. 1816.
Literature: 76
Species:
Carphephorus odoratissimus (J.F. Gmelin) Hebert, Rhodora
70:483. 1968: deertongue (Eng.).

Chamaemelum Mill., Gard. dict. abr. ed. 4. 1754.
Literature and Species: see 178

Chamomilla S.F. Gray, Nat. arr. Brit. pl. 2:454. 1821.
Literature and Species: see 178

Conyza Less., Syn. gen. Compos. 203. 1832.
Literature: 39
Species:
Conyza canadensis (L.) Cronquist, Bull. Torrey Bot. Club 70:632.
1943 (*Erigeron canadensis* L.): fleabane (Eng.), horseweed
(Eng.), erigeron (Fr.), vergerette (Fr.), Erigeron (Ger.).
This species may be divided into 3 varieties, but var.
canadensis is most often encountered.

Eriocephalus L., Sp. pl. 926. 1753.
Species:
Eriocephalus punctulatus DC, Prodr. 6:146. 1838: eriocephalée
(Fr.).

Helichrysum Mill., Gard. dict. abr. ed. 4. 1754 ("*Elichrysum*"); corr.
Pers. Syn. pl. 2:414. 1807.
Literature: see 178
Species: see 178; add:
Helichrysum stoechas (L.) Moench, Methodus 575. 1794.
This species is very variable and can be divided into at least 2
subspecies, with subsp. *stoechas* most commonly encountered.
Helichrysum stoechas is commonly harvested with *H. italicum*
(Roth) G. Don.

Ormenis (Cass.) Cass., Dict. sci. nat. 29:180. 1823.
Species:
Ormenis mixta Dumort., Fl. belg. 69. 1827: Moroccan chamomile
(Eng.).
Ormenis multicaulis Braun-Blanq. & Maire, Bull. Soc. Hist. Nat.
Nat. Afrique N. 16:35. 1925: Moroccan chamomile (Eng.).

Pteronia L., Sp. pl. ed. 2. 1176. 1763.
Species:
Pteronia incana DC, Prodr. 5:358. 1836: pteronia (Eng.), blue dog
(Eng.).

Saussurea DC, Ann. Mus. Natl. Hist. Nat. 16:156, 198. 1810.
Literature: 105
Species:

Saussurea costus (Falc.) Lipschits, Bot. Zurn. (Moscow &
    Leningrad) 49(1):131. 1969 [*Aucklandia costus* Falc., *Aplotaxis
    lappa* Decne., *Saussurea lappa* (Decne.) Schultz-Bip., *S. lappa*
    (Decne) Clarke]: costus (Eng., Fr., It., Sp.), Costus (Ger.).

Solidago L., Sp. pl. 878. 1753.
    Literature and Species: see 178

Tagetes L., Sp. pl. 887. 1753.
    Literature: see 178
    Species: see 178; add:
    Tagetes minuta L., Sp. pl. 887. 1753 (*T. glandulifera* Schrank):
        tagette (Fr.).
    Tagetes patula L., Sp. pl. 887. 1753: French marigold (Eng.).

Tanacetum L., Sp. pl. 843. 1753.
    Literature and Species: see 178.

Acknowledgements

The senior author wishes to acknowledge, in part, the support provided by a grant from the Cooperative State Research Service (#801-15-01C).

V. REFERENCES

1. Amaral Franco, J. do. 1964. *Populus. In* T.G. Tutin, V.H. Heywood, N.A. Burges, D.M. Moore, D.H. Valentine, S.M. Walters, and D.A. Webb, eds. *Flora Europaea.* Vol. 1. University Press, Cambridge. pp. 54-55.

2. Amaral Franco, J. do. 1968. *Acacia. In* T.G. Tutin, V.H. Heywood, N.A. Burges, D.M. Moore, D.H. Valentine, S.M. Walters, and D.A. Webb, eds. *Flora Europaea.* Vol. 2. University Press, Cambridge. pp. 84-85.

3. Amaral Franco, J. do. 1968. *Lupinus. In* T.G. Tutin, V.H. Heywood, N.A. Burges, D.M. Moore, D.H. Valentine, S.M. Walters, and D.A. Webb, eds. *Flora Europaea.* Vol. 2. University Press, Cambridge. pp. 105-106.

4. Amaral Franco, J. do. 1976. *Cynara. In* T.G. Tutin, V.H. Heywood, N.A. Burges, D.M. Moore, D.H. Valentine, S.M. Walters, and D.A. Webb, eds. *Flora Europaea.* Vol. 4. University Press, Cambridge. pp. 248-249.

5. Amaral Franco, J. do. and M.L. da Rocha Afonso. 1972. *Rosmarinus. In* T.G. Tutin, V.H. Heywood, N.A. Burges, D.M. Moore, D.H. Valentine, S.M. Walters, and D.A. Webb, eds. *Flora Europaea.* Vol. 3. University Press, Cambridge. p. 187.

6. Angely, J. 1965. *Flora Analítica do Paraná.* Universidade de São Paulo. 728 p.

7. Arctander, S. 1960. *Perfume and Flavor Materials of Natural Origin.* S. Arctander, Elizabeth, NJ. 736 p.

8. Ashton, P.S. 1981. *Myrtaceae. In* M.D. Dassanayake and F.R. Fosberg, eds. *A Revised Handbook to the Flora of Ceylon.* Vol. 2. Amerind Publishing Company, New Delhi, India. pp. 403-472.

9. Awasthi, D.D. 1965. Catalogue of the lichens from India, Nepal, Pakistan, and Ceylon. Nova Hedwigia 17:1-137.

10. Backer, C.A. and R.C. Bakhuizen van den Brink. 1963-1968. *Flora of Java.* Wolters-Noordhoff N.A., Groningen. 3 vols.

11. Ball, P.W. 1964. *Cheiranthus. In* T.G. Tutin, V.H. Heywood, N.A. Burges, D.M. Moore, D.H. Valentine, S.M. Walters, and D.A. Webb, eds. *Flora Europaea.* Vol. 1. University Press, Cambridge. p. 279.

12. Ball, P.W. 1968. *Robinia. In* T.G. Tutin, V.H. Heywood, N.A. Burges, D.M. Moore, D.H. Valentine, S.M. Walters, and D.A. Webb, eds. *Flora Europaea.* Vol. 2. University Press, Cambridge. p. 106.

13. Barrett, H.C. and A.N. Rhodes. 1976. A numerical taxonomic study of affinity relationships in cultivated *Citrus* and its close relatives. Syst. Bot. 1:105-136.

14. Bates, D.M. 1968. Notes on the cultivated Malvaceae. 2. *Abelmoschus.* Baileya 16:99-112.

15. Bechtel, H., P. Cribb, and E. Launert. 1981. *The Manual of Cultivated Orchid Species.* MIT Press, Cambridge. 444 p.

16. Bogdanov, P.L. 1968. *Poplars and Their Cultivation.* 2nd ed. rev. Transl. by R. Karschon. Israel Program for Scientific Translations, Jerusalem. 89 p.

17. Boivin, B. 1959. *Abies balsamea* (Linné) Miller et ses variations. Naturaliste Canad. 86:219-223.

18. Brickell, C.D., ed. 1980. *International Code of Nomenclature for Cultivated Plants-1980.* Bohn, Scheltema & Holkema, Utrecht. 32 p.

19. Brooker, M.I.H. and D.A. Kleinig. 1983. *Field Guide to Eucalypts, South-eastern Australia.* Inkata Press, Melbourne. 288 p.

20. Browicz, K. 1976. *Lonicera. In* T.G. Tutin, V.H. Heywood, N.A. Burges, D.M. Moore, D.H. Valentine, S.M. Walters, and D.A. Webb, eds. *Flora Europaea.* Vol. 4. University Press, Cambridge. pp. 46-48.

21. Burkill, I.H. 1966. *A Dictionary of the Economic Products of the Malay Peninsula.* Ministry of Agriculture and Co-operatives, Kuala Lumpur, Malaysia. 2 vols.

22. Burtt, B.L. 1977. The nomenclature of turmeric and other Ceylon Zingiberaceae. Notes Roy. Bot. Gard. Edinburgh 35:209-215.

23. Burtt, B.L. and R.M. Smith. 1983. Zingiberaceae. *In* M.D. Dassanayake and F.R. Fosberg, eds. *A Revised Handbook to the Flora of Ceylon.* Vol. 4. Amerind Publishing Company, New Delhi. pp. 488-532.

24. Callen, G. 1977. *Les Conifères Cultivés en Europe.* J.-B. Ballière, Paris. 2 vols.

25. Campbell, M.S. 1968. *Myrtus. In* T.G. Tutin, V.H. Heywood, N.A. Burges, D.M. Moore, D.H. Valentine, S.M. Walters, and D.A Webb, eds. *Flora Europaea.* Vol. 2. University Press, Cambridge. pp. 303-304.

26. Carvalho, A., F.P. Ferwerda, J.A. Frahm-Liliveld, D.M. Medina, A.J.T. Mendes, and L.C. Monaco. 1969. Coffee (*Coffea arabica* L. and *Coffea canephora* Pierre ex Froehner). *In* F.P. Ferwerda and F. Wit, eds. *Outlines of Perennial Crop Breeding in the Tropics.* Misc. Papers No. 4, Landbouwhogeschool. Wageningen, The Netherlands. pp. 189-241.

27. Carvalho, A., and L.C. Monaco. 1967. Genetic relationships of selected *Coffea* species. Ci. & Cult. 19:151-165.

28. Childers, N.F., H.R. Cibes, and E. Hernández-Medina. 1959. Vanilla—The orchid of commerce. *In* C.L. Withner, ed. *The Orchids: A Scientific Survey*. Ronald Press Company, New York. pp. 477-508.

29. Chinnappa, C.C. 1981. Palynology and systematics of the genus *Coffea*. J. Coffea Res. 11:55-69.

30. Codd, L.E., B. de Winter, H.B. Rycroft, O.A. Leistner, D.J.B. Killick, and J.H. Ross, eds. 1966-1983. *Flora of Southern Africa*. Botanical Research Institute, Department of Agriculture, Republic of South Africa. 33 vols.

31. Coombe, D.E. 1968. *Trifolium*. *In* T.G. Tutin, V.H. Heywood, N.A. Burges, D.M. Moore, D.H. Valentine, S.M. Walters, and D.A. Webb, eds. *Flora Europaea*. Vol. 2. University Press, Cambridge. pp. 157-172.

32. Cope, F.W. 1976. Cacao. *In* N.W. Simmonds, ed. *Evolution of Crop Plants*. Longman, London. pp. 285-289.

33. Cope, T.A. 1982. Poaceae. No. 143. *In* E. Nasir and S.I. Ali, *Flora of Pakistan*. Department of Botany, University of Karachi. 678 p.

34. Correll, D.S. and H.B. Correll. 1982. *Flora of the Bahama Archipelago*. J. Cramer, Vaduz, Liechenstein. 1296 p.

35. Council of Scientific and Industrial Research. 1948-1976. *The Wealth of India*. Publications and Information Directorate, CSIR, New Delhi. 11 vols.

36. Cramer, L.H. 1981. Lamiaceae (Labiatae). *In* M.D. Dassanayake and F.R. Fosberg, eds. *A Revised Handbook to the Flora of Ceylon*. Vol. 3. Amerind Publishing Company, New Delhi. pp. 108-194.

37. Craveiro, A.A., A.G. Fernandes, D.H.S. Andrade, F.J. de Abreu Matos, J.W. de Alencar, and M.I.L. Machado. 1981. *Óleos Essenciais de Plantas do Nordeste*. Fortaleza-Ceará, Universidade Federal do Ceará, Brazil. 209 p.

38. Critchfield, W.B. and E.L. Little. 1966. Geographic distribution of the pines of the world. Forest Serv. Misc. Publ. 991. 97 p.

39. Cronquist, A. 1943. The separation of *Erigeron* from *Conyza*. Bull. Torrey Bot. Club 70:629-632.

40. Cuatrecasas, J. 1964. Cacao and its allies: A taxonomic revision of the genus *Theobroma*. Contr. U.S. Natl. Herb. 35:379-614.

41. Darlington, D.C., J.B. Hair, and R. Hurcombe. 1951. The history of the garden hyacinths. Heredity 5:233-252.

42. Dassanayake, M.D. and F.R. Fosberg, eds. 1980-1985. *A Revised Handbook to the Flora of Ceylon*. Amerind Publishing Company, New Delhi. 5 vols.

43. Davis, P.H., ed. 1965-1984. *Flora of Turkey and the East Aegean Islands*. University Press, Edinburgh. 8 vols.

44. Debazac, E.F. 1964. *Manuel des Coniferes*. M.R. Viney, Nancy, France. 172 p.

45. Den Ouden, P. and B.K. Boom. 1978. *Manual of Cultivated Conifers Hardy in the Cold and Warm-temperate Zone*. Martinus Nijhoff, The Hague. 526 p.

46. Dress, W.J. 1958. Notes on the cultivated Compositae. 2. *Arnica*. Baileya 6:194-198.

47. Dykes, W.R. 1913. *The Genus* Iris. University Press, Cambridge. 245 p.

48. Farr, E.R., J.A. Leussink, and F.A. Stafleu. 1979. *Index Nominum Genericorum (Plantarum)*. Bohn, Scheltema & Holkema, Utrecht. 3 vols.

49. Fassett, N.C. 1945. *Juniperus virginiana, J. horizontalis,* and *J. scopulorum*-V. Taxonomic treatment. Bull. Torrey Bot. Club 72:480-482.

50. Ferguson, I.K. 1976. *Sambucus. In* T.G. Tutin, V.H. Heywood, N.A. Burges, D.M. Moore, D.H. Valentine, S.M. Walters, and D.A. Webb, eds. *Flora Europaea.* Vol. 4. University Press, Cambridge. pp. 44-45.

51. Ferguson, I.K. 1976. *Arnica. In* T.G. Tutin, V.H. Heywood, N.A. Burges, D.M. Moore, D.H. Valentine, S.M. Walters, and D.A. Webb, eds. *Flora Europaea.* Vol. 4. University Press, Cambridge. pp. 189-190.

52. Ferwerda, F.P. 1976. Coffees. *In* N.W. Simmonds, ed. *Evolution of Crop Plants.* Longman, London. pp. 257-260.

53. Fink, B. 1935. *The Lichen Flora of the United States.* University of Michigan Press, Ann Arbor. 426 p.

54. Fish, F., and P.G. Waterman. 1973. Chemosystematics in the Rutaceae II. The chemosystematics of the *Zanthoxylum/Fagara* complex. Taxon 22:177-203.

55. Fontaine, F.J. 1970. Het geslacht *Betula* (bijdrage tot eenmonografie). Meded. Bot. Tuinen Belmonte Arbor. Wageningen 6:99-180.

56. Forty, J. 1980. A survey of hardy geraniums in cultivation and their availability in commerce. Plantsman 2:67-78.

57. Furia, T.E. and N. Bellanca, eds. 1975. *Fenaroli's Handbook of Flavor Ingredients.* 2nd ed. Vol. 1. CRC Press, Cleveland. 551 p.

58. Gentry, H.S. 1961. Buchu, a new cultivated crop in South Africa. Econ. Bot. 15:326-331.

59. Gilberti, G.C. 1979. Las especias argentinas del génera *Ilex* L. (Aquifoliaceae). Darwiniana 22:217-240.

60. Gildemeister, E. and F. Hoffmann. 1956-1968. *Die ätherischen Öle.* 4th ed. rev. W. Treibs. Akademie Verlag, Berlin. 11 vols.

61. Goodspeed, T.H. 1954. *The Genus* Nicotiana. Chronica Botanica Company, Waltham, MA. 536 p.

62. Green, P.S. 1966. Studies in the genus *Jasminum* III. The species in cultivation in North America. Baileya 13:137-172.

63. Guenther, E. 1948-1952. *The Essential Oils.* Van Nostrand Reinhold, New York. 6 vols.

64. Hall, R., D. Klemme, and J. Nienhaus. 1985. *The H&R Book: Guide to Fragrance Ingredients.* Johnson Publishing, London. 144 p.

65. Hansen, A. 1968. *Melilotus. In* T.G. Tutin, V.H. Heywood, N.A. Burges, D.M. Moore, D.H. Valentine, S.M. Walters, and D.A. Webb, eds. *Flora Europaea.* Vol. 2. University Press, Cambridge. pp. 148-150.

66. Hawkes, A.D. 1965. *Encyclopedia of Cultivated Orchids.* Faber and Faber, London. 602 p.

67. Hebert, H.J.-C. 1968. Generic considerations concerning *Carphephorus* and *Trilisa* (Compositae) Rhodora 70:474-485.

68. Hegi, G., ed. 1963-1984. *Illustrierte Flora von Mittel-Europa.* 2nd ed. Verlag Paul Parey, Berlin. 7 vols.

69. Hepper, F.N. 1969. Arabian and African frankincense trees. J. Egypt. Archaeol. 55:66-72.

70. Heywood, V.H. 1968. *Spartium. In* T.G. Tutin, V.H. Heywood, N.A. Burges, D.M. Moore, D.H. Valentine, S.M. Walters, and D.A. Webb, eds. *Flora Europaea.* Vol. 2. University Press, Cambridge. p. 101.

71. Heywood, V.H. 1968. *Daucus. In* T.G. Tutin, V.H. Heywood, N.A. Burges, D.M. Moore, D.H. Valentine, S.M. Walters, and D.A. Webb, eds. *Flora Europaea.* Vol. 2. University Press, Cambridge. pp. 373-374.

72. Heywood, V.H. and A. Regueiro. 1980. *Hyacinthus. In* T.G. Tutin, V.H. Heywood, N.A. Burges, D.M. Moore, D.H. Valentine, S.M. Walters, and D.A. Webb, eds. *Flora Europaea.* Vol. 5. University Press, Cambridge. p. 44.

73. Hirota, N. and M. Hiroi. 1967. The later studies on the camphor tree, on the leaf oil of each practical form and its utilisation. Perfumery & Essential Oil Rec. 58:364-367.

74. Hodgson, R.W. 1967. Horticultural varieties of *Citrus. In* W. Reuther, H.J. Webber, and L.D. Batchelor, eds. *The Citrus Industry.* Vol. 1. Rev. ed. University of California Press, Berkeley. pp. 431-591.

75. Holttum, R.E. 1950. The Zingiberaceae of the Malay Peninsula. Gard. Bull. Straits Settlem. 13:1-249.

76. Howes, F.N. 1949. *Vegetable Gums and Resins.* Chronica Botanica Company, Waltham, MA. 188 p.

77. Hu, S.-y. 1970. *The Compositae of China.* Taipei. 704 p.

78. Hutchinson, J. and J.M. Dalziel. 1954-1972. *Flora of West Tropical Africa.* 2nd ed. rev. R.W.J. Keay and F.N. Hepper. Crown Agents for Oversea Governments, London. 3 vols.

79. Hyland, B.P.M. 1983. A revision of *Syzygium* and allied genera (*Myrtaceae*) in Australia. Austral. J. Bot. Suppl. Ser. 9. 164 p.

80. International Organization for Standardization. 1984. *Essential Oils Nomenclature-First List.* ISO, Geneva. 9 p.

81. International Seed Testing Association. 1968. *A Multilingual Glossary of Common Plant-names. I. Field Crops, Grasses and Vegetables.* I.S.T.A., Wageningen, Netherlands. 371 p.

82. Kariyone, T. and R. Koiso. 1973. *Atlas of Medicinal Plants.* Nihon Rinshosha, Osaka. 151 p.

83. Kartesz, J.T. and R. Kartesz. 1980. *A Synonymized Checklist of the Vascular Flora of the United States, Canada, and Greenland. Volume II. The Biota of North America.* University of North Carolina Press, Chapel Hill. 500 p.

84. Keep, E. 1976. Currants: *Ribes* spp. (Grossulariaceae). *In* N.W. Smmonds, ed. *Evolution of Crop Plants.* Longman, London. pp. 145-148.

85. Kelley, S. 1983. *Eucalypts.* Thomas Nelson Australia, Victoria. 2 vols.

86. Komarov, V.L., ed. 1968-1976. *Flora of the USSR.* Israel Program for Scientific Translations, Jerusalem. 20 vols.

87. Korovin, E. 1947. *Generis* Ferula (*Tourn.*) L.: *Monographia Illustrata.* Academia Scientarum UzRSS, Taschkent. 91 p.

88. Kostermans, A.J.G.H. 1964. *Bibliographia Lauracearum.* Ministry of National Research, Bogor, Indonesia. 1450 p.

89. Kostermans, A.J.G.H. 1968. Materials for a revision of Lauraceae I. Reinwardtia 7:291-356.

90. Kostermans, A.J.G.H. 1969. Materials for a revision of Lauraceae II. Reinwardtia 7:451-536.

91. Kostermans, A.J.G.H. 1970. Materials for a revision of Lauraceae III. Reinwardtia 8:21-196.

92. Koyama, T. 1985. *Cyperaceae. In* M.D. Dassanayake and F.R. Fosberg, eds. *A Revised Handbook to the Flora of Ceylon.* Vol. 5. Amerind Publishing Company, New Delhi. pp. 125-405.

93. Krajina, V.J. 1956. A summary of the nomenclature of Douglas-fir, *Pseudotsuga menziesii.* Madrono 13:265-267.

94. Krüssman, G. 1985. *Manual of Cultivated Conifers.* Transl. M.E. Epp. Timber Press, Portland, OR. 361 p.

95. Landry, P. 1984. Synopsis du genre *Abies.* Bull. Soc. Bot. France, Lett. Bot. 131:223-229.

96. Lawrence, B.M. 1978. *Essential Oils 1976-1977.* Allured Publishing Company, Wheaton, IL. 175 p.

97. Lawrence, B.M. 1979. *Essential Oils 1978.* Allured Publishing Company, Wheaton, IL. 192 p.

98. Lawrence, B.M. 1984. Major tropical spices-ginger (*Zingiber officinale* Rosc.). Perfumer & Flavorist 9(5):1, 3, 6-8, 10, 12-13, 16-18, 20-22, 24-26, 28-40.

99. Lawrence, G.H.M., A.F.G. Buchheim, G.S. Daniels, and H. Dolezal. eds. 1968. *B-P-H: Botanico-Periodicum-Huntianum.* Hunt Botanical Library, Pittsburgh. 1063 p.

100. Li, H.-L. 1963. *Woody Flora of Taiwan.* Livingston Publishing Company, Narbeth, PA. 974 p.

101. Li, H.-l. 1975. Cupressaceae. *In* H.-l Li, T.-s. Liu, T.-c. Huang, T. Koyama, and C.E. DeVol, eds. *Flora of Taiwan.* Vol. 1. Epoch Publishing Co., Taipei. pp. 534-544.

102. Li, H.-l., T.-s. Liu, T.-c. Huang, T. Koyama, and C.E. DeVol, eds. 1975-1979. *Flora of Taiwan.* Epoch Publishing Company, Taipeh. 6 vols.

103. Liberty Hyde Bailey Hortorium, Staff of the. 1976. *Hortus Third.* Macmillan Publishing Company, New York. 1290 p.

104. Lippert, W. 1979. Zur Kenntnis von *Salvia* im westlichen Mittelmeergebiet. Mitt. Bot. Staatssamml. München 15:397-423.

105. Lipschits, S. 1979. *Genus* Saussurea DC. (*Asteraceae*). Academia Scientarum URSS, Institutum Botanicum Komarovianum. 282 p.

106. Little, E.L. 1979. *Checklist of United States Trees* (*Native and Naturalized*). U.S.D.A. Agric. Handb. No. 541. 375 p.

107. Little, E.L. and K.W. Dorman. 1952. Slash pine (*Pinus elliottii*), its nomenclature and varieties. J. Forest. (Washington) 50:918-923.

108. Liu, T.-s. 1971. *A Monograph of the Genus* Abies. National Taiwan University, Taipei. 608 p.

109. Macbride, J.F., B.E. Dahlgren, R. McVaugh, M.E. Mathias, L. Constance, and D.S. Correll. 1936-1967. *Flora of Peru.* Field Mus. Nat. Hist., Bot. Ser. vol. 13, part 1-5.

110. Malik, M.N., R.W. Scora, and R.K. Soost. 1974. Studies on the origin of the lemon. Hilgardia 42:361-382.

111. Marsh, J.A. 1966. *Widdringtonia. In* L.C. Codd, B. de Winter, and H.B. Rycroft, eds. *Flora of Southern Africa.* Vol. 1. Botanical Research Institute, Department of Agriculture, Republic of South Africa.

112. Martinez, M. 1963. *Las Pinaceas Mexicanas.* 3rd ed. Universidad Nacional Autónoma de Mexico, Mexico. 400 p.

113. Mathew, B. 1981. *The Iris.* B.T. Batsford, London. 202 p.

114. McKelvey, S.D. 1928. *The Lilac: A Monograph.* Macmillan Company, New York. 581 p.

115. McVaugh, R. and J. Rzedowski. 1965. Synopsis of the genus *Bursera* L. in western Mexico, with notes on the material of *Bursera* collected by Sesse & Mociüo. Kew Bull. 18:317-382.

116. Meikle, R.D. 1984. *Willows and Poplars of Great Britain and Ireland.* Botanical Society of the British Isles, London. 198 p.

117. Merrill, E.D. 1923-1926. *An Enumeration of Philippine Flowering Plants.* Bureau of Printing, Manila. 4 vols.

118. Merrill, E.D. 1947. The technical name of allspice. Contr. Gray Herb. 165:30-38.

119. Mirov, N.T. 1967. *The Genus* Pinus. Ronald Press Co., New York. 602 p.

120. Moore, H.E. 1955. Pelargoniums in cultivation. I. Baileya 3:5-25, 41- 46.

121. Moore, H.E. 1955. Pelargoniums in cultivation. II. Baileya 3:70-97.

122. Morton, J.K. 1963. Labiatae. *In* J. Hutchinson and J.M. Dalziel, eds. *Flora of West Tropical Africa.* Vol. 2. 2nd ed. rev. F.N. Hepper. Crown Agents for Overseas Governments, London. pp. 450-473.

123. Naves, Y.R. and G. Mazuyer. 1947. *Natural Perfume Materials: A Study of Concretes, Resinoids, Floral Oils and Pomades.* Reinhold Publishing Co., New York. 338 p.

124. Neve, R.A. 1976. Hops: *Humulus lupulus* (Moraceae). *In* N.W. Simmonds, ed. *Evolution of Crop Plants.* Longman, London. pp. 208-211.

125. Ohwi, J. 1965. *Flora of Japan.* Smithsonian Institution, Washington. 1067 p.

126. Ozenda, P. and G. Clauzade. 1970. *Les Lichens: Étude Biologique et Flore Illustrée.* Masson & Cie, Paris. 801 p.

127. Penfold, A.R. and F.R. Morrison. 1950. "Tea tree" oils. *In* E. Guenther, *The Essential Oils.* D. Van Nostrand Company, Princeton. pp. 526-548.

128. Penfold, A.R. and J.L. Willis. 1961. *The Eucalypts: Botany, Cultivation, Chemistry, and Utilization.* Interscience, New York. 547 p.

129. Pillans, N.S. 1950. A revision of *Agathosma.* J. South African Bot. 16:55-183.

130. Portères, R. 1954. Le genre *Vanilla* et ses espèces. *In* G. Bouriquet, ed. *Le Vanillier et la Vanilla dans le Monde.* Paul Lechevalier, Paris. pp. 94-288.

131. Potvin, C., Y. Bergeon, and J.-P. Simon. 1983. A numerical taxonomic study of selected *Citrus* species (Rutaceae) based on biochemical characters. Syst. Bot. 8:127-133.

132. Poucher, W.Q. 1974. *Perfumes, Cosmetics and Soaps. Volume I. The Raw Materials of Perfumery.* 7th ed. rev. by G.M. Howard. Chapmand and Hall, London. 381 p.

133. Pound, F.J. 1938. History and cultivation of the tonka bean (*Dipteryx odorata*) with analyses of Trinidad, Venezuelan and Brazilian samples. Trop. Agric. (Trinidad) 15:4-9, 28-32.

134. Pringle, J.S. 1983. A summary of the currently accepted nomenclature at the specific and varietal levels in *Syringa*. Lilac Newslett. 9(3):1-6.

135. Pryor, L.D. and L.A.S. Johnson. 1971. *A Classification of the Eucalypts*. Australian National University, Canberra. 102 p.

136. Rehder, A. 1949. *Bibliography of Cultivated Trees and Shrubs Hardy in the Cooler Temperate Regions of the Northern Hemisphere*. Arnold Arboretum, Jamaica Plain, MA. 825 p.

137. Richardson, I.B.K. *Achillea. In* T.G. Tutin, V.H. Heywood, N.A. Burges, D.M. Moore, D.H. Valentine, S.M. Walters, and D.A. Webb, eds. *Flora Europaea*. Vol. 4. University Press, Cambridge. pp. 159-165.

138. Rogers, O.M. 1976. Tentative international register of cultivar names in the genus *Syringa*. New Hampshire Agric. Exp. Sta. Res. Rep. 49. 81 p.

139. Röst, L.C.M. 1979. Biosystematic investigations with *Acorus*. 4. Communication. A synthetic approach to the classification of the genus. Pl. Med. 37:289-307.

140. Rouleau, E. 1948. Two new names in *Populus*. Rhodora 50:233-236.

141. Rouleau, E. 1949. *Populus*: A correction. Rhodora 51:149-150.

142. Rudd, V.E. 1980. Fabaceae. *In* M.D. Dassanayake and F.R. Fosberg, eds. *A Revised Handbook to the Flora of Ceylon*. Vol. 1. Amerind Publishing Company, New Delhi. pp. 428-458.

143. Schmid, R. 1972. A resolution of the *Eugenia-Syzygium* controversy (Myrtaceae). Amer. J. Bot. 59:423-436.

144. Scora, R. 1975. Volatile oil components in *Citrus* taxonomy. Int. Flavours 1975:342-346.

145. Scora, R.W., A.B. England, and D. Chang. 1969. Taxonomic affinities within the rough lemon group (*Citrus jambhiri* Lush.) as aided by gaschromatography of their essential oils. Proc. Int. Citrus Symp. 1:441-450.

146. Scora, R.W. and J. Kumamoto. 1983. Chemotaxonomy of the genus *Citrus. In* P.G. Waterman and M.F. Grundon, eds. *Chemistry and Chemical Taxonomy of the Rutales*. Academic Press, New York. pp. 343-351.

147. Scora, R.W., J. Kumamoto, R.K. Soost, and E.M. Nauer. 1982. Contribution to the origin of the grapefruit, *Citrus paradisi* (Rutaceae). Syst. Bot. 7:170-177.

148. Sealy, J.R. 1958. *A Revision of the Genus* Camellia. Royal Horticultural Society, London. 239 p.

149. Shaw, G.R. 1909. The pines of Mexico. Publ. Arnold Arbor. No. 1. 30 p.

150. Silba, J. 1981. Revised generic concepts of *Cupressus* L. (Cupressaceae). Phytologia 49:390-399.

151. Silba, J. 1983. Addendum to a revision of *Cupressus* L. (Cupressaceae). Phytologia 52:349-361.

152. Silba, J. 1986. Encyclopaedia Coniferae. Phytologia Mem. VIII. 217 p.

153. Sinclair, J. 1968. Flora Malesianae Precursores-XLII. The genus *Myristica* in Malesia and outside Malesia. Gard. Bull. Straits Settlem. 23:1-540.

154. Smith, R.E. 1984. *Curcuma. In* S.M. Walters, A. Brady, C.C. Brickell, J. Cullen, P.S. Green, J. Lewis, V.A. Matthews, D.A. Webb, P.F. Yeo, and J.C.M. Alexander, eds. *The European Garden Flora: A Manual for*

the Identification of Plants Cultivated in Europe, both Out-of-doors and Under Glass. Vol. 2. University Press, Cambridge. p. 127.

155. Smith, R.E. 1984. *Alpinia. In* S.M. Walters, A. Brady, C.C. Brickell, J. Cullen, P.S. Green, J. Lewis, V.A. Matthews, D.A. Webb, P.F. Yeo, and J.C.M. Alexander, eds. *The European Garden Flora: A Manual for the Identification of Plants Cultivated in Europe, both Out-of-doors and Under Glass.* Vol. 2. University Press, Cambridge. pp. 128-129.

156. Smith, R.E. 1984. *Zingiber. In* S.M. Walters, A. Brady, C.C. Brickell, J. Cullen, P.S. Green, J. Lewis, V.A. Matthews, D.A. Webb, P.F. Yeo, and J.C.M. Alexander, eds. *The European Garden Flora: A Manual for the Identification of Plants Cultivated in Europe, both Out-of-doors and Under Glass.* Vol. 2. University Press, Cambridge. p. 123.

157. Smith, R.E. 1984. *Hedychium. In* S.M. Walters, A. Brady, C.C. Brickell, J. Cullen, P.S. Green, J. Lewis, V.A. Matthews, D.A. Webb, P.F. Yeo, and J.C.M. Alexander, eds. *The European Garden Flora: A Manual for the Identification of Plants Cultivated in Europe, both Out-of-doors and Under Glass.* Vol. 2. University Press, Cambridge. pp. 124-125.

158. Smith, R.E. 1984. *Elettaria. In* S.M. Walters, A. Brady, C.C. Brickell, J. Cullen, P.S. Green, J. Lewis, V.A. Matthews, D.A. Webb, P.F. Yeo, and J.C.M. Alexander, eds. *The European Garden Flora: A Manual for the Identification of Plants Cultivated in Europe, both Out-of-doors and Under Glass.* Vol. 2. University Press, Cambridge. p. 128.

159. Soenarko, S. 1977. The genus *Cymbopogon.* Reinwardtia 9:225-375.

160. Stafleu, R.A. and R.S. Cowan. 1976-1983. *Taxonomic Literature.* 2nd ed. Bohn, Scheltema & Holkema, Utrecht. 5 vols.

161. Standley, P.C. 1920. Trees and shrubs of Mexico. Contr. U.S. Natl. Herb. 23:1-1721.

162. Stapf, O. 1906. XLVI. The oil-grasses of India and Ceylon. Bull. Misc. Inform. 1906:297-364.

163. Steenis, C.G.G.J., ed. 1948-1983. *Flora Malesiana.* Martinus Nijhoff/W. Junk, The Hague. 9 vols.

164. Steyermark, J.A. 1951-1953. *Contributions to the Flora of Venezuela.* Fieldiana, Bot. 28:1-678.

165. Stone, B.C. 1976. Pandanaceae. *In* C.J. Saldanha and D.H. Nicolson, eds. *Flora of Hassan District, Karnataka, India.* Smithsonian Institution, Washington, D.C. pp. 777-781.

166. Stone, B.C. 1985. Rutaceae. *In* M.D. Dassanayake and F.R. Fosberg, eds. *A Revised Handbook to the Flora of Ceylon.* Vol. 5. Amerind Publishing Company, New Delhi. pp. 406-476.

167. Storey, W.B. 1976. Fig: *Ficus carica* (Moraceae). *In* N.W. Simmonds, ed. *Evolution of Crop Plants.* Longman, London. pp. 205-208.

168. Swingle, W.T. 1967. The botany of *Citrus* and its wild relatives. Rev. P.C. Reece. *In* W. Reuther, H.J. Webber, and L.D. Batchelor, eds. *The Citrus Industry.* Vol. 1. Rev. ed. University of California Press, Berkeley. pp. 190-430.

169. Tanaka, T. 1954. *Species Problem in* Citrus: *A Critical Study of Wild and Cultivated Units of* Citrus *Based upon Field Studies in Their Native Homes (Revisio Aurantiacearum IX).* Japanese Society for the Promotion of Science, Tokyo. 152 p.

170. Torres, A.M., R.K. Soost, and U. Diedenhofen. 1978. Leaf isozymes as genetic markers in *Citrus.* Amer. J. Bot. 65:869-881.

171. Torres, A.M., R.K. Soost, and T. Mau-Lastovicka. 1982. *Citrus* isozymes: Genetics and distinguishing nucellar from zygotic seedlings. J. Heredity 73:335-339.

172. Townsend, C.C. 1968. *Dictamnus. In* T.G. Tutin, V.H. Heywood, N.A. Burges, D.M. Moore, D.H. Valentine, S.M. Walters, and D.A. Webb, eds. *Flora Europaea.* Vol. 2. University Press, Cambridge. p. 229.

173. Townsend, C.C. 1968. *Citrus. In* T.G. Tutin, V.H. Heywood, N.A. Burges, D.M. Moore, D.H. Valentine, S.M. Walters, and D.A. Webb, eds. *Flora Europaea.* Vol. 2. University Press, Cambridge. pp. 229-230.

174. Trelease, W. and T.G. Yuncker. 1950. *The Piperaceae of Northern South America.* University of Illinois Press, Urbana. 2 vols.

175. Trueblood, E.W.E. 1973. "Omixochitl"–the tuberose (*Polianthes tuberosa*). Econ. Bot. 27:157-173.

176. Tsunoda, S., K. Hinata, and C. Gómez-Campo, eds. 1980. Brassica *Crops and Wild Allies.* Japan Scientific Societies Press, Tokyo. 354 p.

177. Tucker, A.O. 1981. The correct name of lavandin and its cultivars [Labiatae]. Baileya 21:131-133.

178. Tucker, A.O. 1985. Botanical nomenclature of culinary herbs and potherbs. *In* L.E. Craker and J.E. Simon, eds. *Herbs, Spices, and Medicinal Plants: Recent Advances in Botany, Horticulture, and Pharmacology.* Vol. 1. Oryx Press, Phoenix, AZ. pp. 20-58.

179. Tucker, A.O. 1986. Frankincense and myrrh. Econ. Bot. (in press).

180. Turrill, E.B. 1920. The genus *Rosmarinus.* Bull. Misc. Inform. 1920:105-108.

181. Turrill, W.B., E. Milne-Redhead, *et al.* 1952-1982. *Flora of Tropical East Africa.* A.A. Balkema, Rotterdam.

182. Tutin, T.G. 1964. *Ficus. In* T.G. Tutin, V.H. Heywood, N.A. Burges, D.M. Moore, D.H. Valentine, S.M. Walters, and D.A. Webb, eds. *Flora Europeae.* Vol. 1. University Press, Cambridge. pp. 66-67.

183. Tutin, T.G. 1968. *Pistacia. In* T.G. Tutin, V.H. Heywood, N.A. Burges, D.M. Moore, D.H. Valentine, S.M. Walters, and D.A. Webb, eds. *Flora Europeae.* Vol. 2. University Press, Cambridge. p. 237.

184. Tutin, T.G. 1968. *Apium. In* T.G. Tutin, V.H. Heywood, N.A. Burges, D.M. Moore, D.H. Valentine, S.M. Walters, and D.A. Webb, eds. *Flora Europeae.* Vol. 2. University Press, Cambridge. pp. 351-352.

185. Tutin, T.G. 1968. *Pastinaca. In* T.G. Tutin, V.H. Heywood, N.A. Burges, D.M. Moore, D.H. Valentine, S.M. Walters, and D.A. Webb, eds. *Flora Europeae.* Vol. 2. University Press, Cambridge. p. 364.

186. Tutin, T.G. 1980. *Anthoxanthum. In* T.G. Tutin, V.H. Heywood, N.A. Burges, D.M. Moore, D.H. Valentine, S.M. Walters, and D.A. Webb, eds. *Flora Europeae.* Vol. 5. University Press, Cambridge. pp. 229-230.

187. Tutin, T.G., V.H. Heywood, N.A. Burges, D.M. Moore, D.H. Valentine, S.M. Walters, and D.A. Webb, eds. 1964-1980. *Flora Europaea.* University Press, Cambridge. 5 vols.

188. United States Department of Agriculture. 1982. *National List of Scientific Plant Names.* Soil Conservation Service SCS-TP-159. 2 vols.

189. van de Walt, J.J.A. 1977. *Pelargoniums of Southern Africa.* Purnell, Cape Town. 51 p.

190. Voss, E.G., ed. 1983. *International Code of Botanical Nomenclature.* Bohn, Scheltema & Holkema, Utrecht. 472 p.

191. Warburg, E.F. 1968. *Cistus. In* T.G. Tutin, V.H. Heywood, N.A. Burges, D.M. Moore, D.H. Valentine, S.M. Walters, and D.A. Webb, eds. *Flora Europaea.* Vol. 2. University Press, Cambridge. pp. 282-284.

192. Ward, D.B. 1974. On the scientific name of the longleaf pine. Rhodora 76:20-24.

193. Waterman, P.G. 1975. New combinations in *Zanthoxylum* L. (1753). Taxon 24:361-366.

194. Watt, G. 1966. *The Commercial Products of India.* Today and Tomorrow's Publishers, New Delhi. 1189 p.

195. Webb, D.A. 1964. *Ribes. In* T.G. Tutin, V.H. Heywood, N.A. Burges, D.M. Moore, D.H. Valentine, S.M. Walters, and D.A. Webb, eds. *Flora Europeae.* Vol. 1. University Press, Cambridge. pp. 382-383.

196. Webb, D.A. 1968. *Prunus. In* T.G. Tutin, V.H. Heywood, N.A. Burges, D.M. Moore, D.H. Valentine, S.M. Walters, and D.A. Webb, eds. Flora Europaea. Vol. 2. University Press, Cambridge. pp. 77-80.

197. Webb, D.A. 1980. *Narcissus. In* T.G. Tutin, V.H. Heywood, N.A. Burges, D.M. Moore, D.H. Valentine, S.M. Walters, and D.A. Webb, eds. *Flora Europaea.* Vol. 5. University Press, Cambridge. pp. 78-84.

198. Webb, D.A. and A.O. Chater. 1980. *Iris. In* T.G. Tutin, V.H. Heywood, N.A. Burges, D.M. Moore, D.H. Valentine, S.M. Walters and D.A. Webb, eds. *Flora Europaea.* Vol. 5. University Press, Cambridge. pp. 87-92.

199. Webb, D.A. and I.K. Ferguson. 1968. *Geranium. In* T.G. Tutin, V.H. Heywood, N.A. Burges, D.M. Moore, D.H. Valentine, S.M. Walters, and D.A. Webb, eds. *Flora Europaea.* Vol. 2. University Press, Cambridge. pp. 193-199.

200. Weberling, F. 1978. Monographie der Gattung *Nardostachys* DC. (Valerianaceae). Bot. Jahrb. Syst. 99:188-221.

201. Weinert, E. 1973. Die taxonomische Stellung und das Areal von *Angelica archangelica* L. und *A. lucida* L. Feddes Repert. 84:303-314.

202. Wells, F.V. and M. Billot. 1981. *Perfumery Technology. Art: Science: Industry.* 2nd ed. John Wiley & Sons, New York. 449 p.

203. Wild, H. 1959. A revised classification of the genus *Commiphora* Jacq. Bol. Soc. Brot. ser. II, 33:67-100.

204. Wright, D. 1983. Climbing honeysuckles. Plantsman. 4:236-252.

205. Wylie, A.P. 1952. The history of the garden narcissi. Heredity 6:137-156.

206. Yeo, P.F. 1964. *Reseda. In* T.G. Tutin, V.H. Heywood, N.A. Burges, D.M. Moore, D.H. Valentine, S.M. Walters, and D.A. Webb, eds. *Flora Europeae.* Vol. 1. University Press, Cambridge. pp. 346-349.

207. Yeo, P.F. 1968. *Glycyrrhiza. In* T.G. Tutin, V.H. Heywood, N.A. Burges, D.M. Moore, D.H. Valentine, S.M. Walters, and D.A. Webb, eds. *Flora Europeae.* Vol. 2. University Press, Cambridge. p. 127.

208. Zanoni, T.A. 1978. The American junipers of the section *Sabina* (*Juniperus,* Cupressaceae)–a century later. Phytologia 38:433-454.

Index

Compiled by Linda Webster

NOTE: Page numbers with a "t" indicate a table; those with an "f" indicate a figure.